From the foreword and the preface to the end of chapter ... this is a fascinating and thought provoking (if very occasionally to this particular reviewer just provoking!) collection of articles. Although the book is about primary care ethics anyone interested in health care ethics-including those who work in hospitals- will find in it interesting and intellectually nourishing material. Whether you dip or devour, you won't regret.

Raanan Gillon
Faculty of Medicine, School of Public Health
Emeritus Professor of Medical Ethics

This book is an excellent mix of ethical theories and exposition combined with practical examples. Written by many of the thought leaders of the collective primary care conscience the chapters cover the reality of the breadth of modern general practice. It is a valuable and accessible resource for everyday GP ethical dilemmas, for educators and for those developing policy.

Simon Gregory
Chair of RCGP Committee on Medical Ethics
Director and Dean of Education and Quality, Midlands and East
Health Education England

This enterprising collection spans the breadth of primary care in multiple ways. Contributions from general practitioners, philosophers, nurses, physiotherapists, dentists, health economists, educationalists, patients and others reflect the rich variety that makes up primary care. Authors do not shy away from the messy complexity of primary care. Instead, they embrace the uncertainty inherent in the day-to-day reality of primary care. Numerous stakeholder perspectives are used to identify and analyse ethical issues, using a diversity of frameworks and models. The theoretical perspectives represented in the book (ranging from Hippocrates to postmodernism) mirror the eclecticism of primary care itself. Practical advice sits alongside heartfelt accounts of issues that challenge practitioners. The book is helpfully organised into four sections, on the primary care interaction, vulnerable patients, teaching and learning, and justice and resources. The section on teaching and learning is particularly valuable, with its strong focus on reflective practice and the practical challenges of combining service delivery with educational goals. The section on the primary care encounter is wide-ranging, including discursive explorations of important concepts as well as discussion of the specific features of primary care that warrant its own ethical analysis. Case studies provide tantalising glimpses into the consultation, thereby showcasing the richness of the primary care environment. Chapters in the section on justice and resources do not shy away from political topics such as funding models and workforce issues.

The *Handbook* focuses on general practice as delivered within the National Health Service, which may limit its appeal to other members of the primary care team. However, there is something here for everyone, whether the reader is looking for guidance on duties in primary care, a framework for analysing a difficult consultation, insights into the voice of the patient, or an understanding of the economics of primary care. Throughout there is a welcome focus on 'ethics of the ordinary' or 'everyday ethics', reflecting the ethical nuances of the millions of interactions that occur each day in primary care.

Wendy Rogers
Professor of Clinical Ethics
Macquarie University

Handbook of
Primary Care Ethics

Edited by

Andrew Papanikitas

John Spicer

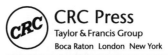

CRC Press
Taylor & Francis Group
Boca Raton London New York

CRC Press is an imprint of the
Taylor & Francis Group, an **informa** business

CRC Press
Taylor & Francis Group
6000 Broken Sound Parkway NW, Suite 300
Boca Raton, FL 33487-2742

International Standard Book Number-13: 978-1-4987-6967-9 (Hardback)
978-1-7852-3090-5 (Paperback)

Library of Congress Cataloging-in-Publication Data

Names: Papanikitas, Andrew, editor. | Spicer, John, 1954- editor.
Title: Handbook of primary care ethics / [edited by] Andrew Papanikitas, John Spicer.
Description: Boca Raton, FL : CRC Press/Taylor & Francis Group, [2018] |
Includes bibliographical references and index.
Identifiers: LCCN 2017033137 (print) | LCCN 2017033901 (ebook) | ISBN
9781315155487 | ISBN 9781785230905 (pbk. : alk. paper) | ISBN
9781498769679 (hardback : alk. paper)
Subjects: | MESH: Primary Health Care--ethics | Family Practice--ethics |
General Practice--ethics
Classification: LCC R724 (ebook) | LCC R724 (print) | NLM W 84.61 | DDC
174.2--dc23
LC record available at https://lccn.loc.gov/2017033137

Visit the Taylor & Francis Web site at
http://www.taylorandfrancis.com

and the CRC Press Web site at
http://www.crcpress.com

Contents

Foreword

From a traditional clinical point of view, community or general practice may not seem to be easy. Where tasks are defined, and challenges have known causes, researched treatments and objective outcomes, it might be said that everyone knows where they are, and problems are largely professional ones. In community practice, however, very few of these descriptions apply. Here, a patient's complaints may be poorly defined and hard to grasp, or multiple, disparate and overwhelming. Whether speaking to a nurse, a physiotherapist, a public health practitioner or any other specialist, the way in which a patient or his/her relative explains the condition may be unfamiliar to the professional, and the key issue may be tangential, unexpressed or even deliberately hidden. Patient's lifestyle or culture may be very different from that of clinician's lifestyle and has different preoccupations or aims from those with which she is familiar. Arriving from the security of hospital practice, the newcomer may feel deprived of skills, in a fog, as if she had suddenly been dropped into a boundary zone, the badlands, where every move seems to provoke more problems. Leaning on such insecure foundations, community public health can seem to share some of these structural faults. As to generalising in terms of planning or politics, well, some might say, best not to try.

In such a situation, many would feel that they have enough to cope with without the additional stress of asking a moral question, such as what is best, what might be better and what is right and wrong? But, the very reverse is the case. Without those questions, confusion is further confounded. Once they begin to be asked, the fog begins at last to clear. Medical ethics started as a discipline over half a century ago when specialist treatments like transplants and dialysis were new, but this book turns the searchlight towards the place where moral issues actually arise. It brings its focus sharply onto what should be done there in the making of ordinary everyday decisions.

Yet here again, if we are not careful, a similar difficulty as we started with above can arise. Ethical issues have come to be described and categorised under clear phrases or labels that are linked to an ill-considered action or (conversely) to an ideal aim. Many of these derive from the struggles in a hospital or teaching context to cope with the bizarre or the impossibly challenging. But, in the press of professional life in primary care, the issues are different; and many decisions simply do not come with familiar headings or indeed with moral headings at all. For instance, where medical practice meets people's ordinary lives, the question in mind may often be less what to do about 'this illness' than whether there is an 'illness' here to be attended to at all. Where health as a concept has various interpretations, the good outcomes desired may not even be expressed in terms of improved health.

Thus, the issues that a person could discuss or encounter with a primary care clinician are both hard to predict and at the same time theoretically almost limitless. A professional in community practice, therefore, should think clearly, discuss with all involved and make good decisions about topics that may be surprising and may well not have any easy labels. And his or her authority will largely reside in being able not just to reach a decision but also explain and justify in terms that satisfy the patient as to why she has reached the conclusions that she has. Both

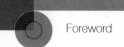
the boundaries and the conclusions will have to be clear, even in a fuzzy field – if only for the sake of the rest of the work that day!

How should we learn to do this? Paul Freeling, an early pioneer in academic practice, was fond of asking 'Give me a case and I'll give you a research project'. The same could very productively be said for thinking in ethics. I would maintain that almost every encounter between individuals or groups in primary care would productively raise a small handful of issues whose discussion would improve that care. But in this rich profusion, where should one start? There are many possibilities, not the least of which is simply realising when on reflection what you are doing or being asked to do is simply wrong, or could have been done a lot better. Also, one of my own surprises as a (relatively!) calm individual was, having often been anxious but never angered as a hospital doctor, how frequently in general practice I had to control my temper. So it has come to be my view that passion of any sort – anger, say, or extreme enthusiasm, disdain or disgust – indicates something that needs urgent ethical examination (as well as management). Therefore, we might also say 'give me a strong emotion (expressed or repressed) in a medical encounter and I'll give you an ethical issue'. Whether we are working as an individual or in a team, in treatment or prevention, in research, teaching, management, advocacy or politics, the resulting analysis should always be cool and clear, but should never deny its origin in a 'hot' topic. Moral medical practice is made for man, not, as sometimes seems to be the attitude within professions, the other way round.

We shall all need the insights of a wide range of disciplines to help us, both in the formulation and in the processing of such work, even though this field of applied ethics may need to start and finish at different points from those disciplines. The challenges are many: somehow we have to bring clear thinking to bear on a charged debate, to make the discussion, whether with others or in our own heads, wider by consciously addressing the arguments against our own cherished opinions as well as for them, and, where medical ethics often parts company with its philosophical advisers, reaching a conclusion which could actually and immediately be put into practice. We shall need to keep a close eye on what we are there to do, and how best to work with others: as one might put it, a good sense of 'self', of 'other' and of 'together'.

At this point, it should be clear how important this book is, perhaps even raising the question about how we have managed without it before. You will find it does not flinch from exploring possible issues, and more. It covers the meeting between patients and their advisers in community care from the beginning of the encounter to the end. It examines the way in which problems come to community practice as well as the minutiae of the doctor's response: and goes out from clinical behaviour to wider issues in public health and community politics. It not only asks what is right but also how to find what is better in the midst of so much demand on the resources of time and energy. Nobody wants the dogmatic or moralistic, and what will always be important in every area will be to lay out clearly the thinking and reasoning that will help us to reach conclusions, the 'why' as well as the 'what'.

Read it carefully but critically: your day may be a bit longer, but I can assure you your nights will be very much more peaceful.

Roger Higgs
Institute of Medical Ethics
St Helens, England

Preface

Handbooks tend to be light on grand concepts. I'll put forth only one.

'The danger of isolation, and the healing power of good connection'.

What I will describe here I would call 'A relational ethics'.

Since 1978, when my first novel, *The House of God*, appeared[1], I have been asked to speak all over the world, and from the start, in a less refined way, this concept has always been what I say, putting it in terms of 'Staying Human in Medicine'. I'm delighted to use it here, in this remarkable scholarly and pragmatic volume put together by my dear and remarkable friends Andrew and John.[2] Note that this guiding phrase is central not just to medicine but also to our lives. My attempt to write about American primary care is a novel, *The Spirit of the Place*, about a doctor going back to his home town to join the old doc who steered him into medicine when he was a lost teenager.[3]

Hints of this concept were present in *The House*, in rudimentary form. Over and over, there is the phrase, 'Being with (x)' – sometime 'x' is the patient, or a family member, or a colleague, or, even oneself. As *The Fat Man*, the hero of the novel who deftly conceals his deep care for patients, docs, and life itself: 'I make them feel that they're still part of life, part of some grand nutty scheme instead of alone with their diseases. With me, they still feel part of the human race'. And at the end of the novel, the African-American intern chuck sums up the main reason that the year in *The House* has been horrific: 'How can we care for patients, if nobody cares for us?'.[4] The tone of any institution comes from the top; the top of the House was unwise and abusive in the way that almost all big power-over systems are such. In my new institutionalisation, New York University Medical School, run by three of my generation who trained at 'The House of God' hospital, there is an aura of 'We were treated badly, and now that we are in a position of power, we will not treat the 'lower-downs' badly'. The institution reflects this kindness from the top, all the way through.

What is a good connection? *(See We have to talk: Healing Dialogues between Women and Men, the novel Mount Misery and the play Bill W. and Dr. Bob).*[5,6,7]

Think of going to lunch with a friend. If the lunch goes well, by the end each of you feels an increase of 'five good things': more energy or zest, more sense of self-worth and worth of the other, more self-knowledge and knowledge of the other, more empowered to take action, and, last, a desire for more connection – 'Hey let's do this again soon!' Note, especially the issue of 'power'. This is not the traditional model of the dominant culture, where 'power' resides in a person. Rather, the power here arises in connecting. You may have felt burnt out, unable to act, disempowered, when you went to lunch, but in the mutual connecting there is an arising of power in both of you. (The gerund is as close as our language gets to describing this.) This is especially helpful for doctors: it means that good connection helps you to take action in your job and your life! It helps you to be a better clinician and person. Note that in this 'relational model', the measure of a person's psychological health and growth does not reside in the 'self'. Rather it resides in the quality of that person's relationships.

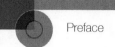

THREE NEW LAWS OF MEDICINE*

A good connection is a mutual connection; a good relationship is a mutual relationship. If it ain't mutual, it ain't good; if it is, it is. A mutual connection is when each person sees the other clearly, and each person senses the other 'feeling seen'. There's a 'click' – like, well, what we call love. We know it when know it.

This leads to three new *Laws of Medicine*, crucial to primary care – and – do see this – to our lives:

1. *The Shift to the 'We', 'The Connection', 'The Relationship'*: We live in an 'I'/'You' world, which implies adversarial relationships, the kind that makes lawyers rich. It is quite easy to introduce the word 'We' into conversations with patients and others in your life. Way back when I was a psychiatrist, I found that if I said to a patient, 'Tell me about your mother', I would hear about the mother, usually in narrowly 'self' terms; if I asked 'tell me about the *relationship* with your mother', all of a sudden the aperture opened up, and the patient would say, 'Well, in the relationship with my mother, there's x, y, z' – which were in fact, the 'qualities of the relationship with the mother', which opened things up for our understanding, and, frankly, healing. Here's the key: if you as a doctor (and person) use the word 'We', the patient will answer using the word 'We' – and the word concretises the fact that there is a relationship here! Old time patriarchal surgeons used to say, 'I did the tests, and I'm going to operate on you'. Now surgeons might say, 'I did the tests, and I suggest operating, but you can get a second opinion'. Both statements are 'I'/'You'. But if the surgeon says, 'I did the tests. Let's talk about what we can do'. The patient will say, 'Well I think we can…' Try it. Oh, and the main reason surgeons get sued is if the patient doesn't feel there is a good relationship there.
2. *Connection Comes First*: With a patient (or, e.g., a spouse or friend), if you are in good connection, you can talk about anything; if you're not in good connection, you can't talk about anything. Connection comes first. And connection with a patient is not really a matter of the time it takes: the good docs can do it quickly, with a look, a hand in a hand or on a shoulder, an attentive listening (most doctors interrupt within 17 seconds and talk 80% of the time thereafter).
3. *It's Not Just What We Do, It's What We Do Next*: In relationships – again, with patients and others – nobody gets it right all the time – it's what you do after you get it wrong that matters. The challenge is, when you are in a disconnect, if you can 'hold the idea that there is a relationship here, with a past and present, you can walk the other through it to a better connection'. In fact, just to say, at that crucial fractious angry or sullen moment: 'We're in a disconnect' – is a connecting statement. Differences can be used in dialogue to turn disconnections into better connections. We describe this work of moving from disconnects to connection in terms of gender difference in *We Have to Talk: Haling Dialogues between Women and Men.*[5]

---

* In 1978, Samuel Shem's novel *The House of God* offered a set of rules of thumb (the 'Laws') that were essential to newly qualified doctors' survival. The 'Laws' of *The House of God*, as espoused by the all-knowing fictional resident *The Fat Man*, were the key to survival for both interns and patients. The novel was recently named on *Publishers Weekly* as the second in the *Ten Best Satires of all Time*, after Don Quixote.

WHAT'S ALL THIS GOT TO DO WITH PRIMARY CARE?

Well, since this admirable specialty is the closest to living your job, in community, all this is central to every aspect: from individual patients to when you turn out the light and go home and in your centrality in your community, your country – hey, your world. And boy does the world need us to know how to connect, and create community and live with others, now. Clinicians are in a great position, through the job we have taken on – not for money or fame or any other of the 'craving' jobs where the process and the product is the same – making money – but for providing care for those who suffer: to be with others at the crucial moments of their lives, the three Buddhist 'heavenly messengers' of 'illness, old age and death', and helping to walk them through. It's a great job – despite the epidemic of all the admin-shit by the financiers.

In my novel *The Spirit of the Place*, about primary care in a small town, at one point the young doctor has to make a decision. He is surprised to hear the words, 'Don't spread more suffering around. Whatever you do, don't spread more suffering around'. And he makes his decision. We clinicians, especially in your specialty, are lucky: we are present at the most crucial moments of our patient's lives – and their families' lives. As we all know, everyone suffers – big suffering, little suffering, it's not optional. If any of us, clinicians or patients, try to walk through it alone, tough it out – we will suffer more and spread more suffering around. But if we walk through the crucible of suffering with others – and that's where we clinicians come in, that's our job, that's why we went into this specialty, not or the big bucks or the fame – if we walk with them through their suffering, we and they will not suffer as much, and will not spread more suffering around, and we will come through it with awareness, and even joy.[8]

Samuel Shem
NYU Langone Medical Center, NY

REFERENCES

1. Shem S. *The house of god*. New York: Richard Marek Publishers Inc.; 1978.
2. Papanikitas A, Spicer J, eds. *Handbook of primary care ethics*. London: CRC Press; 2016.
3. Shem S. *The spirit of the place.* New York: Berkley Publishing Group; 2008.
4. Shem S. *The house of god*. London: Black Swan Edition; 1985: 372.
5. Shem S, Surrey J. *We have to talk: Healing dialogues between women and men.* New York: Basic Books; 1998.
6. Shem S. *Mount misery.* New York: Random House; 1997.
7. Shem S, Surrey J. *Bill W. and Dr. Bob.* New York: Samuel French; 1987.
8. Shem S, Surrey J. *The Buddha's wife: The path of awakening together.* New York: Atria Books; 2015.

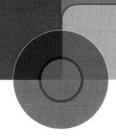

Acknowledgements

The editors would like to thank all of our contributors and reviewers, as well as the publishing team at Taylor and Francis.

We feel fortunate indeed that Elsbeth Manders agreed to grace our cover with her artwork.

We would also like to acknowledge the institutional support that has made this volume possible. The Royal Society of Medicine Open Section and General Practice and Primary Healthcare Section have run an annual Primary Care Ethics conference since 2011 with inputs from a group of clinicians and academics who have from time to time been called The Ethics of The Ordinary group or the Primary Care Ethics Group.

The Nuffield Department of Primary Care Health Sciences, Harris Manchester College, The Collaborating Centre for Values-Based Practice, The Oxford Healthcare Values Partnership and The Oxford Research Centre for the Humanities have all provided support and creative space as we and our contributors developed this project. We would similarly like to acknowledge the Royal College of General Practitioners' committee on medical ethics, and successive RCGP conference organising committees who have provided a much needed forum for the discussion of ethical issues. Much research took place at the British Medical Association library and we thank the staff for their assistance.

Our work with many groups of learners, particularly those centred in primary care, over the years has helped stimulate and evolve our interest in conceiving and developing this book.

We finally thank our colleagues, our patients and our families, for keeping us grounded in the real world and (in the case of the latter) occasional tea and proofreading.

Editors

Andrew Papanikitas is an academic general practitioner currently in an academic clinical lectureship in the Nuffield Department of Primary Care Health Sciences at the University of Oxford. He holds degrees in medicine, the history of medicine, and medical law and ethics, as well as postgraduate diplomas in history, philosophy, child health and higher education teaching. He has taught medical ethics and law at King's College London (KCL) and St George's medical schools. From 2010 to 2017, he has co-led a module on ethics law and professionalism for the KCL Department of Primary Healthcare. He currently co-leads an online MSc module in 'Ethics for the biosciences' at the University of Oxford. He is on the council of the Royal Society of Medicine GP and Primary Healthcare Section and was president of the RSM Open Section from 2012 to 2015. He currently serves as a co-opted observer on the Royal College of General Practitioners' ethics committee. He has been ethics and philosophy editor for the *London Journal of Primary Care* and peer reviews for several journals. He has written several books and chapters themes relating to both clinical examinations and medical ethics, including the 'Crash course in medical ethics and sociology'. In January 2014, he was appointed director for the Society of Apothecaries' Diploma Course in philosophy and ethics of health care. Dr Papanikitas' PhD thesis, 'From the classroom to the clinic: ethics education and general practice', explores ethics education in UK general practice.

John Spicer is a general practitioner in London, and Head of Primary Care Education and Development for Health Education England – South London. He has taught and written on clinical ethics for many years, having previously been a senior lecturer in law and ethics at St George's University of London. He is a member of the UK Clinical Ethics Network board, and a London Arts and Health Forum trustee.

Contributors

Sanjiv Ahluwalia is postgraduate dean at Health Education England – North Central and East London. He was previously Head of Primary Care Education and Development. He led on the development and provision of primary care education and development, including GP training. He is also a practising GP in a deprived community in North London. He has been involved in postgraduate education since 2002, as a GP trainer, programme director, associate director and Head of School for GP Training across London. Sanjiv's interests include the effects of postgraduate GP training on patient outcomes, medical professionalism and complexity theory in healthcare and education.

Stephen Bergman, professor of medical humanities at New York University, writes under the name **Samuel Shem**. Alongside a career in psychiatry, he is an acclaimed author of several novels, plays and textbooks, and his work has been translated into several languages. *The House of God,* his first novel, has sold over 3 million copies. His work exposes the potential moral challenges of the medical workplace and the connection between values, good relationships and healing. Other novels include *Mount Misery* (a darkly comic tale about psychiatric training) and the *Spirit of the Place*, set in the context of American small-town family practice. His most recent play is *Bill W and Dr Bob*, written with partner Janet Surrey about the foundation of Alcoholics Anonymous.

Jay Bowden is a general practitioner in South London with a diverse portfolio including medical education, integrated adolescent health, NHS and private general practice. He has worked with a variety of different patient demographics, ranging from deprived inner city areas to affluent leafy London suburbs and even spent some time at a medium security prison, though not at Her Majesty's pleasure! This diverse experience has enabled him to reflect on some of the enablers and barriers to patient autonomy. He is a strong believer in innovation in healthcare, particularly where this involves integration of services and empowerment of patients to improve outcomes. He has taught medical ethics at undergraduate level and retains a strong interest in this field.

Deborah Bowman is professor of bioethics, clinical ethics and medical law and deputy principal (Institutional Affairs) at St. George's, University of London. She is also the Editor-in-chief of the BMJ journal *Medical Humanities*. She is particularly interested in therapeutic relationships, narrative ethics, mental health, public engagement and the ways in which moral questions can be explored via the arts, particularly theatre and literature. She is a regular broadcaster and has contributed to, and presented, a wide range of programmes, particularly for radio, including Inside the Ethics Committee, Test Case, Inside Health, Night Waves and Start the Week.

Chris Caldwell is executive director of Nursing at Tavistock & Portman NHS Foundation Trust in London and programme director for the CapitalNurse Programme, working with Health Education England (HEE), NHS England and NHS Improvement. Chris was previously

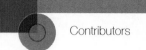

dean for Healthcare Professions at HEE working across North Central East London. Other past roles include Assistant Director of Nursing, Education and Organisational Development at Great Ormond Street Hospital for Children in London as well as a range of roles in education, clinical practice and policy at local and national level. She is an honorary visiting professor at City, University of London, vice chair of the London Perinatal Mental Health Network and a member of the London Mental Health Programme's Clinical Leadership Group. Chris is a registered nurse in adult and children's nursing and a nurse teacher. She has a Masters in Health Psychology and gained her Doctorate from Ashridge Business School focusing on transformational organisational change.

Dennis Cox is a GP based in Cambridge with 35 years of clinical experience. He has an MA in medical law and ethics and has taught at the medical school in Cambridge. He is an experienced expert witness for the courts and was a member of the Liverpool Care Pathway Review Panel for the Department of Health. He is a current member of the RCGP ethics committee.

Clare Delany is an associate professor in medical education at Melbourne Medical School, The University of Melbourne. Clare also works as a clinical ethicist at the Royal Children's Hospital Children's Bioethics Centre in Melbourne conducting clinical ethics consultations, education and research in paediatric bioethics. Clare's research and publications have mostly centred on physiotherapy; however, she reaches beyond the profession to teach and research in clinical ethics, health professional education and higher education more broadly. Clare has served as vice president of the Physiotherapists' Registration Board in Victoria and chair of the Australian Physiotherapy National Professional Standards Panel and is current chair of the Humanities and Applied Sciences Human Research Ethics Committee at the University of Melbourne. Her most recent book as co-editor is titled: *When Doctors and Parents Disagree: Ethics, Paediatrics and the Zone of Parental Discretion.*

Surendra Deo has a background in general medical practice, forensic medicine, and professional regulation. He is a case examiner and employer liaison advisor with the General Medical Council in the UK, and an associate director for the Health Education England in North London. In the past, he was an adjudicator for the Solicitors Regulation Authority in the UK. The chapter was prepared in a personal capacity. The opinions expressed in this book are the author's own and do not reflect the views of the GMC or Health Education England.

Sharon Dixon is a general practitioner in Oxford, UK. She is a medical adviser with the Health Experiences Research Group within the primary care department at the University of Oxford. She is a tutor on the clinical communication skills course in the Oxford University Clinical School. Sharon is the Oxfordshire primary care lead for Female Genital Mutilation and is a member of the Oxfordshire FGM multi-agency operations group.

Michael Dunn is a lecturer in health and social care ethics at the Ethox Centre, University of Oxford. He is also the director of Undergraduate Medical Ethics and Law Education, and the director of the Ethox Centre's Graduate Research Training Programme. Michael's academic research interests span a range of issues in healthcare ethics and bioethics, and he is the author of over 50 peer reviewed journal articles and book chapters. The predominant focus of his current work seeks to address ethical questions presented by the development and expansion of community-based and long-term care practice, law and policy – both in the UK and internationally. Michael is a senior fellow of the Higher Education Academy (SFHEA), an associate editor of the *Journal of Medical Ethics*, a member of the editorial board of *Ethics and Social Welfare*, and a member of both clinical and research ethics committees.

Hilary Engward is a senior research fellow in the Veterans and Families Institute at Anglia Ruskin University, where she leads on research into veterans and families living with limb loss. Hilary is a senior lecturer on PhD/EdD courses, with a specific interest in interprofessional learning and working across the medical and health professions. She also leads on research exploring organisational understandings of incident and serious incident reporting in NHS organisations and teaches health care ethics across medical and nursing undergraduate and postgraduate courses at various organisations.

Bill (KWM) Fulford is a fellow of St Catherine's College and member of the Philosophy Faculty, University of Oxford; emeritus professor of philosophy and mental health, University of Warwick Medical School; and director of the Collaborating Centre for Values-based Practice, St Catherine's College, Oxford (valuesbasedpractice.org). His previous posts include honorary consultant psychiatrist, University of Oxford, and special adviser for Values-based Practice in the Department of Health. His publications include *Moral Theory and Medical Practice*, *The Oxford Textbook of Philosophy and Psychiatry* and *The Oxford Handbook of Philosophy and Psychiatry*. He is lead editor for the Oxford book series International Perspectives in Philosophy and Psychiatry and founder editor and chair of the Advisory Board of the international journal *Philosophy, Psychiatry, & Psychology (PPP)*. His *Essential Values-based Practice* (2012), co-authored with Ed Peile, is the launch volume for a new series from Cambridge University Press on values-based medicine.

John Gillies was a rural general practitioner in Scotland for 28 years after working in Africa. He is interested in ethics and philosophy of medicine. He is now an honorary professor of general practice at the University of Edinburgh, deputy director of the Scottish School of Primary Care and co-director of the Global Compassion Initiative of the University Global Health Academy.

Benedict Hayhoe is a general practitioner in central London, and NIHR clinical lecturer in primary care at Imperial College London. He qualified from University College London in 2005 and was awarded an LLM in Legal Aspects of Medical Practice from Cardiff University in 2009. Having completed his MD on the subject of advance care planning in primary care in 2014, he remains interested in the interaction of law and ethics with medical practice and in dementia, elderly and end-of-life care.

Iona Heath worked as an inner city general practitioner in Kentish Town in London from 1975 until 2010. She is a past president of the UK Royal College of General Practitioners. She has written regularly for the *British Medical Journal* and has contributed essays to many other medical journals across the world. She has been particularly interested to explore the nature of general practice, the importance of medical generalism, issues of justice and liberty in relation to healthcare, the corrosive influence of the medical industrial complex and the commercialisation of medicine, and the challenges posed by disease-mongering, the care of the dying and violence within families.

Roger Higgs worked for over 30 years in south London as general practitioner and academic. He founded a single-handed practice that went on to be a major multidisciplinary group and started the Department of General Practice and Primary Care at King's College School of Medicine (now King's College). Awarded MBE as service developer and educator, he has

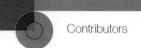

published in these areas as well as medicine and bioethics. His particular interests in the latter are case analysis, truth telling and narrative approaches, and books include *In That Case* with Alastair Campbell and *The New Dictionary of Medical Ethics* with Kenneth Boyd and Anthony Pinching. He teaches on the Society of Apothecaries' Diploma Course in philosophy and ethics of healthcare.

Joshua Hordern is associate professor of Christian ethics in the Faculty of Theology and Religion at the University of Oxford and a fellow of Harris Manchester College. He leads the multi-disciplinary Oxford Healthcare Values Partnership (www.healthcarevalues.ox.ac.uk) and serves on the Royal College of Physicians Committee for Ethical Issues in Medicine. Before taking up his post in Oxford, he was a research fellow at Wolfson College in the University of Cambridge, associate director of the Kirby Laing Institute for Christian Ethics and a local authority councillor with St Edmundsbury Borough Council. His publications include *Political Affections: Civic Participation and Moral Theology* (Oxford University Press, 2013). He is married to Claire, a doctor.

Jeremy Howick received his PhD from the London School of Economics in 2008. He was a lecturer at University College London, and he is currently a senior researcher at the University of Oxford, where he does both philosophical and epidemiological research on placebos and the value of empathy. He has published widely on evidence based medicine and the placebo effect. Dr. Howick is also the founding director of the Oxford Empathy Programme

Carwyn Rhys Hooper was born in Wales and currently lives in London. He is a senior lecturer in medical ethics and law at St George's, University of London. He is also the course director for a number of different global health degrees at the same institution. After completing a medical degree he studied philosophy. He then completed a PhD in law. Carwyn has a particular interest in global health ethics and public health ethics. He is also very interest in public engagement and he regularly discusses ethico-legal issues on television and radio. He is the general and company secretary of the Institute of Medical Ethics and he has served as an *ex officio* member of the clinical ethics committee at St George's University Hospitals NHS Foundation Trust for seven years.

Jonathan Ives is a senior lecturer in biomedical ethics and law in the University of Bristol's Centre for Ethics in Medicine, having previously worked at the University of Birmingham. His primary research interests are the Ethics and Sociology of fatherhood and families, and methodology in Bioethics, but he has published on a variety of topics including research ethics, end of life ethics, and ethics and medical education. He is editor of the book *Empirical Bioethics: Theoretical and Practical Perspectives*, published by Cambridge University Press, and is a co-opted member of the Royal College of General Practitioners Medical Ethics Committee.

Bridget Kiely is a general practitioner, with a background in Public Health and Tropical Medicine. Working with King's Sierra Leone Partnership at Connaught Hospital in Freetown, Sierra Leone, she witnessed the consequences of poor access to quality primary care on a daily basis, from unnecessary deaths due to vaccine preventable illnesses such as tetanus to renal failure from untreated hypertension. She worked with the Ministry of Health and Sanitation in Sierra Leone on their post Ebola recovery plan that aimed to significantly increase access to basic essential services. Currently she works with SafetyNet Primary care, a charity dedicated to bringing primary care to marginalised and vulnerable populations in Ireland.

She is passionate about the importance of primary care at a global level and universal access to health care and takes every opportunity to advance these causes.

Selena Knight is a GP Registrar at Chelsea and Westminster Hospital and an academic clinical fellow in the Department of Primary Care and Public Health at King's College London. She has BSc in Medical Ethics and Law from King's College London. She has continued her interest in ethics through establishing an ethics teaching programme for medical students at Imperial College London, being a member of the Imperial College Clinical Ethics Committee, and working as an intern at the World Health Organisation's Global Health Ethics Unit. Her main areas of interest are ethics education, clinical ethics and public health ethics.

John Launer is a doctor, family therapist, educator and writer. He was a general practitioner in Edmonton, north London, for over 20 years, and is an honorary consultant at the Tavistock and Portman NHS Trust. He is currently lead programme director for educational innovation at Health Education England. He has written extensively on narrative medicine and its applications in primary and secondary care.

Pekka Louhiala is a lecturer in medical ethics at the University of Helsinki. He has degrees in both medicine and philosophy, and he also works as a part-time paediatrician in private practice. He has published on various topics in medical ethics, philosophy of medicine and epidemiology. His current academic interests include conceptual and philosophical issues in medicine, such as evidence-based medicine and placebo effects.

Margaret McCartney is a general practitioner in Glasgow who writes about evidence-based medicine. She is the author of *The Patient Paradox: Why Sexed Up Medicine is Bad for Your Health* and *Living with Dying: Finding Care and Compassion at the End of Life*.

Emma McKenzie-Edwards is a general practitioner and medical educator in Oxford. She teaches undergraduates at Oxford University and runs a course at Magdalen College School in Oxford for sixth formers considering studying medicine. Emma has previously taught at the Peninsula College of Medicine and Dentistry in Exeter and the Australian National University in Canberra.

Nevin Mehmet is the senior lecturer in healthcare ethics at the University of Greenwich. She runs the undergraduate and postgraduate ethics teaching for the Paramedic Science and Applied Health Science programmes. Following her BSc in Complementary Therapies, she pioneered integrated healthcare by instigating an aromatherapy clinic within a GP surgery in North London while also co-ordinating a Complementary Therapy Clinic in a large south London family practice that was also the training centre for Aromatherapy and Complementary Therapy students. She also participated in preparation for the voluntary regulation of Aromatherapists for the CNHC. While participating in the development of Health and Well-being programmes at the university, she completed her MA in healthcare ethics and law at Keele University and is currently researching ethics education for paramedic practice for her doctoral studies.

David Misselbrook was a South London GP for 30 years. He was involved with GP training, CPD development and medical ethics. He is dean emeritus of the Royal Society of Medicine, past course director of the Society of Apothecaries diploma course in philosophy applied to medicine

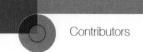

and is senior ethics advisor to the *British Journal of General Practice*. He now teaches family medicine and ethics for RCSI Bahrain, where he is associate professor of family medicine.

David Molyneux is a general practitioner and GP educator who works in East Lancashire. He is involved in GP education throughout the north of England and runs medical ethics courses for GPs and GP registrars. He has been a clinical skills (CSA) examiner for the Royal College of General Practitioners since the examination began. He also works at the University of Leeds as a medical ethics tutor and a personal tutor. His research interests concern the nature of autonomy and the relationship between autonomy and welfare. He has been awarded a doctorate in professional medical ethics at Keele University and is currently completing a BA in philosophy at London University.

Roger Neighbour is a past president of the Royal College of General Practitioners. He is the author of *The Inner Consultation, The Inner Apprentice* and *The Inner Physician*. Now retired from clinical practice, he teaches and lectures in the UK and worldwide on the general practice consultation.

Roger Newham is a senior lecturer at Buckinghamshire New University teaching research methods and professional ethics. He is a registered nurse (California and UK), where he worked primarily in HIV and AIDS care from 1989 to 1995. He has an MA Philosophy from Birkbeck College (University of London) and a doctorate in Bioethics (University of Keele).

David Obree is a practising dentist and medical ethics teacher. He is a fellow in medical ethics and medical education at the University of Edinburgh and honorary lecturer in social and community medicine at the University of Bristol.

Michael Paschke is a medical device patent analyst with Landon IP and the United States Patent and Trademark Office as well as regulatory and ethics board member at the University of Michigan Medical School. He has an educational background in biomedical engineering and kinesiology from the University of Michigan and is presently a Master's student at Oxford University. Michael has years of experience serving on the boards for the University of Michigan and Yale University Medical School Institutional Review Regulatory Boards, NuPath Community Credit Union and Downtown Windsor Business Accelerator. Concurrent with his work in healthcare regulations and healthcare ethics, he is the City Planning Commissioner for the city of Riverview, Michigan, where he is heavily engaged with local business entrepreneurs and executives.

Ed Peile is professor emeritus in medical education, University of Warwick, a fellow of three Royal Medical Colleges in the UK, and was awarded the 2009 President's Medal of the Academy of Medical Educators for his lifetime achievement in medical education. He has now retired from clinical practice but remains active in academic life, researching and publishing on values-based practice. He was recently appointed chair of the Education, Training and Standards Committee of the Academy of Healthcare Sciences.

Ioanna Psalti is a strategy advisor with long-term interests on the dynamics between micro-level processes and macro-level events. She is extensively involved in the review and development of EU policies for health, research and security and a regular contributor to the events organised by the Oxford Healthcare Values Partnership, a network of academics, educators and clinicians with an interest in policies for primary healthcare. She is currently working on the methodology of national healthcare reforms including a framework for exploring associated ethical issues. Ioanna completed her DPhil studies in inorganic chemistry as the holder of the EPA Florey Studentship at Queen's College, Oxford, under Professor Allen Hill, the 2010 recipient of the Queen's Medal for his protein electrochemistry work which revolutionised glucose monitoring. Ioanna is also trained in creative action methods and sociodrama and has additional research interests in organisational change, identity, diversity and trust surfacing in family business and multinational organisations. Ioanna has written extensively from language books to scientific research and history of policies, and she is the author of *Across the Bridge*, a chronicle of the impact of policies on the development of ocean sciences in North Wales. She is co-editor of the *British Journal of Psychodrama and Sociodrama* and a regular workshop leader in the Baltic Moreno Days, the international practical psychodrama conference. Since 2007, she is the director of Dime Limited, a UK-based communications company.

Imran Rafi is a general practitioner principal and senior lecturer in primary care education at St George's, University of London. He is chair of the Royal College of General Practitioners (RCGP) Clinical Innovation and Research Centre (CIRC), providing leadership to oversee the clinical priority programme, contributing to programmes that support research and promote quality improvements in general practice. He has an interest in genetics for at least 10 years and has been a member of the Health Education England Genome Advisory Board and the Human Genome Strategy Group Service working group. He was a founder member of the Primary Care Genetics Society and the World Organisation of Family Doctors specialist interest group in primary care genetics, as well as the Society for Academic Primary Care specialist group on primary care genetics. He is currently funded by the HEE on the Masters Medical Genomics course at the University of Cambridge. He is a member of the RCGP and fellow of the Royal College of Physicians.

Helen Salisbury did a degree in philosophy and psychology before training in medicine. She is a GP in Oxford and runs the communication course for medical students there. Helen is also medical director of the Health Experiences Research Group at the Nuffield Department of Primary Care Health Sciences.

Suzanne Shale works as an independent consultant in the fields of healthcare ethics, patient safety and healthcare leadership. She is Ethics Advisor to the NHS England Patient Safety Steering Group and a member of the DH Independent Reconfiguration Panel. During 2013, she chaired the 'Surgical Never Events Task Force' on behalf of NHS England and is now a member of the group implementing its major recommendations. She is a former Oxford University legal scholar with training in counselling, group facilitation and conflict resolution. Her consultancy has a strong focus on restoring trust and improving support for patients and professionals following harm in care settings. She presents lectures and masterclasses on trust, disclosure, human factors and patient safety throughout the UK, Australia, Europe and Japan. Suzanne is the chair of Action Against Medical Accidents (AvMA). AvMA is the leading organisation for justice and patient safety, and campaigned for many years for a legal duty of candour. She was previously vice chair of Compassion in Dying, and chair of the mental health service provider Umbrella. Suzanne is the sole author of *Moral Leadership in Medicine: Building Ethical Healthcare Organizations* (Cambridge University Press 2012).

Rosamund Snow (1971–2017) lived with chronic disease since she was a teenager. Described by colleagues as 'A true ethnographer', her PhD thesis was entitled, 'The role of patient expertise inside and outside the health system: patient education in diabetes'. As *The British Medical*

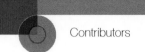

Journal's patient editor, she worked with patient authors from all backgrounds on the journal's educational series 'What Your Patient Is Thinking'. She also worked at the University of Oxford medical school, developing and researching patient involvement in medical education. She died on 2 February 2017.

Christine Stacey was a senior lecturer in nursing and stress management at the University of Greenwich following 18 years of working on all five continents and in 17 developing world countries. During her overseas career, she was involved in a range of health-related projects and interventions including the health and well-being of volunteers working for the United States Peace Corps. Returning to the UK in 1999, she decided to further her knowledge of other health systems undertaking a degree in Complementary Medicine, followed by a Masters in Education. Her research interest was in psychoneuroimmunology, particularly the role of Complementary Medicine for Health and Well-being. She is currently happily retired and studying genomic medicine as a hobby.

Rafik Taibjee trained as a general practitioner in Birmingham and the Black Country before becoming a GP principal in Merton. He is the chairman of Merton Health Federation and of Health Education England [South London]. He is a GP trainer and a GP training programme director at King's GP Scheme, London. He has an interest in Equality and Diversity, and Gay and Trans Healthcare. His ethical interest was developed through studying for a Master's in Public Health, at King's College, London.

Jonathon Tomlinson is general practitioner, trainer and undergraduate tutor at The Lawson Practice, London, UK. He writes a blog about the relationships between doctors and patients at https://abetternhs.wordpress.com/ and is on twitter https://twitter.com/mellojonny.

Peter Toon practised as a general practitioner for 30 years. He also held academic posts at University College London, Queen Mary University of London and the GP Deanery, where he worked mainly on postgraduate and continuing education. He has written many academic papers, particularly on the ethics of medical reports, preventive healthcare and virtue ethics in medical practice, as well as his three major works, *What Is Good General Practice?, A Flourishing Practice, and Towards a Philosophy of General Practice.*

Malcolm Torry is a visiting senior fellow in the Social Policy Department at the London School of Economics. His research interests include the reform of the UK's benefits system, and the characteristics and management of religious and faith-based organisations. He is married to a South London GP.

Andrew Trathen currently practises as a public health specialty registrar in London. His previous roles have been as a primary care dentist, and a Wellcome Trust clinical research fellow in the medical humanities. He teaches ethics to undergraduate and newly qualified dentists, and he is interested in professionalism and developing ethics curricula.

Michael Weingarten was born in England and educated at Oxford University. He was a GP in a Yemenite immigrant town in Israel for 35 years, and author of *Changing Health and Changing Culture – The Yemenite Jews in Israel.* As professor of medicine at Tel-Aviv University, he chaired the Departments of Family Medicine and Behavioural Sciences. In 2011, he moved to the Galilee as founding Dean of Education at the Faculty of Medicine in Galilee, of Bar Ilan

University. He was 2015–2016 visiting scholar at the Centre for Ethics in Healthcare (ETHOX) and Green Templeton College, Oxford University.

Paquita de Zulueta is a sessional London general practitioner (GP) with a special interest in clinical ethics, mental health, migrant health and professional well-being and development. She is honorary senior clinical lecturer at Imperial College and a cognitive behavioural therapist (CBT) in private practice, as well as coach and mentor for clinicians. She has been involved in GP education for many years as programme director and educational supervisor. She is a member of the Nuffield Council on Bioethics, the executive committee of the Worshipful Society of Apothecaries of London as well as the Imperial College Healthcare NHS Trust clinical ethics committee. She was the programme director for the applied clinical ethics course (ACE) at Imperial College for several years and runs seminars on ethics and law for medical students, postgraduates and established practitioners. She has written articles and book chapters on a broad variety of topics in clinical ethics, and her current area of research is compassion in healthcare and compassionate resilience. She is president-elect of the Royal Society of Medicine Open Section, the section concerned with the interface between healthcare and society.

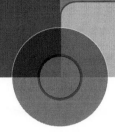

How to use this book

ASSERTIONS

The editors (hereinafter the first person plural – we) of this book are both active general medical practitioners in the UK, both possessed of an academic 'genome' and both passionate about primary care (wherever and by whoever it is practiced).

We both have been involved in various ways with the development of an ethical discourse particular to the practice of primary healthcare. While the term 'primary care' is often taken to mean community medicine or public health,[1] our scope is more interdisciplinary and interprofessional. Therefore, this book is offered as a means of pushing that discourse on, in an accessible and robust fashion. To that end, we have selected chapter authors for their writing facility and their experience in the field, covering a range of topics that is as wide as primary care itself. All have a particular style and preferred methods, which we have valued and have not sought to necessarily streamline into uniformity.

The chapters are grouped thematically into four sections:

1. The primary care interaction
2. On vulnerable patients
3. Teaching and learning
4. On justice and resources

We start with the place where patients and clinicians first come together: a place where the transaction is convened to address the suffering, or perceived suffering, that drives that interaction. It is important to note the key ethical importance of that suffering. It not only underlies the meaning of the word 'patient' but represents a distinctive feature of the meeting of moral agents, both at point of first access and beyond.

Vulnerability is at the root of ethical discussions in many healthcare contexts. While some patients may be conceptualised as of special (or unusual) need, others' needs are more usual but overlooked. In the second theme, we deal with some of those groups of patients: children, the elderly, the dying, among others. The ethics literature is full of texts considering the particular issues of these groups of persons (or more specifically, the philosophy arising from consideration of their situations). Here we seek to apply such philosophy to primary care, where it may be considered differently. Vulnerability implies that someone can be in a position of relative power. It implies a duty to advocate for those who are vulnerable – for example, to act in their interests or to empower them to act in their own.

The third section of this book concerns ethics in the context of teaching and learning in primary healthcare. The original meaning of doctor is 'teacher', and we endorse that ancient meaning. We also apply such an understanding to the many professions that have come to work within a modern primary care team. Moreover, we recognise that primary healthcare is not necessarily a physician-led and increasingly rarely a uniprofessional enterprise. Where the chapters of this book appear primarily to concern general practice (family medicine) or any other particular healthcare profession, we ask the reader to treat this as a case study and consider how the insights apply in the reader's milieu. We similarly ask our readers in different parts of the world to consider similarity and difference, as well as what ethical issues and learning can span geographical and cultural boundaries.

As may be evident, we are not slow to assert the value of primary care to the health and well-being of populations, and further claim that this value is under recognised in the fair distribution of healthcare resources. Such an assertion is shot through with ethical importance and justifies the inclusion of a suite of chapters in this area. In this section, we have explicitly included many of the non-clinical or para-clinical aspects of primary healthcare, such as business ethics, rationales for particular types of healthcare system and a discussion of the ethics of practice administration. In this last section, we have considered clinician self-care, integrity and conscience as well as the meaning of 'professionalism'.

ASSUMPTIONS

If a reader has got this far into the book, it is reasonable to assume that he or she is interested in, as a minimum, primary care, ethics, philosophy or any of the chapter headings on offer. We take a fairly broad interpretation of the title and include much material which may be considered 'standard' clinical ethics, springing as it does from its roots in Western philosophy, as well as some of the newer related issues such as the humanities, clinical empirical research, management theory and much else besides.

We assume that the reader is interested in these connections, as are we, and that the natural home of modern philosophy is the community, the clinic or the patient's home rather than the slightly abstracted, protected environment of the Higher Education (HE) Institution. Many of our authors have a role in HE bodies – a necessary function – but at root we take these essays to be of the real world, and drawn from it.

We suggest that the power relations in healthcare, as elsewhere, are not equal: between clinician and patient, between doctors and other healthcare professionals, between primary and secondary care, by way of example. Therefore, to determine what is the 'right' way of determining consequences of actions in a moral sense must take account of these power relations and the effect they have on decision-making.

As hinted at above, a modern primary healthcare team is just that – a team gathered together to deliver care of a quality better than if it had been delivered by one profession alone. Historically, it has been doctors who have led that delivery: our assumption is that as time goes on, multi-professional primary care will expand to patients' benefit. Nonetheless, some of the chapters do have a mainly medical content, recognising the historical context already mentioned.

While this book has global reach and authorship, there is a predominant reference to primary healthcare in the National Health Service of the United Kingdom. This is a feature because it is where the editors and many of the authors originate, but also because the primary care system is highly developed in the UK, in common with many other countries. Nonetheless, the themes identified in this volume are ethically universalisable and thus of potential relevance to the practice of primary care anywhere in the world. The reader is invited to consider, wherever they sit to read the book, whether that is the case. Furthermore, we invite the reader to reflect on similarities and differences of context throughout this book, both in terms of geography (what might Finnish and British clinicians in the community learn from each other?), or profession (what might physiotherapists, dentists and general medical practitioners have to teach one another?). This diversity of context affords the reader considerable insight into how primary care could be, or may yet be, depending on when and where they explore the essays in this volume.

APPARATUS

At this stage, for those readers not previously engaged in the fascinating world of moral theory, we offer something of an introduction. Philosophers, amateur or professional, can potentially leap over this section to the red meat of the text. However, as clinicians and ethicists, we have noticed colleagues occasionally struggle with the area, so offer a brief introduction to the subject, a toolbox if you will, as it will be useful in navigating the rest of this book.

In healthcare generally, clinical and non-clinical work are complicated because practice is characterised by a potentially confusing and conflicting array of philosophies. A clinician may have a Hippocratic duty to treat the patient in front of them as their first and only concern, or be mindful of general duties for professional conduct laid down by a professional body such as the UK's General Medical Council or the Nursing and Midwifery Council. Simultaneously, clinicians are expected to decide which patient should have priority, whether in terms of time or of healthcare resources and maximise the welfare of their patient-list, the community or indeed the country. Welfare maximisation measures can be described as utilitarian and include public health initiatives such as vaccination, or the incentivised prophylactic treatment of groups who are at risk of chronic disease. Services are judged on their ability to deliver measurable targets at the lowest possible unit-cost. Utilitarian philosophy is often implicit in 'best' or 'evidence-based' practice.

Overlaid on duty and utility is a rhetoric of, 'Excellence and flourishing', as a practitioner. This may be connected with Aristotelian virtue ethics, and virtues are sometimes an explicit component of medical education – especially clinical postgraduate education, where the characteristics of an 'excellent' general practitioner (GP) or a 'Compassionate' nurse are at issue. Clinicians are enjoined to encourage patients to flourish, with illness models based on ideas of disability rather than pathology.[2] A 'Contractarian' discourse of patient, civic or human rights is ever-present in from the mid- to late-twentieth century onwards. To enlarge slightly:

1. *Deontology (duty-based ethics)*
   There are many examples of explicit duties in society. Many are codified in law and take the form of prohibitions, such as a duty to refrain from committing murder. Historical examples include the 10 commandments of the Judeo-Christian tradition. A more medical set of commandments that are often quoted without much reflection are those in the Oath of Hippocrates. As a school of philosophy, contemporary deontology stems from the writings of Immanuel Kant (1724–1804). There are two core ideas that can be put very simply: Firstly, there are categorical duties – moral duties that are right in and of themselves without appeal to a higher authority such as a deity or the law. Secondly, the way of spotting such duties is that they are universalisable – they should be true for all people at all times, for example, we might consider truth-telling to be a universal moral duty – even lying relies on people generally telling the truth! One categorical imperative that might resonate more with readers of this book is the duty to respect persons, treating them always an ends in themselves and never purely as a means. This has immediate relevance for healthcare workers in primary care in that patients are represented as an ethical 'ends', and there is much celebrated duty to respect patient autonomy. However, as

well as being an ethical 'ends', patients are a means to being paid, healthcare education, healthcare research and even practitioner job satisfaction. The explicit nature of duties can be linked to their rightness, and their codification in law can be seen as a way of incentivising healthcare workers to do the right thing; however, rules can also be born out of other philosophical approaches – for example, a rule may be produced which aims to maximise welfare. Problems with deontological theories include the difficulty of conflicting duties, a common problem in medicine today when many different demands are made of doctors. They also struggle with the problem of bad outcomes arising from medical actions performed with good intentions

2. *Utilitarianism (consequences)*

Consequentialist theories are based on the idea that the right action in any situation should be based on the consequences of that action. Most influential of these approaches is 'Utilitarianism ': maximising utility (the good) or happiness. The right action in any situation is therefore that which produces the greatest good for the greatest number. This theoretical approach stems from the work of Jeremy Bentham and John Stuart Mill. Bentham advocated 'Act utilitarianism': we should act to maximise predicted overall benefit/pleasure in each situation. His intellectual successor Mill, however, advocated 'Rule Utilitarianism': We should enact rules to maximise benefit overall. As a contemporary example explored in this volume by Shale, a duty of candour healthcare could be based on consequentialist justifications – such a rule might help patients and relatives recover from a severe medical mistake and could contribute to valuable learning to promote patient safety. Mill also suggested that utility (good) was more complex than pleasure and pain in their simplest forms. 'Maximising welfare' is explicit in public health initiatives such as vaccination, or the incentivised prophylactic treatment of groups who are at risk of chronic disease. Utilitarian thinking is often implicit in 'best' or 'evidence-based' practice and where services are judged on their ability to deliver measurable targets at the lowest possible unit-cost.

3. *Virtues*

The Royal College of Physicians of London (RCP) lists the following as necessary for professionalism in the twenty-first century[3]:

   a. Integrity
   b. Compassion
   c. Altruism
   d. Commitment to continuous improvement
   e. Excellence
   f. Commitment to teamwork

   What the RCP is doing here is defining aspects of professional practice that are, or should be, intrinsic to clinicians' work. Therefore, the 'answers' to ethical dilemmas in everyday work are defined not by a numerical outcome, as in utilitarianism, or a fixed rule, as in deontology, but by the inner personality attributes of the practitioner. What, it may be asked, would the person of these six attributes do in a given situation? Such a way of looking at ethics goes back to Aristotle and has been developed by later thinkers such as MacIntyre[4] and Toon.[5,6] It seems to be having a resurgence in recent years. In this book, this area is described in some depth in Chapter 15, in a discussion of the ethics of migrant care. In the context of a mainly primary care discipline, but with a more regulatory mien, the UK Chartered Society of Physiotherapy define some key attributes of professional practice.[7] This includes integrity, honesty and openness among other things. We suggest that the professional attributes described by these and other professional bodies' despite their differences are all representing virtues in a similar way, common to the clinicians of primary care.

4. *Rights theory*

A more recent exhibition of moral theory, rights are, again, about the relationships between persons; and how there may be entitlements between those persons. Therefore, in a clinical context, a patient might require something of his clinician because that entitlement could be described as a right. It could be treatment for a particular illness perhaps. If we agree that such an entitlement is real, then clearly a duty is created on the clinician to provide the service. For obvious reasons, this is termed a correlative duty. Rights as a moral driver are associated with younger nations around the world, particularly including the United States, whose legal system is built on a scaffolding of rights. In a clinical sphere, we are dealing more with moral rights than necessarily legally enforceable rights.

Therefore, the patient claiming, for example, a right to a particular treatment – when access to it is constrained for financial reasons – is asserting a moral right.

5. *Other moral approaches and epistemic positions*

These first four moral 'spanners' in the toolbox are not the only ones on offer: the keen reader will note references to other ethical tools throughout the book. It is hard to ignore the four principles of Beauchamp and Childress,[8] adapted in the UK by Raanan Gillon.[9] The ethical 'Esperanto' of beneficence, non-maleficence, respect for autonomy and justice is recognised by many who have received a clinical qualification at an British or American HE institution in the last three decades – and is used by some of our authors. Contractarian ethics, care ethics[10] and feminist ethics[11] all are examples of more recent ways of looking at the moral world, which can and do impinge on primary care. Overarching all of them is the issue of moral relativism: the comparison of moral positions around the world. It is not difficult to see how this matters to the primary care clinician: what may count for acceptable practice in one country may not in another. Therefore, for example, a termination of pregnancy has been legally acceptable in the UK since 1967 (and in rare cases before that), but the legal change was founded on a moral shift among the public and healthcare practitioners at the time. Such a moral shift is not evident in other countries, and may even be going backward in yet more. Numerous other examples abound, and the salient point is that what defines moral primary care is more than anything else about the contextual moral climate, as well as professional standards and the law.

A serendipitous outcome of bringing together the authors for this book has been a clear demonstration that ethics is only a part of the philosophy of primary care. Despite its title, the book veers into what practitioners, patients and other moral agents believe, what a person is, what shapes the subsequent moral debates, and what can make them intractable. Several chapters then discuss evidence-based medicine and its role in moral decision-making, whether on an individual basis or in commissioning healthcare services.

ASPIRATIONS

We hope that this book will be a useful resource for anyone who is seeking a better appreciation and understanding of the ethics 'in', 'of' and 'for' primary healthcare. We recommend that readers look beyond their index chapter: for example, someone interested in complementary and alternative medicine is invited to read the chapters on the ethics of placebo, on commissioning and on conscience. Similarly, someone who is interested in how belief and clinical background might shape ethical approaches to practice might find new insights from the chapters on interprofessional ethics, commissioning, omnipractice and physiotherapy. This is a book to be explored, critiqued, agreed and disagreed with. The authors' views are their own but reflect a community of scholars, educators and practitioners who are tapping into a body of literature – we invite readers to look up references and judge their interest and coherence for themselves. With this collection of essays, we hope to inform, educate and occasionally inspire. We hope that the reader will get as much from exploring this book as we have from editing it.

REFERENCES

1. Braunack-Mayer A. The ethics of primary health care. In: Ashcroft R, Draper H, Dawson A, McMillan J, eds. *Principles of healthcare ethics*. 2nd ed. London: Wiley; 2007: 357–64.
2. Misselbrook D. Aristotle, Hume and the goals of medicine. *J Eval Clin Pract* 2016; 22(4): 544–9.
3. Working Party of the Royal College of Physicians. Doctors in society. Medical professionalism in a changing world. *Clin Med (Lond)* 2005; 5(6 Suppl 1): S5–40.
4. MacIntyre A. *The nature of the virtues. After virtue*. London: Duckworth; 2007: 181–203.
5. Toon PD. Towards a philosophy of general practice: A study of the virtuous practitioner. *Occas Pap R Coll Gen Pract* 1999; (78): iii–vii, 1–69.
6. Toon PD. What is good general practice? A philosophical study of the concept of high quality medical care. *Occas Pap R Coll Gen Pract* 1994; (65): i–viii, 1–55.
7. CSOP. Code of member's professional values and behaviour. Chartered Society of Physiotherapy. http://www.csp.org.uk/publications/code-members-professional-values-behaviour (accessed 20 September 2016).
8. Beauchamp TL, Childress JF. *Principles of biomedical ethics*. New York: Oxford University Press; 1979.
9. Gillon R. Ethics needs principles—Four can encompass the rest—And respect for autonomy should be 'first among equals'. *J Med Ethics* 2003; 29(5): 307–12.
10. Held V. The ethics of care as moral theory. In: *The ethics of care: Personal, political and global*. Oxford: OUP; 2006: 9–28.
11. Sherwin S. Feminist approaches to health care ethics. In: Ashcroft R, Dawson A, Draper H, McMillan J, eds. *Principles of health care ethics*. 2nd ed. London: Wiley; 2007: 80–5.

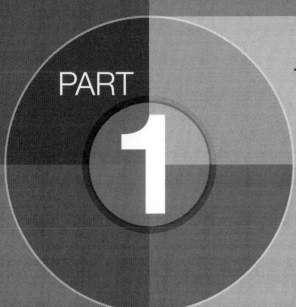

THE PRIMARY CARE INTERACTION

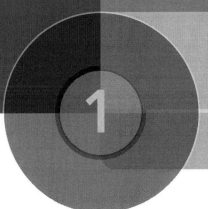

Autonomy and consent in family medicine

IONA HEATH AND JAY BOWDEN

DEFINING AUTONOMY

The word 'autonomy' has its origins in Greek (*auto* meaning 'self' and *nomos* meaning 'law'). Whilst the philosophical concept of autonomy is often traced back to Kant, there have been many important contemporary contributors, each of whom brings their own particular perspective. Perhaps as a result, there is no uniformly agreed definition.

For Kant, autonomy was a moral concern, relating to the ability to govern one's actions through rational judgement.[1] As such an autonomous person would be able to behave in a morally correct manner without the need of external laws. More recently, others such as Lévinas have argued that autonomy is selfishly grounded entirely in one's own personal interests and the contemporary dialogue has moved towards consideration of 'personal autonomy', that is, our ability to pursue the direction of our choosing in life, without such moral obligation.[2]

Dworkin defined 'autonomy' as an ability to make decisions that are grounded in our overall objectives and aspirations in life.[3] He separated our desires into first-order (our desire to commit an act, e.g. smoking during pregnancy) and second-order desires (our overall preferences, goals and values, e.g. to be a good parent). According to Dworkin, an autonomous individual would be able to critically reflect on his/her first-order desires and only choose to act if they were in agreement with his/her second-order desires. Ekstrom took a similar position, but instead of considering each second-order desire in isolation, he theorised that an autonomous individual would have a coherent position across all desires, which reflects his/her sense of 'self'.[4] Whilst this is more difficult for an external agent (such as a clinician or a lawyer) to determine, the concept is helpful when we consider the preservation of the autonomy of individuals who have lost the ability to express it, for example, when making decisions on behalf of patients with cognitive decline.

Substantive accounts of autonomy, such as that proposed by Wolf, build on theories of personal autonomy by revisiting Kant's concern with moral responsibility. For Wolf, an autonomous individual must be able to revise his/her actions based upon an ability to identify what is morally correct.[5] Within a resource-constrained health system, one could argue that this includes individuals taking responsibility for their own proportionate use of resources. However, accounts in biomedical ethics are usually less bold and are guided by the intimate relationship between autonomy and the ability to provide valid consent.

Beauchamp and Childress are prominent biomedical ethical theorists, whose principle-based approach has been firmly embedded within healthcare education. They suggest that even an autonomous individual can fail to self-govern in certain situations, for example, if they are depressed, coerced or even if they place a high level of trust in others.[6] They therefore focus on the autonomy of individual choices and propose that an autonomous decision is:

1. Intentional
2. Based upon 'adequate' understanding
3. Without controlling influences

Each of these points poses a myriad of challenges in modern-day primary care, particularly in the context of the current sociopolitical climate, which we will explore in detail.

One of the problems with a principle-based approach is the tendency to present autonomy as a self-evident good irrespective of context and other competing goods. Definitions of autonomy that include moral responsibility are very different from those that do not, and arguably the use of a definition within healthcare that excludes a moral perspective is potentially detrimental. The danger is that the idea of autonomy is used instrumentally merely to negotiate consent.

INFLUENCES IN THE PRIMARY CARE CONSULTATION

To develop a comprehensive view of autonomy in the primary care consultation, we must first consider its influences and stakeholders. Elwyn identified the potential voices in what he described as the 'postmodern consultation' (see Table 1.1).[7]

Thus, we can see that clinical decisions are not only influenced by patients and their clinicians but also by the people and organisations that inform them. The contribution of evidence-based medicine and guidelines deserves some elaboration. In resource-constrained health systems, such guidelines are not only concerned with clinical effectiveness but also cost-effectiveness. The socio-democratic nature of healthcare in many western societies (e.g. the National Health Service (NHS) in the UK and Medicare in the USA) has resulted in governments becoming huge stakeholders in healthcare and thus guidelines may also reflect political motivations.[8]

Table 1.1 A selection of the potential voices in the postmodern consultation

The patient	The pharmaceutical industry
The patient's family	Patient groups
The clinician	The internet
The clinician's social network	Media (TV, magazines, newspapers)
The continuing medical education system	Direct to consumer advertising
Evidence-based medicine and guidelines	Medical technology industry: investigations, procedures and 'screening' lobby
Independent consumer organisations	

Source: Modified from Elwyn, G., *Eur. J. Gen. Pract.*, 10, 93–97, 2004.

POLITICAL INFLUENCE ON AUTONOMY IN THE UK

Kant maintained that the protection of autonomy from political subversion was through the determination of rights.[1] In the UK this has been enacted through the creation of the NHS constitution, which aims to set out the rights of patients to certain treatments, to choose services and to complain and obtain redress.[9] In parallel with this, an internal market has been set up within the NHS in England, with services competing for 'business' in a drive to increase efficiency, responsiveness, quality of services[10] and, many would argue, to facilitate the privatisation of services. General practitioners' income has become linked to performance against specific clinical and organisational indicators. The government has also set out to further empower patients by enabling them to write 'trip advisor' style reviews of primary care services. The combination of factors has resulted in patients increasingly adopting the role of consumers of healthcare, entitled to certain rights.

However, rights are only valid so long as they do not conflict with the rights of others.[1] In a resource-constrained health system, the rights of one individual to avail, for example, an expensive cancer treatment may compromise the affordability of treatments and services for other patients. Whilst (Kantian) citizens have rights and responsibilities, consumers only have rights and the political response has been to create heteronomous rationing systems.[11] In England, this is the role of the National Institute for Health and Care Excellence (NICE) and Clinical Commissioning Groups (CCGs), whose guidelines recommend and limit treatments not only on the basis of clinical evidence but also on the basis of cost.

The consequence has been the replacement of clinical paternalism with bureaucratic and political paternalism, which compromises the autonomy of both clinicians and patients. Such paternalism is unresponsive to the individual circumstances and best interests of the patient and may therefore be even more detrimental to their autonomy. Patients may be confused with and frustrated by the conflicting messages, which may undermine the clinician–patient relationship, further challenging the expression of either party's autonomy.

With this in mind, the extent to which political interventions have enhanced patient autonomy remains unclear.

CASE STUDY

Abdul came to the UK from Pakistan with his parents. His parents speak little English and a relative acts as an interpreter. Abdul is diagnosed with a serious medical condition and his consultant recommends and prescribes a course of treatment. The next week the family present to their general practitioner (GP), having attended the pharmacy and discovered that the only available preparation contains pork gelatine. His parents are Muslims and are very concerned about the prospect of giving him a non-halal medication. They have spoken to family members and their Imam, who advised them to seek an alternative medication. The GP reads the specialist letter, does some research and identifies that there are three possible treatments. Of the two remaining options, one is not approved by NICE and the other is not recommended for prescribing by the CCG medicines management team (due to poor efficacy and high cost).

Immediately, we can identify multiple voices that could affect the autonomy of both Abdul's parents and his GP:

- NICE and CCG guidelines
- Opinions of religious leaders and family
- The clinicians involved in Abdul's care, their information sources and social network

We will explore the case further as the chapter progresses.

POWER RELATIONSHIPS AND CONSULTATION STYLE

Power relationships in the consultation can be broadly divided into three groups.[12]

1. Clinician centred (paternalism), where the healthcare practitioner makes decisions without patient input, or clinician-as-agent, where decisions are based on the patients' perceived preferences
2. Patient centred (informed decision-making), where the patient is provided with the available options and relevant information, but makes the decision independently
3. Patient centred (shared decision-making), where the patient is provided with relevant information, their individual situation is explored and, ideally, both the patient and the practitioner agree on the best course of action[13,14]

In Abdul's case, it could be tempting for the GP to make a further paternalistic 'clinician-as-agent'-type decision, for example, assuming that initial treatment is unacceptable and switching to the alternative less efficacious treatment. However, this medical approach is not in Abdul's best interests and makes a number of assumptions about his parents' preferences and values.

Taking the other extreme, an 'informed decision-making' approach could be taken. The GP could organise a professional interpreter and provide them with the details of the available options, their side effects, efficacy and the implications of treatment failure and allow Abdul's parents to select which course of action to pursue. The GP can thus discharge his or her duty-based ethical responsibility to ensure that Abdul's parents are informed, to listen to their concerns and to respect their right to reach decisions about their treatment, but remain completely neutral with respect to the decision itself.

Informed decision-making may reduce the chance of the practitioner's own values influencing the decision, but how much autonomy does this approach truly promote? We have learnt that autonomous decisions must be 'rational', 'in keeping with patient's (parents) second-order desires' and 'free from controlling influences'. In this particular situation, Abdul's parents may well have conflicting second-order desires, such as promoting their child's physical well-being versus being good Muslims or good children (i.e. respecting their own parents' views). They may find it difficult to make a 'rational' decision. Leaving patients to choose in such situations can leave them feeling abandoned rather than autonomous.[15] We are also assuming an adequate degree of health literacy, a subject to which we will return later.

Thus, whilst models that maximise patient power may satisfy a politically driven consumerist model of healthcare, they have been criticised for resulting in an abdication of doctor responsibility.[8] With the most recent generation of clinicians training in a culture of consent forms and defensive medicine, promoted by the threat of rising medical litigation, care is needed to ensure that decision-making responsibility is not excessively deferred to patients. Yet, although the sharing of decision-making responsibility may feel protective to healthcare practitioners, there is currently insufficient evidence to determine whether shared decisions actually reduce medical litigation.[16] Conversely, some have argued that litigation hinders collaborative decision-making by promoting 'neo, paternalism' that encourages practitioners to be responsible 'for' rather than 'to' patients, hence making them anxious to relinquish any decision-making power.[12] In either case, the fear of litigation presents a potential threat to patient autonomy, and we must be mindful to minimise its impact.

RELATIONAL ACCOUNTS OF AUTONOMY

Relational accounts of autonomy offer an alternative approach to patient-centred care. From a relational perspective, the empowerment of patient autonomy is achieved not only by enabling informed decisions but also by promoting a sense of self-identity. It is argued that our identity is constructed through our social environment (e.g. family, work, religion, culture, politics and economics) and the vast web of relationships within it. However, these relationships may support or limit the development of our own sense of self, and thus our ability to act autonomously.[17] To be autonomous, we must also trust ourselves to make the right judgements/decisions and to have the ability to act on these, even if those around us may disagree.[15] Yet, these 'skills' can only be developed if we are given opportunities to express our autonomy. In an environment with strict obedience to others (e.g. elders, husbands and religious guidance), autonomy may be much harder to achieve. Abdul's parents may have had little opportunity to consider their own position, beliefs and values in relation to those around them. The new relationships that they have developed since moving to UK may also have changed their perspective or made it uncertain.

As clinicians, we can facilitate relational autonomy by developing respectful adult–adult relationships with patients.[15] Whilst relational accounts tend to focus on the personal autonomy of the patient, we would argue that such relationships should also promote mutual moral commitment within the consultation. This may be achieved by:

- Careful listening and enquiry, to both their description of the situation and the opinions of others around them
- Inviting them to consider alternative perspectives, to determine their own position and think through the potential consequences, including the deliberation of any moral issues
- Providing honest, meaningful explanations, but enabling them to question what they are told[15]
- Making recommendations, clearly identifying how their personal circumstances have been considered, but inviting personal assessments of appropriateness and being clear about the scope to choose an alternative[15]
- Being honest about the external factors that contribute to your recommendations or that may limit their choice, for example, cost, efficacy, guidelines and policy, including any scope to appeal or circumnavigate these, but inviting consideration of their personal proportionate use of resources

The development of the trusting clinician–patient relationship required for patients to enact relational autonomy may take time, and continuity of care is therefore an important potential enabler. In primary care, we are fortunate to have the opportunity to develop longitudinal relationships with patients; however, recent changes to primary care in the UK appear to have adversely affected continuity and as clinicians we may need to argue its benefits with more determination and conviction.[18]

HEALTH LITERACY

Let us first assume that Abdul's parents are recent immigrants to the UK with poor English language skills. They have a limited social network within the UK and limited understanding of the health system. They may have had a limited education and be used to paternalistic models of care. Secondly, let us consider that Abdul's parents were born in the UK, are university educated and work as researchers. They follow the health media and research about their health online. They are aware of the NICE guidelines and have heard of cases where these guidelines have been challenged. They wonder whether Abdul's case may represent a loophole in the guidelines and ask the doctor to prescribe the medication that has been restricted by NICE.

It is not hard to imagine that a different decision could be made in these two situations, a key factor being the differential health literacy, that is, the

"cognitive and social skills which determine the motivation and ability of individuals to gain access to, understand and use information in ways which promote and maintain good health".[19]

From this definition, we can see that health literacy is not only limited by access to information and intellect but is also socially and relationally defined. As clinicians we may seek to improve patients' health literacy by providing health advocates and information leaflets in multiple languages, by allowing time for explanations, using decision aids, eliciting understanding and addressing health beliefs. However, in some cases, the layers of educational, social and cultural determinants of health literacy may make meaningful change unrealistic even in the presence of the most skilled consulter and wider social and educational interventions may be required.

Patient empowerment groups call to 'move beyond participatory medicine and focus on educating patients with the tools necessary to master autonomy and the art of self-care'.[20] In an increasingly stretched health system, this concept may be sociopolitically seductive; however, in the presence of such variable health literacy, this approach may differentially enhance autonomy and exacerbate health inequalities. It is also possible to argue that the aspiration to self-care is being used to enable the state to abdicate its responsibility to provide care for the weakest and the most vulnerable.

Yet, although knowledge and information undoubtedly help to promote the autonomy and agency of patients, the experience of sick healthcare professionals suggests that knowledge and information only go so far and can be all too easily undermined by the effects of fear which saps autonomy and paralyses the exercise of choice. The challenge for the practitioner is to provide information without exacerbating fear. Furthermore, it is important to remember the extent to which language determines the understanding and presentation of symptoms. Healthcare professionals can promote autonomy if they

"notice the subtle ways in which language orders perceptions and how language constructs social interaction. Symptoms are situated in culture and context, and trends in modern everyday life modify symptom understanding continuously. ... a symptom can only be understood by attention to the social context in which the symptom emerges and the dialogue through which it is negotiated".[21]

TENSIONS IN THE PRIMARY CARE CONSULTATION

As Sumner describes, the increasing concern of our society with its rights produces tensions, such as 'consumers against producers' and 'everyone against the state'.[22] It is not difficult to feel this in the consultation room, as health-literate patients feel that their rights (set out in the NHS constitution[9]) are being oppressed by clinicians and external regulation. The consultation is becoming an increasingly contested interaction, with trust sometimes eroded by the perception of healthcare practitioners as double agents, working not only for their patients' interests but also as agents of distributive justice and potentially for their own financial interests.[7,12]

Some argue that respect for autonomy represents a 'moral trump' for patients, creating a power imbalance and potentially resulting in healthcare practitioners acting outside of their professional judgement.[17] Practitioners may feel threatened by patients who behave as informed, empowered consumers of healthcare, a matter which has recently caused open conflict between doctors and patient empowerment groups on social media, prompted by the sale of a mug labelled *'Don't confuse your Google search with my medical degree'*.[23] They may also feel both intellectually and morally compromised by the increasingly rule-bound context within which they are supposed to provide care and by politically imposed priorities with which they do not agree.

Regrettably, much of the rhetoric, which portrays medical paternalism as bad and patient autonomy as an unequivocal good, seems to interpret the distribution of power within the clinician–patient relationship as a zero sum. Anything which increases the practitioner's power must necessarily reduce that of the patient, and vice versa. However, it is important to remember that human relationships always have the potential to augment the power of both parties. Facing the challenges of illness and suffering brought on by the inevitable heteronomy of the body, both patients and healthcare practitioners have the capacity to combine and so enhance their separate powers. In Abdul's case, his parents' 'refusal' to give him the non-halal medication may have loosened the doctor's bureaucratic shackles, enabling him or her to act against the NICE guidelines and prescribe a more effective and acceptable treatment. The autonomy of both parties is thus enhanced. Yet, primary care is being delivered by an increasingly multi-professional team, with ever greater overlap in roles and responsibilities. In comparison with doctors, the practice of nurses and allied health professionals is traditionally more confined by protocols and guidelines, and the ethical dimensions of these must be considered pragmatically if we are to empower all professionals to promote patient autonomy.

Finally, we consider that the quality of the clinician–patient relationship remains the key to the promotion of patient autonomy.

REFERENCES

1. Kant, I. *Practical Philosophy,* ed. and trans. Gregor, M. Cambridge, 1996.
2. Lévinas, E. *Totality and Infinity*, trans. Alphonso Lingis, Pittsburgh, PA: Duquesne University Press, 1969.
3. Dworkin, G. *The Theory and Practice of Autonomy,* Cambridge: Cambridge University Press, 1988.
4. Ekstrom, L. A coherence theory of autonomy, *Philosophy and Phenomenological Research,* 1993; 53: 599–616.
5. Wolf, S. *Freedom within Reason,* New York: Oxford University Press, 1990.
6. Tom, B. L., Childress, J. F. *Principles of Biomedical Ethics,* 7th ed., Oxford: Oxford University Press, 2013.
7. Elwyn, G. Arriving at the postmodern medical consultation, *European Journal of General Practice,* 2004; 10(3): 93–97.
8. Balint, J., Shelton, W. Regaining the initiative. Forging a new model of the patient-physician relationship. *JAMA,* 1996; 275(11): 887–891.

9. UK Government, Department of Health. *The NHS Constitution*. Available at: http://www.nhs.uk/choiceintheNHS/Rightsandpledges/NHSConstitution/Pages/Overview.aspx. Accessed July 10, 2017.

10. Dixon, A., Robertson, R., Appleby, J., Burge, P., Devlin, N., Magee, H. *Patient Choice*. King's Fund, 2010. Available at: http://www.kingsfund.org.uk/sites/files/kf/Patient-choice-final-report-Kings-Fund-Anna_Dixon-Ruth-Robertson-John-Appleby-Peter-Purge-Nancy-Devlin-Helen-Magee-June-2010.pdf. Accessed July 10, 2017.

11. McDonald, R., Mead, N., Cheraghi-Sohi, S., Bower, P., Whalley, D., Roland, M. Governing the ethical consumer: Identity, choice and the primary care medical encounter, *Sociology of Health & Illness*, 2007; 29(3): 430–456.

12. Goodyear-Smith, F., Buetow, S. Power issues in the doctor-patient relationship, *Health Care Analysis*, 2001; 9: 449–462.

13. Emanuel, E. J., Emanuel, L. L. Four models of the physician-patient relationship, *JAMA*, 1992; 267(16): 2221–2226.

14. Mol, A. *The Logic of Care: Health and the Problem of Patient Choice*, Abingdon: Routledge, 2008.

15. Entwistle VA et al., Autonomy and the clinician patient relationship. *JGIM*, 2010; 25(7): 742–745.

16. Durand, M.-A., Moulton, B., Cockle, E., Mann, M., Elwyn, G. Can shared decision-making reduce medical malpractice litigation? A systematic review, *BMC Health Services Research*, 2015; 15: 167.

17. Ells, C., Hunt, M., Chambers-Evans, J. Relational autonomy as an essential component of patient-centered care. *International Journal of Feminist Approaches to Bioethics*, 2011; 4(2): 79–101.

18. Freeman, G., Hughes, J. *Continuity of Care and the Patient Experience*, Kings Fund, 2010. 18–20. Available at: http://www.kingsfund.org.uk/sites/files/kf/field/field_document/continuity-care-patient-experience-gp-inquiry-research-paper-mar11.pdf. Accessed July 10, 2017.

19. Nutbeam, D. Health literacy as a public health goal: A challenge for contemporary health education and communication strategies into the 21st century, *Health Promotion International*, 2000; 15: 259–267.

20. De Bronkart, D. From patient centred to people powered: Autonomy on the rise, *BMJ*, 2015; 350: h146.

21. Malterud, K., Guassora, A. D., Graungaard, A. H., Reventlow, S. Understanding medical symptoms: A conceptual review and analysis, *Theoretical Medicine and Bioethics*, 2015; 36(6): 411–424.

22. Sumner, W. 'Rights', in *The Blackwell Guide to Ethical Theory*, H. Lafollette (ed.), Oxford: Blackwell. 2000; 288–305.

23. De Bronkart, D. Googling is a sign of an engaged patient. *MedPage Today Professional*. 2015; Available at: http://www.kevinmd.com/blog/2015/12/googling-sign-engaged-patient.html. Accessed July 10, 2017.

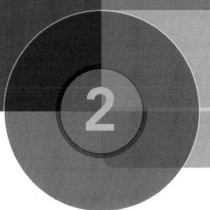

Benefits, harms and evidence – Reflections from UK primary healthcare

MARGARET McCARTNEY

INTRODUCTION

Benefits and harms are wedded like horses and carriages, or bows and arrows. Interventions we (clinicians) offer often give us some of something useful, but rarely include none of something either useless or harmful. In primary care, these qualities are immutably tied together. Naturally, to make decisions as good as possible, we need to know, 'What is the benefit relative to harm?'

Firstly, I will examine: 'What is a benefit and what is a harm?' Secondly, what should we know about where the balance of risk and benefit appear to lie? Thirdly, what should we do with this knowledge, particularly in the context of the biopsychosocial gaze of primary care?

WHAT IS A BENEFIT AND WHAT IS A HARM?

Many studies have examined the harm of treatments, and death as a comparative measurement in particular. This is an obvious, binary outcome to measure, and is naturally of great importance. It is particularly important in screening studies, where the harm caused by treatment of overdiagnosed conditions can result in death – for example, the surgery for a screening-detected aortic aneurysm incurs a mortality rate – however, the aneurysm being operated on may have been destined never to rupture. When we talk of using statins to reduce the risk of future heart disease or stroke, we can compare the expected numbers of heart attacks and strokes in statin-treated against untreated groups.

Then there are other benefits and harms which may be less obvious. For people considering a statin for primary prevention, reasons for not wishing to take it can range from a feeling that one is already consuming too many tablets; that friends or neighbours have had problems; that one would prefer to avoid side effects, visits to the doctor or pharmacist, or, as one person as put it to me 'I'd rather die of a heart attack than cancer'. Or, in choosing between two antico-agulants, one requiring regular blood tests at a clinic and the other needing no monitoring, the latter would seem more convenient and therefore obviously preferred. However, some people prefer the former, often because regular contact with a health professional and the social inter-action of a clinic visit is viewed as an advantage. Some people may have beliefs about inter-ventions that are changed after a discussion about evidence (e.g. the purpose and evidence for preventative vaccination). However, many other people have views on interventions that are essentially clashes of competing values and priorities: a guideline whose purpose is to reduce future strokes using tablets is of little value when the person's stated aim is to avoid tablets.

WHAT SHOULD WE KNOW ABOUT WHERE THE BALANCE OF RISK AND BENEFIT APPEAR TO LIE?

However, what should that evidence which the doctor presents, and which is capable of chang-ing minds, consist of? Judging what is a benefit and what is a harm requires the opinion of the individual to whom the intervention is being offered. Benefits and harms are, in the eye of the doctor, often medico-legal tabulations that must be cited correctly, in purpose to ensure informed consent and legal protection. In practice, our reckonings may be mere inexact gam-bles, and benefits and harms of the interventions we propose may be more subtle and unquan-tified. The problem, as we will come to see, is that professionals may present risks and benefits in such ways as to make doing more elaborate or invasive medical interventions seem like the more appealing option. Further, unequivocal harms – such as death or damage from needless surgery – are often framed by using a toxic combination of misleading or incomplete statistics and emotion, making it hard for contemplative citizens to make choices on the basis of clean facts and personal priorities.

In order to place the values held by individuals about risks and benefits, we therefore need to know what outcomes, and in what quantity, we can reasonably expect from medical inter-ventions on offer. These outcomes need to include things that patients would like to know about. In the UK, the General Medical Council (GMC) says that doctors should 'not make assumptions' about '(1) the information a patient might want or need, (2) the clinical or other factors a patient might consider significant or (3) a patient's level of knowledge or understand-ing of what is proposed'. They go on to say that patients should be given information they want or need about 'the potential benefits, risks and burdens, and the likelihood of success, for each option'.[1]

This is where the problems really start to accumulate. Firstly, we know that not all the evi-dence gathered in clinical trials are published, meaning that even the most thorough systematic reviews are capable of reaching misleading conclusions.[2,3] This is not the only bias, but may be ethically challenging. If ethical decisions should be fully informed, selective publication, for example, may prejudice a fully informed state of knowledge. When data are independently analysed, rather than by the drug company sponsoring, very different conclusions may be reached. Initial trials of antidepressants in teenagers found them to be 'generally well tolerated and effective',[4] but independent scrutiny found them to be not effective and overall harmful.[5] Publication bias means that more trials are published which find benefit than harm.[6] All of these issues would point towards medical interventions being perhaps not as good in reality as they might appear in research papers.

One might therefore expect some caution when translated into real world practice. Yet, when asked about some of these binary outcomes, doctors tend to not only overestimate the cardiovascular risk patients have,[7] and overestimate the benefits of treatment.[8] Doctors overestimate the lifespan of people with type 2 diabetes and overestimate the effect of treatments.[9] No wonder that citizens, too, overestimate the benefits of screening tests and underestimate the harms.[10] The biases in how we interpret research continue. If we don't know about lead-time bias, we assume that finding more occurrences of cancer in screened populations is always a good and useful thing. And of course, doctors are very good at using another form of bias, confirmation bias, to justify what we do by seeing only what suits the internal narrative we construct. Naturally, we think that what we offer does more good than harm; we underplay risk, we exaggerate benefits: it's easier all round if we continue to believe in the medicine, and don't examine the nasty underbelly of unpublished trials, our own and other biases, and bad statistics. But, of course, we must not.

There are ways to do it better. It is here, in how we reckon with benefit and harm, that we can make useful differences to how we perceive them. When we are told that we can reduce our risk of disease by 50%, a treatment might seem very useful. When we are told that a treatment can reduce our risk of disease from 0.05% to 0.025%, it seems less impressive. This is the difference between the relative and the absolute risk, and is the cause of recurrent irritability on my behalf when listening to media reports about alleged medical breakthroughs. This – framing – does not necessarily lie, but may mislead. There is evidence that presenting the same data in more favourable ways results in people overestimating treatment effects – with doctors and patients getting it wrong in very similar ways.[11] Not surprisingly, presenting data using absolute numbers makes it more likely for doctors to report risk and benefit accurately.[12] Similarly, decision aids – often computer-aided – can help people gain greater knowledge about the choices they have – and notably reduce the numbers of people wishing elective surgery.[13]

This of course takes time, and our rapid appointment systems, with emphasis on throughput rather than the quality of decision-making, make for a poor starting point.

And even then, what about our unknown unknowns? What about the things we didn't ask to begin with: my second question. If we want to help people make good decisions about healthcare options, we need to ensure that we have information about benefits and harms that matter. For example, researchers want to do more drug trials; patients are more interested in better information about non-drug treatments.[14] When people with arthritis were asked about their priorities for research, they were not so keen on knowing the impact of treatments on pain, but on fatigue – yet, this was not something that researchers were routinely asking about.[15] When patients are not involved in setting up research trials, the benefits and harms we end up knowing about are the ones that doctors identified as being important, not patients. This means that when the findings of the research (which need patients to take part in, or else it is not done) are made known, they do not give the answers patients wanted. This is wasteful – and essentially unethical. Certainly, there are outcomes in trials which doctors should be keen to study (not least, harms), but until researchers and patients work together to find the valuable unknown unknowns, we will guddle around in the dark when we could have turned the lights on.

Or take, for example, the risk of negative psychological effects following screening tests. This was hardly examined in the research evidence leading up to the beginning of many screening programmes in the UK.[16] Who would have thought that the steep rise in early breast 'cancer' of the type 'DICS' (ductal carcinoma, detected by screening) would be mainly due to overdiagnosis?[17] Overdiagnosis is a harm, because the associated sequelae – surgery or radio or chemotherapy – can never benefit the individual, because the underlying problem was not destined to ever do damage to the person. Yet, unless the person has the knowledge that overdiagnosis is possible or likely, the medical experience is likely to be seen as overall beneficial. There may have been painful, time-consuming, difficult treatments – but these harms are balanced by the benefit of being alive. If we knew that our life was not under threat, we would be more likely to view the treatments as harmful. Women activists have eloquently reminded doctors that this is not about more information, but better information – and the opportunity to exercise real autonomy.[18,19]

WHAT SHOULD WE DO WITH THIS KNOWLEDGE? A KEY CONTRIBUTION OF THE PRIMARY HEALTHCARE SETTING

Being able to present benefits and harms accurately and with as little bias as possible is not the end of the story. Medical decision-making is not simply to do with weighing up one against the other, but about the burdens of healthcare, the priority it has, ones' family, work and interests, philosophy of life, view of death, quality of living, purpose, spirituality and mental health. Decisions can unfold over time, and a discussion of benefit and harm for most doctors will not involve the exchange of digested numbers needed to treat or harm for a binary yes or no deal. General practice is richer and more subtle than this. At the pinnacle of general practice, it realises a mutual regard and appreciation for values. A study in a journal explained that for 100,000 women being screened for breast cancer, every year from age 40 to 75 (more frequent than in the UK), 11 deaths due to radiation would be expected. However, because they felt more deaths would be stopped through breast cancer, they concluded, 'The risk of radiation-induced breast cancer should not be a deterrent from mammographic screening of women'.[20] Another study about how to control blood sugar strictly in people with diabetes found that lower sugar levels result in less later complications from the diabetes. However, there was a bigger risk of hypoglycaemia. Nevertheless, the authors wrote that 'Although we are mindful of the potential for severe injury, we believe that the risk of severe hypoglycemia… is greatly outweighed by the reduction in microvascular and neurologic complications'.[21] Each of these conclusions is unhelpful because it denies both the values and autonomy of the person at the receiving end. It is not for the researchers to say which of these outcomes is a benefit relative to harm and which intervention is worthwhile to accept. Even perfect knowledge about benefits and harms requires to be translated in the context of the individual patient: it also requires to be interpreted according to what those persons' wishes are.

How do we get there? Much work is underway in articulating patient views and values in research and decision aids. This is welcome, but we need more. Clearly, systematic imperatives that push compliance with targets to treat patients rather than offering considerate discussion on options must go. In the real, messy frontline world of general practice, we will always have uncertainty about where the balance of risk and benefit might lie. By reiterating again and again how biases are stacked in favour of recommending treatments and interventions well beyond their rational evidence, my hope is that more honest medicine will result in less but higher value medicine. Stopping doing things that don't work, or work rarely or come with an unacceptable burden of side effects or appointments should make room for the pleasure of practicing medicine. As I wrote, in 2016, that joy has been buried under nearly two decades of tedious target culture. By shifting our focus away from the computer, and back onto the person, talking about risks and harms, sharing uncertainties and talking about priorities – the reason that general practitioners like me consider that general practice is the best job in the world which will surely re-emerge.

REFERENCES

1. General Medical Council Consent Guidance. http://www.gmc-uk.org/guidance/ethical_guidance/consent_guidance_sharing_info_discussing_treatment_options.asp (accessed 27 April 2016).

2. Beth Hart, Doris Duke, Andreas Lundh, Lisa Bero. Effect of reporting bias on meta-analyses of drug trials: Reanalysis of meta-analyses. *BMJ* 2012; 344: d7202. http://www.bmj.com/content/344/bmj.d7202 (accessed 27 April 2016).

3. Dwan K, et al. Evidence for the selective reporting of analyses and discrepancies in clinical trials: A systematic review of cohort studies of clinical trials, June 24, 2014. http://journals.plos.org/plosmedicine/article?id=10.1371/journal.pmed.1001666 (accessed 27 April 2016). http://dx.doi.org/10.1371/journal.pmed.1001666.

4. Doshi P. No correction, no retraction, no apology, no comment: Paroxetine trial reanalysis raises questions about institutional responsibility. *BMJ* 2015; 351. http://www.bmj.com/content/351/bmj.h4629 (accessed 21 August 2016). doi: http://dx.doi.org/10.1136/bmj.h4629.

5. Le Nour J, et al. Restoring study 329: Efficacy and harms of paroxetine and imipramine in treatment of major depression in adolescence. *BMJ* 2015; 351. http://www.bmj.com/content/351/bmj.h4320 (accessed 21 August 2016). doi: http://dx.doi.org/10.1136/bmj.h4320.

6. The James Lind Library 2.7 Dealing with biased reporting of the available evidence. http://www.jameslindlibrary.org/essays/2-7-dealing-with-biased-reporting-of-the-available-evidence/ (accessed 21 August 2016).

7. Pignone M, Phillips CJ, Elasy TA, Fernandez A. Physicians' ability to predict the risk of coronary heart disease. *BMC Health Serv Res.* 2003; 3: 13. http://bmchealthservres.biomedcentral.com/articles/10.1186/1472-6963-3-13 (accessed 21 August 2016). doi: http://dx.doi.org/10.1186/1472-6963-3-13.

8. Schroen AT, et al. Beliefs among pulmonologists and thoracic surgeons in the therapeutic approach to non-small cell lung cancer. *Chest* 2000; 118(1): 129–137. http://www.sciencedirect.com/science/article/pii/S0012369215390139 (accessed 02 September 2016).

9. Price HC, Thorne KI, Dukát A, Kellett J. European physicians overestimate life expectancy and the likely impact of interventions in individuals with type 2 diabetes. *Diabetic Med.* 2009; 26(4): 453–455. http://onlinelibrary.wiley.com/doi/10.1111/j.1464-5491.2009.02702.x/abstract (accessed 02 September 2016).

10. Hoffmann TC, Del Mar C. Patients' expectations of the benefits and harms of treatments, screening, and tests: A systematic review. *JAMA Intern Med.* 2015; 175(2): 274–286. http://archinte.jamanetwork.com/article.aspx?articleid=2038981 (accessed 03 September 2016). doi: http://dx.doi.org/10.1001/jamainternmed.2014.6016.

11. Perneger TV, Agoritsas TJ. Doctors and patients' susceptibility to framing bias: A randomized trial. *Journal of Gen Intern Med.* 2011; 26(12): 1411–1417. http://www.ncbi.nlm.nih.gov/pmc/articles/PMC3235613/ (accessed 03 September 2016).

12. Girgerenzer G, Edwards A. Simple tools for understanding risks: From innumeracy to insight. *BMJ* 2003; 327. http://www.bmj.com/content/327/7417/741?hwoasp=authn%3A1460920033%3A4130220%3A1366167283%3A0%3A0%3AeBsTDc%2FQrMpZPXH9IsFojQ%3D%3D (accessed 21 August 2016). doi: http://dx.doi.org/10.1136/bmj.327.7417.741.

13. Stacey D, et al. Decision aids to help people who are facing health treatment or screening decisions. *Cochrane Library* 2014. http://www.cochrane.org/CD001431/COMMUN_decision-aids-to-help-people-who-are-facing-health-treatment-or-screening-decisions (accessed 21 August 2016).

14. Crowe S, et al. Patients', clinicians' and the research communities' priorities for treatment research: There is an important mismatch. *Res Involv Engag.* 2015; 1: 2. http://researchinvolvement.biomedcentral.com/articles/10.1186/s40900-015-0003-x (accessed 21 August 2016). doi: http://dx.doi.org/10.1186/s40900-015-0003-x© 2015.

15. Presentation by Iain Chalmers to the Comet Initiative, 2011. http://www.comet-initiative.org/assets/downloads/2nd-meeting/day-2/Day2_Iain_Chalmers.pdf – Conference Presentation (accessed 21 August 2016).

16. Heleno B, et al. Quantification of harms in cancer screening trials: Literature review. *BMJ* 2013; 347: f5334. http://www.bmj.com/content/347/bmj.f5334?ijkey=046ffd3c3b2e3b9dd06b99f98acea85ef61cc1b5&keytype2=tf_ipsecsha (accessed 21 August 2016).

17. Bleyer A, Welch HG. Effect of three decades of screening mammography on breast-cancer incidence. *N Engl J Med.* 2012; 367: 1998–2005. http://www.nejm.org/doi/full/10.1056/NEJMoa1206809 (accessed 21 August 2016).

18. Pryke M, et al. How should screeners respond to women's distress about unexpected DCIS uncertainties? *J Med Screen.* 2011; 18(2): 104–105. http://msc.sagepub.com/content/18/2/104.full (accessed 21 August 2016).

19. Rogers WA. Whose autonomy? Which choice? A study of GPs' attitudes towards patient autonomy in the management of low back pain. *Fam Pract.* 2002; 19(2): 140–145.

20. Yaffe MJ, Mainprize JG. Risk of radiation-induced breast cancer from mammographic screening. *Radiology* 2012; 264(1): 306. http://www.ncbi.nlm.nih.gov/pubmed/21081671 (accessed 21 August 2016).

21. Greenhalgh T, Snow R, Ryan S, Rees S, Salisbury H. Six 'biases' against patients and carers in evidence-based medicine. *BMC Med.* 2015; 13: 200. http://bmcmedicine.biomedcentral.com/articles/10.1186/s12916-015-0437-x (accessed 21 August 2016). doi: 10.1186/s12916-015-0437-x.

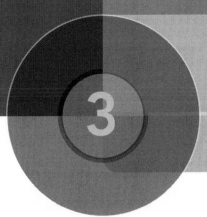

Why it can be ethical to use placebos in clinical practice

JEREMY HOWICK

INTRODUCTION

Placebo treatments are often prescribed by clinicians.[1,2] Widespread use, of course, does not imply that such use is ethical, but merely that clinicians appear to be willing to prescribe them in spite of any potential ethical concerns. Placebo treatments are claimed to be unethical for two reasons. Firstly, they are supposedly ineffective (or less effective than 'real' treatments), so the ethical requirement of beneficence (and 'relative' non-maleficence) makes their use unethical. Secondly, they allegedly require deception for their use, which violates patient autonomy. Here, I will argue that in cases where placebos are effective options and do not require deception, they are arguably ethical. Importantly, questions about the magnitude of placebo effects and about whether placebos require deception are *empirical* questions with ethical implications rather than purely ethical ones.

The arguments for the ethics of placebos are also intertwined with at least two other issues: alternative medicine and the rationality of science. One of the reasons so many patients choose to visit alternative practitioners is that many alternative practices spend more time with patients and thus could be better than conventional medicine at eliciting placebo effects.[3] This relates arguments about the ethics of placebos to arguments about the ethics of alternative medicine. Although the relationship between the ethics of placebos and the ethics of alternative medicine is interesting, it is beyond the scope of this chapter to consider in any detail. Secondly, placebos seem to question the rationality of science. If, as many seem to believe implicitly or explicitly since Descartes, the body is a complex machine, then it is difficult to see how placebo effects (e.g. thinking positively) could benefit anyone. According to David Morris': 'this way of thinking … makes as much sense as filling up the gas tank with Earl Grey tea'.[4] To many people, therefore, acknowledging placebo effects puts on a slippery slope whereby irrational forms of healing ranging from remote prayer to spiritual healing could be considered acceptable. However, it is possible to avoid the slippery slope and use the tools of evidence-based medicine to separate effective therapies from ineffective ones.[5] And besides, the fact that the body and mind can be separated is not currently accepted by the current scientists, with neurological mechanisms of placebo effects becoming increasingly well understood.[6] The thoughts of good food, a negative past event or sex are all 'mental' phenomena, yet they cannot be separated from their physiological correlates. Hence, Moerman's reply to the Earl Grey tea quip is: 'Does this mean that we might double our gas mileage if we wished for it hard enough? Well, no. But people are not machines, and we shouldn't treat them as such'.[7]

WHAT IS A PLACEBO?

Before we delve into the debate about whether placebos are ethical, it is useful to say a few words about what placebos *are*. Many people have claimed that placebos are 'inactive', 'inert' or 'nonspecific', which is false. Assuming for the moment that placebos are effective – somewhat effective at least for some ailments – then they cannot be inactive or inert. Inert and inactive things do not have effects. Similarly, placebo analgesia seems to work by activating the brain's reward system, releasing endogenous opioids into the bloodstream.[6] This seems just as specific as, say, taking an analgesic drug. Others claim that placebos are 'psychological', which is partly true but inadequate; antipsychotic drugs and psychotherapy are also 'psychological', yet are not necessarily placebos. For the purposes of this chapter, I will assume, following recent philosophical research,[8] that if a treatment is a placebo, it is relative to a disorder. So, a sugar pill might be a placebo for some things like pain, but not necessarily for a diabetic patient. The placebo should also work because the patient *expects* it to work (either consciously or, as we shall see below, subconsciously). On this view, an antibiotic is *not* a placebo for treating bacterial pneumonia, but *is* a placebo for treating a viral cold.

HOW EFFECTIVE ARE PLACEBOS?

Three factors are of major importance in the suffering of badly wounded men [during World War II]: pain; mental distress; and thirst. Therapy has been almost entirely directed to pain, and this usually limited to the administration of morphine in large dosage.

The requirement of beneficence bounds clinicians to provide the best available treatment for a given disorder. If placebos are not effective, and there are other effective treatments available, then it would appear that placebos are unethical. On the contrary, if placebos are effective, and they have a superior cost–benefit profile than other options, then it seems a barrier to their ethical use has been removed. In fact, the effectiveness of placebos is the subject of ongoing controversy. Henry Knowles Beecher was one of the first investigators to attempt to quantify placebo effects. Beecher was a Harvard Medical School graduate who was a doctor in Europe during World War II. Morphine was sometimes in short supply, and he noticed that some soldiers did not require any painkillers, even if they had serious wounds. After the war was over, he conducted one of the first 'systematic reviews' by examining 15 studies (with over 1000 patients) that compared 'real' drugs with placebos together. He found that a third of the patients who had only received placebos got better a third of the time, and concluded that placebos were as effective as 'real' treatments in a third of cases.[9]

However, in the 1990s, researchers began to question Beecher's results. After all, most people suffering from most diseases get better whether or not they are treated. So, the people who got better after taking the placebos might have recovered even if they had not taken the placebo. In medical-research-speak, the fact that most people recover with or without medication is called *natural history*. In philosophy-speak, the possibly mistaken inference that the placebo caused the cure is called the *post hoc ergo procter hoc* (after, therefore, because of) fallacy.[10] To test whether placebos really make people get better, we have to compare people who take placebos with people who take no treatment at all.

Taking up the task, Peter Gøtzsche and Asbjorn Hróbjartsson conducted a systematic review and 'meta-analysis' of trials that comprised three groups of patients (see Figure 3.1):

1. One group of patients was not treated at all (often people in these groups were placed on waiting lists).
2. One group of patients was given a placebo.
3. One group of patients was given a 'real' treatment.

They then compared what happened to patients who received the placebo with patients in the untreated groups (groups 2 and 3 in Figure 3.1). They found that on average, placebos only have small effects. For a few conditions (especially pain, but also anxiety and depression), they found that placebos had small effects. Based on what they found, they recommend that doctors should not use placebos unless they were part of a clinical trial. (As we saw in the introduction, doctors commonly prescribe placebo interventions.)

Unfortunately, Hróbjartsson and Gøtzsche's sceptical conclusions about placebo effects are mistaken. Irving Kirsch asks us to imagine a systematic review not of placebos, but of all *treatments* for any condition ranging from the common cold, alcohol abuse, smoking, poor oral hygiene, herpes simplex infection, infertility, mental retardation, marital discord, faecal soiling, Alzheimer's disease, carpal tunnel syndrome and 'undiagnosed' ailments.

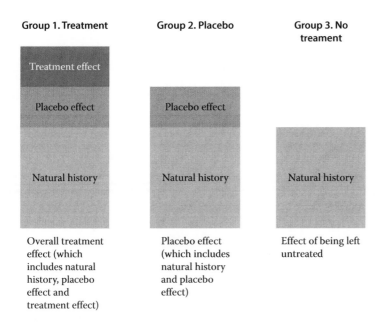

Figure 3.1 Treatment, placebo and no-treatment groups.

Imagine further that medical treatment 'is difficult to define satisfactorily', so the authors of this fictitious study 'defined medical treatment practically as an intervention labelled as such in the report of a clinical trial'. This led to a diverse range of medical treatments included in the review such as psychotherapy, homeopathy, acupuncture, meditation, chiropractic and faith healing. The fictitious review then found that medicine overall has no significant benefit. Kirsch claims, correctly, that such a trial would not be accepted by a reputable journal. Yet, that is just what Hróbjartsson and Gøtzsche did. Their hodge-podge of placebos included relaxation (classified as a treatment in some of the studies and as a placebo in others); leisure reading; answering questions about hobbies, newspapers, magazines, favourite foods, and favourite sports teams; and talking about daily events, family activities, football, vacation activities, pets, hobbies, books, movies, and television shows (finding a small but significant 'placebo effect'). The main problem with the Hróbjartsson and Gøtzsche study is that it is unfair to lump *all* placebos into the same group, because the placebos were too different (the fancy medical term for difference is 'heterogeneous').

I recently turned Kirsch's imaginary example into a real study. To accomplish this, I examined the same trials Hróbjartsson and Gøtzsche did. However, instead of measuring the difference between placebo and untreated control groups, I compared average treatment effects (from group 1 in Figure 3.1) with the average placebo effects (from group 2 in Figure 3.1). This analysis yielded the average *treatment* effect size in the same trials used by Hróbjartsson and Gøtzsche. I then compared the treatment effect estimate with the placebo effect estimate. The study had two interesting outcomes. Firstly, the average effect of treatments wasn't very big either. Secondly, the size of the placebo effect was sometimes bigger than the size of the treatment effect.

What can we conclude about the power of placebos from these studies? The first thing is to acknowledge the obvious fact that placebos won't work for everything. If someone has a leg amputated, believing it will grow back is unlikely to have any effect. The second thing is that many ailments, especially the most common ones people visit their primary care clinicians for such as mild to moderate pain, depression, anxiety, flu, colds, and so on, will go away on their own. The body usually heals itself without medication, or we remain ill no matter what they give us despite of the medication. Thirdly, just as 'real' treatments are exceptionally powerful for treating some conditions (e.g. antibiotics for meningitis), placebo treatments can be highly effective for treating some conditions, especially mild to moderate pain and depression, anxiety and smoking cessation, and they can generally improve quality of life.

Yet, even if placebos are effective, using them still could violate the principle of beneficence if there is a more effective option. A practitioner should not prescribe a placebo, even if the placebo is effective, if there is a more effective option. However, in some cases, there is no more effective option. For example, until recently, there was no accepted treatment for irritable bowel syndrome (IBS). Hence, some researchers have prescribed placebos within the context of a clinical trial and found it to be effective.[11] Some patients who found the placebos to be effective in the trial allegedly asked for the placebos to be prescribed in routine practice, but have been denied on ethical grounds even though no other treatment is available! In other cases such as non-steroidal anti-inflammatory drugs, they may be more effective than placebos; however, they also carry the risk of serious side effects, causing an estimated 16,000 deaths in the United States alone each year.[12] So, although placebos may not be as effective, they may carry a more favourable benefit/harm ratio. Moreover, the question of whether there is a more effective treatment applies if we have to choose *either* a placebo *or* another treatment. However, this is not always the case. Placebo treatments, broadly construed, can be delivered alongside 'real' treatments in order to reduce the dose (and hence the risk of adverse events) or simply to boost effectiveness.

However, even if placebos turn out to be the most effective or beneficial option in some cases, one might claim that they remain unethical because they require deception. Whether placebo treatments are, in fact, an acceptable effective option will depend on the ailment and the individual patient.

DO PLACEBOS REQUIRE DECEPTION?

If a doctor must lie to a patient about the nature of a placebo (telling the patient that it is a 'real' treatment when it is not), then this arguably violates the principle of autonomy. While Bennett Foddy makes what might be a good argument that deception is sometimes legitimate,[13] deception remains controversial and I will take it as given here that it is generally not a good thing to lie to patients. However, numerous trials have shown that placebos still work in spite of patients being told they are placebos.[14–20] These 'open label' placebos typically demonstrate similar effects to standard (deceptive) placebos.

In one of these interesting trials, Ted Kaptchuk et al. at Harvard randomised patients suffering from IBS into two groups. One group was assigned to a waiting list, whereas the other group was given placebo pills presented as 'placebo pills made of an inert substance, like sugar pills, that have been shown in clinical studies to produce significant improvement in IBS symptoms through mind–body self-healing processes'. The symptoms among patients receiving the open-label placebos reduced by 20% compared with the control patients.

The mechanisms of action of open-label placebos are becoming increasingly well understood, but are currently speculative. Classical conditioning, a 'bottom-up' mechanism, is perhaps supported by the most evidence: the conditioned expectation of a reward has been shown to activate the brain's conditioning mechanism.[6] Supporting the conditioning hypothesis, a recent study of open-label placebos for treating pain showed that the open-label placebo effect persisted in patients who had been conditioned for longer periods (4 days) but not shorter (1 day) durations.[21] If the open-label placebo is accompanied by a suggestion that the placebo is or might be effective, then conscious expectancy – a 'top-down' mechanism – could also play a role. Clinical studies have shown that the expectation of a positive outcome may cause pain relief, lowered anxiety and reduction in Parkinson's disease symptoms.[17] Conversely, negative expectations have been shown to adversely affect health, most notably by increasing pain.[22] An expectation of pain relief has been found to activate neurological systems involved in regulating pain such as the dopamine reward system and the endogenous opioid system.[23] Prescription for repeated consumption of open-label placebos acts as a daily positive auto-suggestion, and positive expectations have benefits for the ailment being treated. It is also possible that the social interaction with a healthcare practitioner plays a role in explaining the effects of open-label placebos. Social support – of which healthcare practitioner support could be considered a component – is a well-established determinant of health. Not only can social networks provide support in the form of care and advice,[24] but social networks have also been shown to influence the neuroendocrine response.[25] Since encounters with a healthcare practitioner are social events, we might expect such encounters to enhance the benefits of social networks and to mitigate the negative effects associated with a lack of social networks. While the hypothetical mechanisms could all work independently, they are more likely to operate together, producing variable effects depending on the individual and the condition.

CONCLUSIONS

The ethical principles of beneficence and autonomy suggest that if placebos are not effective or if they require deception, they are unethical. However, since they are sometimes effective and they do not always require deception, it is not the case that they are always unethical. For treating some ailments such as IBS, they could be the best available treatment, and for other ailments such as pain, they might have the most desirable benefit–harm ratio. Therefore, placebo use in clinical practice can be ethical and any regulatory restrictions against their use should be revised. Finally, belief that placebo treatments can be ethical in some cases does not imply a commitment to the effectiveness of alternative medicine or any irrational practice.

REFERENCES

1. Fassler M, Meissner K, Schneider A, Linde K. Frequency and circumstances of placebo use in clinical practice – A systematic review of empirical studies. *BMC Med* 2010; **8**: 15.
2. Howick J, Bishop FL, Heneghan C, et al. Placebo use in the United Kingdom: Results from a national survey of primary care practitioners. *PLoS One* 2013; **8**(3): e58247.
3. Kaptchuk TJ. The placebo effect in alternative medicine: Can the performance of a healing ritual have clinical significance? *Ann Intern Med* 2002; **136**(11): 817–25.
4. Morris DB. Placebo, Pain, and Belief: A Biocultural Model. In: Harrington A, ed. *The Placebo Effect: An interdisciplinary exploration.* Cambridge, MA: Harvard University Press; 1997: 187–207.
5. Howick J. *The Philosophy of Evidence-Based Medicine.* Oxford: Wiley-Blackwell; 2011.
6. Benedetti F. *Placebo effects: Understanding the Mechanisms in Health and Disease.* Oxford: Oxford University Press; 2009.
7. Moerman DE. Meaningful placebos – Controlling the uncontrollable. *N Engl J Med* 2011; **365**(2): 171–2.
8. Howick J. The relativity of placebos: Defending a modified version of Grünbaum's scheme. *Forthcoming* 2015.
9. Beecher HK. The powerful placebo. *J Am Med Assoc* 1955; **159**(17): 1602–6.
10. Kienle GS, Kiene H. The powerful placebo effect: Fact or fiction? *J Clin Epidemiol* 1997; **50**(12): 1311–8.
11. Kaptchuk TJ, Friedlander E, Kelley JM, et al. Placebos without deception: A randomized controlled trial in irritable bowel syndrome. *PLoS One* 2010; **5**(12): e15591.
12. Singh G, Triadafilopoulos G. Epidemiology of NSAID induced gastrointestinal complications. *J Rheumatol Suppl* 1999; **56**: 18–24.
13. Foddy B. A duty to deceive: Placebos in clinical practice. *Am J Bioethics* 2009; **9**(12): 4–12.
14. Aulas JJ, Rosner I. Efficacy of a non blind placebo prescription. *L'Encephale* 2003; **29**(1): 68–71.
15. Bergmann JF, Chassany O, Gandiol J, et al. A randomised clinical trial of the effect of informed consent on the analgesic activity of placebo and naproxen in cancer pain. *Clin Trials Metaanal* 1994; **29**: 41–7.
16. Dahan R, Caulin C, Figea L, Kanis JA, Caulin F, Segrestaa JM. Does informed consent influence therapeutic outcome? A clinical trial of the hypnotic activity of placebo in patients admitted to hospital. *Br Med J* 1986; **293**(6543): 363–4.
17. Kirsch I, Weixel LJ. Double-blind versus deceptive administration of a placebo. *Behav Neurosci* 1988; **102**(2): 319–23.

18. Park LC, Covi L. Nonblind placebo trial: An exploration of neurotic patients' responses to placebo when its inert content is disclosed. *Arch Gen Psychiatry* 1965; **12**: 36–45.

19. Pollo A, Amanzio M, Casadio C, Maggi G, Benedetti F. Response expectancies in placebo analgesia and their clinical relevance. *Pain* 2001; **93**(1): 77–84.

20. Sandler AD, Bodfish JW. Open-label use of placebos in the treatment of ADHD: A pilot study. *Child Care Health Dev* 2008; **34**(1): 104–10.

21. Schafer SM, Colloca L, Wager TD. Conditioned placebo analgesia persists when subjects know they are receiving a placebo. *J Pain* 2015; **16**(5): 412–20.

22. Bingel U, Wanigasekera V, Wiech K, et al. The effect of treatment expectation on drug efficacy: Imaging the analgesic benefit of the opioid remifentanil. *Sci Transl Med* 2011; **3**(70): 70ra14.

23. Price DD, Finniss DG, Benedetti F. A comprehensive review of the placebo effect: Recent advances and current thought. *Annu Rev Psychol* 2008; **59**: 565–90.

24. Cohen S, Janicki-Deverts D. Can we improve our physical health by altering our social networks? *Perspect Psychol Sci* 2009; **4**(4): 375–8.

25. Ozbay F, Johnson DC, Dimoulas E, Morgan CA, Charney D, Southwick S. Social support and resilience to stress: From neurobiology to clinical practice. *Psychiatry (Edgmont)* 2007; **4**(5): 35–40.

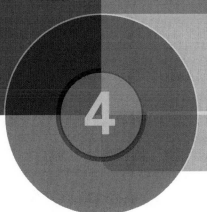

Compassion in primary and community healthcare

4

JOSHUA HORDERN

COMPASSION IN PRIMARY AND COMMUNITY HEALTHCARE

Compassion is an attribute of a person's affective understanding, which aims to enable, so far as possible, shared experiences of the world's ills and some alleviation of those ills' effects. Such an attribute is thus of great value within healthcare institutions such as general practices and other primary and community healthcare settings. It may characterise the people who participate in those institutions; or, it may not so characterise them. The appearance of compassion, under certain conditions and even in fragile and incomplete forms, is a kind of human excellence, a way of being for the good in community.* Compassion is not, therefore, a commodity, to be bought, sold and traded. Although time can be costed, there is no line for compassion in any budget. Were compassion to be thought a commodity, one could imagine trading it off against some more measurable factor (efficiency, cost-effectiveness, etc.). However, our human capacity for compassion, though fragile, tends to resist such marginalisation and reductionism.

As an attribute of human *affective understanding* aiming at shared experience amidst life's illness, compassion is *cognitive, participative* and *alleviative*. As an affection, compassion is not reducible to mere sensation, although it may coincide with physical expressions such as weeping or reassuring touch. Rather, compassion is centrally an affective attitude towards someone's suffering, a core dimension of the 'partnership-working' crucial to patient–practitioner relationships in the 'new professionalism' of health and social care.[1] The affectivity of compassion does not entail that it is somehow non-rational or anti-rational. Rather, compassion is directed towards situations, people or things with which it is concerned. This directedness or 'aboutness' of compassion indicates that we can ask questions about its intelligibility and reasonableness – whether understanding of an individual's suffering is being appropriately grasped and communicated in this case. This ability to assess compassion strongly suggests

---

* For this account of fragile virtue, see Ref. 2.

that it is in some way cognitive, involving a kind of belief or mental attitude. Precisely as cognitive, it can initiate reasoning towards action which will constitute the alleviation of suffering.

If this is so, compassion cannot be reserved or detached. Compassion alleviates suffering by participating in it. As an essentially alleviative affection, it reaches out in understanding and embodied service to engage with persons in need. In compassion, one person relates their self to the other, seeking to share in understanding of that other's experience of the suffering human condition.* Just because of its quality as a kind of intelligent understanding rather than an inscrutable sensation, compassion may constitute an experience which is intelligibly shared by both sufferer and carer, leading to shared decision and action. However, this participative, alleviative sharing in suffering is not automatic. It is a goal to be achieved in the everyday encounters of healthcare.

Since compassion is like this, its content is not fixed but filtered through the circumstances and beliefs of those concerned. Accordingly, compassion is quite different from a healthcare professional's self-indulgent emoting, which signals his or her own self-regard instead of aiming at shared experience. *More* emotion does not equate to better compassion; ill-focussed emoting is worse than detached but efficient practice. However, intelligent, well-directed affection can enable practice that is humane and effective.

This description of compassion focusses compassion not chiefly on specific practical manifestations of concern important though they are – the accessibility of an elderly person's home, the practicability of contacting a general practitioner (GP) out of hours and the glass of water within reach – but on persons' deeper experiences of illness, disease and care. Participation by compassion in that deeper level is cognitive and affective, and only thus can it be alleviative. For the logic of compassion is that suffering involves loss of some goodness in human life. In healthcare, alleviation of suffering might not involve action beyond kindly presence aimed at reassurance of solidarity and relief of fear: the health visitor or GP having that second cup of tea with the lonely person so that their story is properly heard. Or, it may involve extensive activity aimed at diagnosis and healing of disease. However, both of these forms of alleviation are initiated by an affective, cognitive participation in suffering, aiming at the shared experience both of suffering and of some goodness by the one who has lost or never known it.

Compassion is, therefore, not an optional extra but a necessary and in some fashion ever-present quality of healthcare, central to its goals. To construe the term 'concordance', a term which complements 'compliance' or 'adherence', in terms of the moral psychology of shared decision-making, compassion involves being united affectively with another in their experience of the world's ills, in their suffering.† As a systematic review of evidence has shown (Box 4.1), such 'emotional rapport and support [are] … associated with improvements in emotional health,

> ### BOX 4.1: Elements of compassion
>
> - *Cognitive* – We understand each person's experience of suffering, listening and loving.
> - *Participative* – We seek, so far as possible, to share that experience, working alongside.
> - *Alleviative* – We think about how to make things better, looking forward in hope.
> - *Civic* – We encounter each other as citizens, meeting with respect and solidarity.
> - *Persuasive* – We talk with each other, helping one another understand suffering differently and better.

---

* For this account of affectivity in more detail, see Refs. 3 and 4.
† For a brief introduction to these terms, see Ref. 5.

symptom resolution, physical functioning and quality of life assessments, as well as … measures … such as physiological indicators of disease management … and pain control'.[6]

Primary and community healthcare's practices such as listening, visiting, discussing, advising, comforting, recommending, prescribing and referring concern encounters between persons amidst life's drudgery, drama and hypochondria. Persons engaging in such every-day practices encounter one another in ways which bear witness to their profound human unity amidst vulnerability and suffering. For these practices enflesh human solidarity as some-body inclines ear, mind and whole person towards somebody else in time of need. Through these practices, primary and community healthcare (hereafter 'primary care') workers often act as 'gatekeepers' to healthcare services: as district nurses identifying medical needs among the housebound, occupational therapists enabling someone to access help needed for daily tasks and GPs discerning whether specialist care is appropriate.

Primary care, characterised by its generalism and by these specific practices of encounter, is the beginning of a road down which patients may travel, a hospitable entry point on a jour-ney towards specialist avenues of care they may require.[7] The task of primary care is then a demanding one, requiring clinical understanding leavened with compassion so that 'the vast undifferentiated mass of human distress and suffering'[8] may be ordered, personalised and then alleviated. To continue welcoming sufferers' faces in the all-too-brief encounters of counte-nances that embody compassion requires perseverance, not only through each long day but also, where continuity of care is maintained, over the long years during which trust may grow amidst the sometimes frightening but often fertile trials of life.

COMPASSION FOR PATIENTS IN PLURAL POLITIES

In practice, the character of encounters between primary care workers and patients cannot be generalised beyond a certain level because compassion is for *this person* at *this time* and because forms of primary care vary. Nonetheless thinking about compassion can be disci-plined by understanding its nature as irreducibly concerned with personal subjects seeking shared experience and understanding. In many present-day societies, a complication arises. Although in traditional societies, a relative homogeneity of culture was common, in modern nation-states, this has been widely, though not universally, replaced with overlapping, inter-secting networks of diverse, heterogeneous cultures. These multiple cultures nonetheless share a common political identity and, in many European contexts at least, a socialised healthcare system, albeit to varying degrees. Health, being 'a basic socio-personal good',[9] valued variously by all cultures, therefore provides a point of reference in political life, in which the beliefs and practices of plural societies can meet in disciplined conversation.

Since health is both social and personal, compassion is necessarily a civic matter as an individual's suffering becomes a matter of public concern, mediated through the persons of primary care workers. However, since present-day civic life is plural, a new understanding of compassion in primary care is needed. Those who seek to exercise compassion, as a form of affective, cognitive, participative understanding aimed at alleviating subjective suffering and attentive to cultural factors, must grasp the diverse ways that individual and community values concerning health and illness shape people's outlook. Sharing experience involves 'the ability to identify imaginatively'[10] with the way that a particular patient perceives their condition and its significance.

Patient perception will of course include expectations about what should be done, if anything, about their condition, a trend entrenched by access to medical information online and 'shared decision-making'.* More generally, personalisation of healthcare relating to

> a patient with respect, at least ideally, means treating their experiences, perceptions and preferences not just as relevant data for professional decision-making but as matters worth taking seriously in their own right including within decision-making partnerships.[11]

However, taking patient perceptions seriously does not mean that compassion involves *uncritical* affirmation of such perceptions. One might be tempted to think this if one failed to grasp compassion's affective, cognitive, participative, alleviative nature and role in decision-making. Such a failure would make it harder to say 'no' to a patient for it allows compassion to become mere acquiescence not only to a patient's perception but also to that patient's demands. However, for two reasons, this uncritical notion of compassion as acquiescence should be resisted.

Firstly, while a person's condition is *their* condition and they are in an important sense an *expert* in it – it is *their* experience and no one else's[†] – conditions are not absolutely unique because persons are not absolutely unique. Persons are members of the species of persons, characterised by observable regularities of health and disease. Those who have knowledge of such regularities, formulated as evidence which then informs the cognitive understanding that constitutes compassion, are better placed than those who do not to assess diagnoses, interpretations and expectations regarding health conditions and so to resist, kindly and respectfully, certain patient perceptions and demands.

Secondly, a patient's perception of their condition and best interests may be challenged, gently and transparently, in order for the alleviative dimension of compassion to be realised. Compassion's cognitive quality is ordered to seeking all patients' good, from those patients who are demanding and confident about their wishes to those who do not grasp or care about their interests to those who, for example, feel that nicotine or alcohol use is all that makes life bearable but are afraid to clash with the official view, represented by the doctor, that such behaviour is in some way wrong. In short, how a patient perceives their circumstances may have much to do with culturally mediated or individually constructed values and beliefs which may require open, if tender, challenge.

While the paternalistic 'doctor/nurse knows best', presupposition is rightly no longer prevalent partly due to a diminution of unstudied deference in society, it is also right that primary care provides a context in which patient perceptions of their situation can be kindly, respectfully, gently and transparently but critically discussed. Inasmuch as compassion involves a cognitive participation in the feelings of another – in particular their experience of suffering – then, compassion must incorporate this element of critical analysis and even persuasion, whereby suffering may be interpreted by both patient and healthcare practitioner differently and better. Primary healthcare workers' 'power to do good' and 'relational expertise' amount to social authority to know and pursue goodness even amidst the flat landscape of liberal political life that tends to discourage others' 'interference' in the lives individuals are building or destroying for themselves.[12] Such a landscape may, without the wise mediation of primary care workers, end up populated by people abandoned to loneliness and ill health.[‡]

---

* For a multi-perspectival analysis of this trend, see Ref. 13. For discussion of how technology will and perhaps should displace the face-to-face encounter in parts of healthcare, see Ref. 14.

† For weaknesses in the idea of the 'expert patient', see Ref. 15.

‡ As one commentator on Edmund Pelligrino's work puts it, 'One cannot abandon persons to their autonomy when they are in difficult straits'.[16]

POWER, CRITIQUE AND THIS 'SECULAR' TIME

Yet, there is a dark side to compassion's critical dimension in which persuasion or encouragement becomes domination and oppression and in which professional power undermines the patient's own reasoning and ignores their interests. Beware the idealisation of the doctor as moral saint! Humanities disciplines, such as theology, have been at pains to analyse the fragility of individuals' moral quality and unmask the self-deceptiveness which attends status and power.

Moreover, cultural wisdom garnered through engagement with patients and their cultures may itself function to critique a professional's own prejudice or vice and improve the way he or she understands suffering and compassion. However, far from diminishing the social authority of healthcare professionals, this two-way street in compassion actually reinforces their role as mediators in between and advocates for the individuals and cultures they serve and indeed between those cultures and professional, regional or government policy. This is a position of influence in which primary care workers are called to moral discernment in critical service of the population among whom they practice. Cribb and Gewirtz note this critical edge and its relation to justice when they comment that healthcare practitioners:

> … will need an awareness that respecting the autonomy of individuals, by trying to respond to their needs and preferences, is not only potentially in conflict with beneficence to that individual, but may also exact some 'cost' on wider groups or populations – and thus may be in tension with other important concerns such as social justice or population effectiveness.[17]

The possibility of critique signals a continuing professional development need for those in primary care. For while the individual encounter is basic to general practice, wider cultural factors require primary care workers' critically compassionate understanding. Culture is of course not simply local, especially in the digital age where beliefs and communities are formed online in dispersed networks. Nonetheless, local cultural practice remains a decisive influence on the lives of many. GP practices and community healthcare teams, such as church ministers, local authority councillors and national politicians, typically have some sense of defined geographical responsibility. Just so, primary healthcare workers must mediate between local and cultural expectations regarding health and what is practically possible, bearing in mind regional and national factors. On this point at least, there is a similarity between the account here and 'values-based practice' as 'a less prescriptive and more local approach [which] aims to introduce a greater variability of viewpoints and greater recognition for individually specific values.'[18]

To deploy a term in its traditional rather than its contemporary usage, this culturally astute compassion may be best dubbed 'secular', not at all in the sense of being 'anti-religious' but rather in its native theological sense in which 'secular' is a word for a Christian idea – that of the quality of the time in *this age*, when ultimate questions of the meaning of human life have not been finally answered and when cultures live side by side in shared 'penultimate' civic life. The 'secular', on this view, is the time in which diverse philosophies, theologies, religions, values and moral outlooks contribute respectfully and critically to a plural society's public good. Inasmuch as time allows space for conversation, the secular may be thought of as the forum for differing forms of thought to meet in sometimes critical conversation.* Compassion, understood

---

*See e.g. Ref. 19.

as a cognitive, affective, critical, alleviative participation in suffering, is the proper beginning of the moral understanding of suffering, shaping discourse, deliberation and policy, a basic feature of this secular time in plural polities.

Thus, what is required is a morally substantial, affectively rich notion of 'secular' citizenship and discourse, embedded within professional training and development and benefitting society at large. Primary and community healthcare services, rooted in locality and conversant with that locality's cultures, are well placed to cultivate such civic discourse as the context in which compassion may be richly practised and experienced. A primary healthcare worker's understanding of and participation in local cultural life are key to the realisation of compassion in practice and so a proper focus for ongoing professional education. Inasmuch as deep understanding of multiple cultures is not itself a cultural norm, primary care workers must be countercultural if they are to be compassionate. They must be places of resistance to ways of perceiving cultural difference which are characterised by either impatient ignorance or uncritical acquiescence.

TIME, COMPASSION AND JUSTICE

Compassion has now been considered in terms of time in the sense of the secularity of the age in which political identity is now constituted. However, compassion also concerns time in the equally down to earth but more intuitive sense that time available to participate compassionately in suffering is scarce as primary care workers move from patient to patient and home to home. Time is often too pressured to engage in depth with each person encountered, share properly in decisions or pursue 'the search for meaning'.[20]

An important factor shaping this experience is the way that time and compassion are bound up with justice. One attitude to their interrelation is 'to perceive healthcare rationing problems as involving an explicit opposition between justice and caring'.[21] GPs in particular increasingly have responsibilities for considering how the needs of each one should be justly related to the needs of the very many.* The daily challenge appears in the widely attested experience of 'no time' or 'very little time' for compassion. Ten-minute (or briefer) appointments seem inadequate to create shared experience between patients and practitioners, the goal towards which compassion aims: a man with heart disease and depression, the teenager *only* needing a prescription and the domiciliary visit which is *just* 'social'. Although continuity of care may mitigate this problem, the dearth of time is a constant challenge which requires transparency in dialogue so that issues which the patient wants to address come into the open. The primary care worker can aid this transparency by honestly specifying how few minutes are available, thus focussing the conversation supportively rather than foreclosing it and avoiding difficult dialogue by handing out a prescription or by some other means.

However, filling the day to capacity militates against the kind of care which is required and leads to an 'appointment book that lies to us about the properties of time', precisely in its

---

* Carlsen and Norheim suggest that this resource allocation responsibility involves significant challenges to maintaining a compassionate practice, as patients become 'demanding consumers' or 'shared decision-makers', thus reshaping – perhaps unhelpfully – societal respect for healthcare workers' professional standing (Ref. 22). Over against the changing nature of general practice, Iona Heath mounted a passionate argument in favour of general practitioners' 'partisan' advocacy for patients and against such doctors taking financial responsibility for allocation of scarce resources. For, so Heath argued, the doctor's very responsibility for allocation will be understood by patients as a threat and so undermine the trust necessary for his or her relationship with the doctor (Ref. 23).

deceptive 'visual representation of time, setting out the day in appointment-sized chunks',[24] which do not measure up to patient needs. That which is visible, the schedule of appointments, attempts to give structure to the underlying shared purpose upon which the patient–practitioner relationship is premised, that purpose of making space for compassionate shared experience. However, a lack of or misuse of time may result in failing to reach the goal of shared experience and so do injustice to some in favour of others. In this situation, time spent which is not answerable to a metric or budget, is the time which it may feel harder to justify.

This scarcity paradigm regarding compassion bears witness to important truths: that time is limited and that the GP's appointment book and its equivalents in other forms of primary care are full of a weight of human need that stretches the capacities and waking hours of healthcare workers to breaking point. And yet, the paradigm may occlude the way that compassion is a participative, cognitive, alleviative affection. Compassion is not a 90-second feature of a 10-minute appointment in which one asks an 'extra' question about the patient's experience or family situation. Such a question is important in enabling shared understanding but compassion is not hermetically sealed within that segment of an appointment or visit. Rather, as an attribute of understanding, compassion may infuse the whole encounter, focussing attention in listening, assessment and diagnosis, consideration of the proper use of time and resources *and* engagement in underlying personal or cultural factors. Compassion also properly includes a justice consideration which can grasp that another patient further down the list will suffer if the current appointment goes on too long. Thus, compassion is not in opposition to justice – a thoughtless implication of the scarcity paradigm – but rather a constitutive feature of the realisation of justice. For compassion, as a cognitive, alleviative affection, is competent to understand not only suffering but also any injustice which may cause further suffering.

CONCLUSION: FOSTERING COMPASSION

For compassion to be realised in practice requires a supportive organisational ethos. Compassion is certainly basic to the shared experiences of patients and healthcare workers in primary care settings. However, such experiences should be supported by compassion between primary care colleagues. For those who care for the suffering are themselves vulnerable members of the human community. The GP who provides continuous long-term care to a local community may journey with the population through the challenges which life inevitably throws up, sharing something of his or her own life and suffering in a way which benefits patients.[25] Similarly, the experience of sharing vulnerability prudently with those with whom one works can support compassionate practice. Endurance in compassion towards patients will be enabled by a shared concern for colleagues, which is intelligent, participative and alleviative, renewing and refreshing collegiality on a regular basis.

Such supportive workplace cultures rarely happen by accident and are easily endangered by the commodification of one's colleagues as units of production – efficient and lauded or inefficient and stigmatised. Teams in general practices, district nursing or health visiting, for example, need to sustain a compassionate ethos if people are to see colleagues in depth, building long-term, stable, working relationships. Each primary care worker needs regular personal refreshment, deep drinking from some well of meaning and purpose to be sustained for the next stage of the journey.

Offered as one such source of refreshment in a plural polity, the motto of the Royal College of General Practitioners, *cum scientia caritas*, emphasises the greatest of the 'three theological virtues', love. It stands as a reminder to those in primary care of what Health Education

England's Simon Gregory called the need 'to regain, or not be afraid to admit to, our love of our patients'.[26] *Caritas*, in its theological sense, speaks of the participative, merciful and hopeful love of God as revealed in Jesus Christ, enabling humanity's peaceful friendship with God and others. Such love serves sick and lonely persons that they might be accompanied in suffering and made better. Such love seeks this mercifully, never allowing the ascription of fault, however just, to stand in the way of that care and company. Informed by this *caritas*, the real knowledge of primary care may become true wisdom. This is love which deploys up-to-date clinical evidence, seeks justice, rejoices in mercy and shows critical sensitivity to locality and culture. It is a love which, participating in the suffering human condition, becomes that intelligent compassion that unites in solidarity patients, professionals, managers and policymakers, fellow travellers all on the journey through the world's real sorrows, deep fears, enduring hopes and great joys.

ACKNOWLEDGEMENTS

This work was supported by the University of Oxford Wellcome Trust Institutional Strategic Support Fund (grant number 105605/Z/14/Z); and the Arts and Humanities Research Council (grant number: AH/N009770/1). The author gratefully acknowledges this funding and also that of the Sir Halley Stewart Trust. The views expressed within this chapter are those of the author and not necessarily those of the Sir Halley Stewart Trust.

REFERENCES

1. Cribb A and Gewirtz S. *Professionalism*. Cambridge: Polity Press; 2015. p. 33.
2. Adams RM. *A Theory of Virtue: Excellence in Being for the Good.* Oxford: OUP, 2006.
3. Hordern J. *Political Affections: Civic Participation and Moral Theology.* Oxford: OUP; 2013. Chapters 1–2.
4. Hordern J. What's wrong with 'compassion'? Towards a political, philosophical and theological context. *Clin Ethics* 2013; **8**(4): 91–7.
5. Bell JS, et al. Concordance is not synonymous with compliance or adherence. *Br J Clin Pharmacol* 2007; **64**(5): 710–11.
6. Roter DL, et al. Effectiveness of interventions to improve patient compliance: A meta-analysis. *Med Care* 1998; **36**(8): 1138–61.
7. Papanikitas A and Toon P. Primary care ethics: A body of literature and a community of scholars? *J R Soc Med* 2011; **104**: 94–6.
8. Heath I. *The Mystery of General Practice.* London: Nuffield Provincial Hospitals Trust; 1995, 27.
9. Maxwell B. Just compassion: Implications for the ethics of the scarcity paradigm in clinical healthcare provision. *JME* 2009; **35**: 219–23.
10. Heath, 1995, *op. cit.*, 35.
11. Cribb and Gewirtz, 2015, *op. cit.*, 36.
12. Cribb and Gewirtz, 2015, *op. cit.*, 56, 66–7, 97.
13. Edwards A and Elwyn G, editors. *Shared Decision-Making in Health Care: Achieving Evidence-Based Patient Choice.* Oxford: OUP; 2009.
14. Susskind R and Susskind D. *The Future of the Professions: How Technology Will Transform the Work of Human Experts.* Oxford: OUP; 2015.

15. Badcott D. The expert patient: Valid recognition or false hope? *Med Health Care Philos* 2005; **8**(2): 173–8.
16. Thomasma D. Establishing the moral basis of medicine: Edmund D. Pellegrino's philosophy of medicine. *J Med Philos* 1990; **15**(3): 245–67.
17. Cribb and Gewirtz, 2015, *op. cit.*, 81.
18. Petrova M, et al. Values-based practice in primary care: Easing the tensions between individual values, ethical principles and best evidence. *Br J Gen Pract* 2006; **56**(530): 703–9.
19. Biggar N. Why religion deserves a place in secular medicine. *JME* 2015; **41**(3): 229–33.
20. Heath, 1995, *op. cit.*, 20.
21. Maxwell B. Just compassion: Implications for the ethics of the scarcity paradigm in clinical healthcare provision. *JME* 2009; **35**: 219–23.
22. Carlsen B and Norheim O. 'Saying no is no easy matter'. A qualitative study of competing concerns in rationing decisions in general practice. *BMC Health Serv Res* 2005; **5**: 70.
23. Heath, 1995, *op. cit.*, 42–4.
24. Senior T. The strange time-bending properties of the appointment book. *Br J Gen Pract* 2014; **64**(625): 416.
25. Malterud K, et al. When doctors experience their vulnerability as beneficial for the patients. *Scand J Prim Health Care*, 2009; **27**: 85–90.
26. Gregory S. William Pickles Lecture 2014: *Cum Scientia Caritas* compassion with knowledge. *Br J Gen Pract* 2015; **65**(630): 36–7.

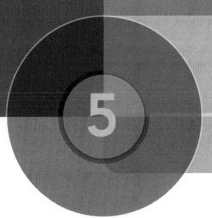

The ethics of the family in primary care

5

MICHAEL WEINGARTEN

For centuries, individual autonomy has been deeply ingrained in western culture and in bioethics in particular. The autonomous patient needs to know all about his or her medical problems and their management in order to decide themself whether to consent or not. To prevent undue interference in the exercise of autonomous choice, the patient needs privacy and confidentiality.

In primary care, it is often difficult to claim that all patients always benefit from autonomy, understood in this way. Beyond issues of reduced competency for one reason or another, there is often a family that seeks to intrude into the moral space of the patient that autonomy so respects. At least, that is how the family's presence is often perceived by the practitioner or even the patient, as a challenge to autonomy, misconstruing concerned interest as interference. The family's search for involvement often comes from a laudable position of offering support to the patient.[1] This then is the basic tension, between the independence of autonomy and the intimacy of family. Autonomy can be a lonely place, and the family can be suffocating. As ever, in primary care, it is not always clear to the practitioner, and often not even to the patient, how to resolve this tension in any particular case or at any particular time. In this chapter, I will present the components of this predicament, hoping to help the practitioner to think through the various issues at stake and to consider the various philosophical positions that the literature offers us. Firstly, I will discuss what we mean when we speak of 'the family'. Then I will propose a simple ethical framework for dilemmas in family care, and continue to consider in some detail the rights and duties of families. There follows a discussion of family relationships and of coping styles, before returning to the patient's rights and concluding with the family doctor's predicament.

DEFINITION OF FAMILY

I will use Levine's definition, which is appropriately flexible for our use:

> Family members are those who by birth, adoption, marriage, or declared commitment share deep, personal connections and are mutually entitled to receive and obligated to provide support of various kinds, to the extent possible, especially in times of need.[2]

Or, as Robert Frost puts it, in 'The death of the hired man',

Home is the place where, when you have to go there, They have to take you in.

This definition begs the question of the families whose personal connections are not deep. Sometimes they are frankly dysfunctional or even destructive, but more of this later.

For the purposes of the present discussion, we should highlight a few frequent family constellations. Babies and children brought to the clinic by their parents are the most straightforward case; the child patient is deemed incompetent and the parents are charged with the duty to act in their children's best interests.* Adolescents are a different matter as they gradually separate from their parents, eventually attaining their independence as they mature into adulthood.[3] At the other end of life, when adult children become involved in the care of their old parents, the decline of a parent into incompetence, though not inevitable, may be just as difficult for the child as adolescence was agonising for the parent. Then, there are spouses or other partners who may agree on the limits of privacy within the relationship, or not. Adult siblings are yet another group who may see themselves as legitimately involved in one another's medical care, more so in traditional cultures. Each of these family situations needs consideration in order to identify the potential for resolution of the tensions between the patient and the family, that is, the tension between individual and relational autonomy, a distinction that I will discuss. My discussion here centres on adult patients with other adult family members involved in their care.

ETHICAL FRAMEWORKS

For everyday clinical use for someone who has to make immediate ethical decisions, in real time and alone, an accessible ethical frame of reference is needed. For use in daily clinical work with patients and their families, I propose a set of ethical domains which together aim to preserve and promote the dignity† of everyone involved, including the practitioner's justice, compassion and humility.

Dealing justly with patients, broadly defined, requires the healthcare practitioner's due attention to their rights and duties, and his or her own, as well as concern for the well-being of others who may be involved and affected by his or her actions – the family, the healthcare system, the community and the society at large. By the nature of the work, he or she will more often than not be faced with competing interests and rights, and the function of justice is to weigh them fairly against each other. Other than the directives of the law, which cover only a minority of contingencies, there are no guidelines exactly on how to do this, but it is imperative that we are conscious of all the competing claims.‡

Compassion enables us to respond supportively and therapeutically to the human suffering of our patients as sensitive human beings ourselves, using both our emotional and our

---

* Modified models have been proposed: the 'constrained parental autonomy' model, which I do not discuss, is presented in Friedman Ross[4]; the 'relationship goods' model, based on the balanced rights of children and their parents as described below, is presented in Brighouse and Swift.[5]
† Dignity-based accounts of medical ethics offer ways of solving complex problems where autonomy-based accounts fail. Respect for persons goes beyond respect for the rights of persons, see Ref. 6. Recent full-length discussions include Barilan[7] and Foster.[8]
‡ An ethic of justice is at the core of a liberal philosophy of life and has been applied to the family by Brighouse and Swift.[9]

cognitive professional skills.[10] As compassionate practitioners, we act to protect and sustain the dignity of our patients, treating them no worse than we would like to be treated ourselves.*

Humility implies that we remain aware of the limits of our knowledge of medical science[11,12] and of the patient's inner and social lives. In particular, humility requires us to respect and take into consideration the diversity of cultures that our patients represent. A western ethnocentric stance is a sure way of distancing ourselves from the patient and the family.

Our task, then is to check for ourselves that we are caring humanely for patients and their families, taking due consideration of their rights and interests, and of the wider context of our interactions with them. What we decide to do will be an idiosyncratic balance, for no two situations are the same and no two doctors are the same. We can justify our actions only insofar as we can claim to have taken everything into account and that we truly care about what happens next.

RIGHTS AND DUTIES OF FAMILIES

Insofar as the family has any moral right at all to be involved, this right has been derived from their function in supporting the patient. This support may be physical and technical, nursing care, financial, and not least, emotional. Parents of small children are required to do this by law, reflecting a seemingly natural duty of parents to protect and nurture their children. In face of the dramatic changes in the structure of families, such as second marriages, adoptions and surrogacy, parenthood, etc., we have seen proposals to revise the justification for parents' rights to decide about the welfare of their children.[13] Rather than seeing this right as natural, the parents must earn it, in return for what they invest materially and emotionally in the family (Brighouse and Swift call these 'relationship goods'). The corollary is that where this investment is deemed unsatisfactory, the state will and should step in to protect the best interests of the child. Perhaps, this approach invites and justifies primary care practitioners too to challenge some parents over their medical choices.

As for filial duties, the duties of children towards their parents, a similar mechanism has been suggested, derived from 'the special respects in which the parent–child relationship makes lives go better'.[14] Others have seen filial duties as arising from indebtedness or gratitude for the parenting the child received earlier in life, or from simple friendship.

Even if we take the position that children do not have a positive duty to do so, sometimes they, or other family members, have to support the patient even if they really do not want to do so, and that is where there are no other available sources of support. Siblings may become supporters, but their duty to provide it is weaker than for parents or children, hence, also their rights to become involved in sharing of information and in decision-making is that much weaker. Often, these rights simply do not exist. The situation with spouses is perhaps clearer; the right of a spouse to be involved is totally dependent on the assent of the patient. Partnerships and marriages come from outside the genetic or nuclear family, with its *a priori* duties, and the arrangements in each individual case are a matter of negotiation, agreement and reassessment.

Duty or not, legislators often assume they may depend on a certain amount of family support when allocating public resources to medical, especially nursing care. The family may indeed be motivated by emotional attachment, or more cynically, by expectation of a cut of the inheritance. Whatever the motives, when families assume responsibility, they do need to be involved in the management of the patient – access to necessary information, discussion of options and decisions regarding action. They earn this involvement by contributing to supporting the

---

* An ethic of care is at the core of a feminist philosophy of life and has been applied to the family by Mackenzie and Stoljar.[15]

patient; it is not an unconditional right.[16]* It is also limited to what is necessary for the patient's care. Furthermore, it is contingent on the patient's expressed or implied consent that this is the way it should be. The patient retains the right of veto at any stage over the family's involvement, or the extent of it.

This, at least, is how it looks to a secular western liberal culture and law that strives to protect individual autonomy and to restrict incursions into it.[17] This is not the way it looks to other cultures where individual identity is indivisible from family membership, as is discussed elsewhere in this book.[18–21] This account of individual autonomy has also been challenged by feminist ethicists, who urge a more relational approach to autonomy. Their understanding is that we are not atomised individuals but we are constituted by the family and the nexus of social relations within which we exist. Our thoughts, judgements and feelings, hence our choices and our actions, are formed in relation to other people. It has been argued most compellingly that the family even in contemporary western culture, is the critical arena for personal growth; it realises a particular structure of human goodness and sustains the necessary conditions for core areas of human flourishing, as Mark Cherry puts it.[22] The Lindemann Nelson lists some specific features that make it important to take families into consideration. Parents who caused their children to exist bear responsibilities and are therefore ethically involved even after their children grow up. Virtues are learned at our mother's and father's knees, and this intimacy also produces special responsibilities. In families, motives matter a lot, and not just actions, again providing grounds for involvement. At a purely pragmatic level, family members are stuck with each other, and family members are not replaceable by similarly, or better, qualified people. As an ongoing story, the family has an intrinsic moral identity independent of specific nomination by the patient, and family opinions should therefore be taken seriously *a priori* in medical decisions.[23] Another view is that patients are vulnerable and need to trust their families to care for them. This trust is based partly in shared interests, but often simply in love.[24] Seen like this, it is difficult to isolate the patient's autonomy from his or her family relations.

A theoretical structure that has been proposed to take account of these aspects of the ethics of family is 'relational autonomy', which in its most general form encompasses the political, social and intersubjective influences on the way we formulate our ideas, on how we want to live our lives.[25] We do not make our decisions in a rationalistic vacuum, but rather in relational contexts that foster our competency to develop and exercise our autonomy.[26] The Nuffield Council for Bioethics subscribes to this approach:

> [Autonomy] should not be equated simply with the individual's ability to make and communicate rational decisions. Rather, [...] a person's autonomy is found also in how they express their sense of self, in their relationships with those important to them, and in their values and preferences.[27]

It has recently been well summarised and applied in the field of family law.[28] In the moderate form of the theory, family relationships are seen as highly significant influences on personal choice, which remain the basic feature of autonomy,[29] but in a more extreme version the family is seen as an entity in its own right, as an end in itself and not merely as a means to support its individual members. Subscribing to this version, the philosopher John Hardwig envisages situations where the wishes of the family rightly prevail over the wishes of the patient, when the other family members are affected particularly severely by the decision.[30] He sees the family as an end in itself and not merely a means to support the patient.

---

* Friedman Ross[31] calls this 'proportionate respect'.

The general consensus of contemporary philosophical and legal literature is that there is an expectation of support that rests on families in general, and that it is their collaborative and reciprocal actions that give them the moral right to become partners in medical decision processes.[32] The primary care practitioner will have to decide how far to acknowledge and realise these rights depending on the individual case. To deal justly will be to recognise the legitimate rights of all the parties involved, even when it is impossible to fulfil them all. Although in this act of balancing one set of rights against another, the practitioner cannot be non-judgemental, he/she can strive to take them all into account, rather than rejecting the family out of hand.

PATIENT–FAMILY RELATIONS

Family practitioners are not starry-eyed about family relations. We understand only too well the psychological mesh, the ambivalences, the repressed unfinished businesses, the expectations and the disappointments, the pride and the frustrations, the altruism and the egoism and the love and the hatred that go into making most families into a creative and reproductive environment, recognising too that some degenerate into a destructive and dispersive mess.[33] The family is always present in the consultation, whether in person or in the inner world of the patient.[34] Patients come to us with an internalised version of their families, forged out of their emotional experience with them. The full array of psychological mechanisms becomes apparent in looking after patients and their families: coalitions, projection, transference, repression and suppression. Much of this is unconscious, and many practitioners too are not consciously aware of what is going on beneath the surface. Balint has shown us the path to understanding by analysis of our own reactions to patients and the various members of the family: in technical terms, the analysis of counter-transference.[35] However, even the most skilled and experienced practitioners cannot give a full account of the patient-in-family, and what they does understand is only a personal account from their particular perspective, and reflects only those parts of themselves the family choses to reveal. There is no objective account, no view from nowhere. Hence the need for humility.

A particularly tough challenge is posed by families whom the primary care practitioner perceives as dysfunctional in one way or another. Children who were treated badly by a parent in early life might not have resolved their relationships by adulthood, and may not be best placed to make critical medical decisions for the parent. Brothers and sisters may have old rivalry scores to settle. Another common example would be discussions around the end-of-life care of an elderly parent. Pressure to keep the parent alive as long as possible may come from one child, while the other may express more concern not to extend the length of the suffering life. Is the latter truly altruistic when the will stipulates an unequal distribution of the estate among the children, and is he or she the one who stands to benefit most who does not want to lengthen the process? Second marriages sometimes create similar challenges, where the children of the first marriage may feel deprived by the diversion of property to the step-parent and family. The primary care team is unlikely to know much of this information, so that any claims of dealing justly with the family must be tempered by doubt.

FAMILY COPING

Whatever its biography, the family is exposed to the psychological and material stresses of coping with the illness of one of their members, depending on the severity, chronicity and the prognosis of the medical condition. We know a fair amount about the different coping styles of families, and attention to them will help the practitioner to maintain his compassion and empathise even with some quite unlikeable families. One useful schema is known as the Circumplex Model.[36] Families are considered on three dimensions: cohesion, flexibility and communication. On each dimension, there is a spectrum of recognised styles. Looked at for cohesion, the family may be too low on the scale, that is, 'disengaged', or too high, that is, 'enmeshed', or somewhere more functional in the middle. Similarly for flexibility, the spectrum runs from chaotic, through flexible, structured, to rigid. Family communications are observed for listening skills, self-disclosure and respect. Combinations of extremes of behaviour on these scales predict a poor capacity for coping, and these families will pose particular challenges to the practitioner. Thus, a rigid but highly enmeshed family with poor listening skills will find it very difficult to reorganise around a medical catastrophe of one of its members.

Over and above the family's resilience, coping with illness calls upon their resources, including finance, available time, intelligence, literacy, social support and language skills. In these aspects, the practitioner is faced not so much with a challenge to his/her sense of justice, but with the need to work with the family with greater understanding and compassion. In selected cases, the doctor might consider offering the family the help of a professional social worker or a family counsellor. This would not seem to be the remit of the doctor, whose responsibility is clearly towards the patient, but in the long run it is in the patient's interest that the family should function as well as it can in the circumstances. It is the doctor's compassionate concern that gives him/her the right to offer intervention at the family level.

BACK TO THE PATIENT'S RIGHTS

What if the patient, say, does not want to know his diagnosis but the adult children think he ought to know, in order to make reasoned decisions about his future, for example? Although lawyers and philosophers may define the patient's rights, it is the patient who chooses how far to exercise these rights and it is not the primary care practitioner's task to impose them on him or her. We have already mentioned the cross-cultural situations where the patient defines his/her rights vis-a-vis the family quite differently from the dominant culture. In any culture, however, medical need implies increased dependency. Patients who find themselves thrown back on the support of their family may often regress psychologically into earlier dependency patterns and behave in a more child-like way. Alongside the dilution of autonomy that this regression implies, it also redefines the patient's expectations of the family. He or she may simply ask too much from the family, placing on them a burden too great for them to bear. Or he or she may prefer one family member over another, and make this preference contingent on receiving help and support from them. These expectations may be welcome or unwelcome to the family, but it is not for the practitioner to adjudicate even if it looks as if some demands are unreasonable, unnecessary or unjustified. The practitioner must always act in the patient's best interest, but this should not extend beyond the boundaries of immediate medical management, and there is no reason to become involved in family power struggles that are extraneous to the medical context. The practitioner has to act to the best of his or her ability in the context that the patient provides.

Life is easiest if the patient simply and clearly devolves medical decisions on a nominated and consenting member of the family, for then the patient's rights are preserved and the family's rights derive from the patient's free will. Life is rarely that easy and patients may legitimately change their minds at some point, leading us back to all the considerations we have discussed.

The concept of relational autonomy may help us practitioners navigate these difficult situations, positively welcoming the family into the deliberations around the patient's care.

This approach preserves the dignity of our patients, advances their best interests and is consistent with the social reality of family relationships.[37]

THE FAMILY DOCTOR

There are a number of special professional implications in the care of families in the specific context of general practice.* Where the GP is a family doctor, in that several members of the family share the same doctor, the model of the designated patient inside the professional relationship, and the family outside, does not work. The doctor is just as committed to the well-being, the interests and the rights of those other members of the family as to those of the present patient. Although that makes the theoretical analysis just too complex to cope with, in reality it has the potential to make real-life resolutions much easier. The doctor may already have considerable tacit knowledge about the family and its dynamics, as well as an existing relationship, hopefully a trusting one, with the people involved. This is a very different setting from that where the family descends out-of-the-blue with its demands, anxieties and opinions. The family who shares a doctor lends itself quite naturally to collaborative and open conversations. Indeed, choosing not to share a doctor where this is possible, all things being equal may be interpreted as a sign of family difficulties, where they are concerned not to expose themselves as a family unit to professional scrutiny.

In the other direction, the intrusion of the family on the dyadic therapeutic space of practitioner and patient may well be perceived as a threat to the professional authority of the practitioner. Sometimes this is precisely what is happening. The approach, I suggest, should be similar to that when a patient presents with a sheaf of internet print-outs. This is another case where we have to come to terms with the fact that we no longer work in an authoritative vacuum, but we are part of a nexus of information and advice.[38] As long as we retain the trust of the patient, this should not be seen as a challenge but as an opportunity – to learn from the family and to improve the patient's care.[39] In many cases, the perceived threat is simply an erroneous interpretation imposed on the situation by an insecure practitioner. I am hopeful that the analysis in this chapter will help reduce that insecurity.

ACKNOWLEDGEMENTS

I thank Bar Ilan University for the sabbatical leave during which this was written, and my hosts at Oxford – ETHOX and Green Templeton College – for their generous hospitality.

REFERENCES

1. Levine C, Zuckerman C. Hands on/hands off: Why health care professionals depend on families but keep them at arm's length. *Journal of Law, Medicine & Ethics.* 2000; 28: 5–18.
2. Ibid.
3. Walker JK, Friedman Ross L. Relational autonomy: Moving beyond the limits of isolated individualism. *Pediatrics.* 2014; 133 Suppl 1: S16–23.

* In this chapter, I have not touched on the issue of the family in decisions around genetics. There is already an extensive literature on this subject, for example, see Ref. 40.

4. Friedman Ross L. *Children families and health care decision making.* Oxford: OUP; 1998.

5. Brighouse H, Swift A. *Family values: The ethics of parent-child relationships.* Princeton, NJ: Princeton University Press; 2014.

6. Brody B. *Life and death decision making.* New York: OUP; 1988.

7. Barilan YM. *Human dignity, human rights, and responsibility.* Cambridge, MA: MIT Press; 2012. pp. 91–127.

8. Foster C. *Human dignity in bioethics and law.* Oxford: Hart Publishers; 2011. pp. 2–22.

9. Brighouse and Swift, 2014, *op. cit.*

10. de Zulueta P. Compassion in healthcare. *Clinical Ethics.* 2013; 8: 87–90.

11. Coles C. Learning about uncertainty in professional practice. In: Sommers L, Launer J editors. *Clinical uncertainty in primary care: The challenge of collaborative engagement.* New York: Springer; 2013. pp. 47–69.

12. Greenhalgh T. Uncertainty in clinical method. In: Sommers L, Launer J editors. *Clinical uncertainty in primary care: The challenge of collaborative engagement.* New York: Springer; 2013. pp. 23–46.

13. Brighouse and Swift, 2014, *op. cit.*

14. Keller S. Four theories of filial duty. *Philosophical Quarterly.* 2006; 56: 254–274.

15. Mackenzie C, Stoljar N. Autonomy refigured. In: Mackenzie C, Stoljar N, editors. *Relational autonomy: Feminist perspectives on autonomy, agency and the social self.* New York: OUP; 2000. pp. 3–31.

16. Cherry MJ. Re-thinking the role of the family in medical decision-making. *Journal of Medicine and Philosophy.* 2015; 40: 451–472.

17. Levine and Zuckerman, 2000, *op. cit.*

18. Fan R. Self-determination vs. family determination: Two incommensurable principles. *Bioethics.* 1997; 11: 309–322.

19. Frank G, Blackhall LJ, Michel V, Murphy ST, Azen SP, Park K. A discourse of relationships in bioethics: Patient autonomy and end-of-life decision making among elderly Korean Americans. *Medical Anthropology Quarterly.* 1998; 12: 403–423.

20. Candib LM. Truth telling and advance planning at the end of life: Problems with autonomy in a multicultural world. *Family Systems and Health.* 2002; 20: 213–228.

21. Gilbar R, Miola J. One size fits all? On patient autonomy, medical decision-making, and the impact of culture. *Medical Law Review.* 2015; 23: 375–399.

22. Cherry, 2015, *op. cit.*

23. Lindemann Nelson H, Lindemann Nelson J. *The patient in the family: An ethics of medicine and families.* New York: Routledge; 1995.

24. Nys T. Autonomy, trust and respect. *Journal of Medicine and Philosophy.* 2016; 41: 10–24.

25. Dodds S. Choice and control in feminist bioethics. In: Mackenzie C, Stoljar N, editors. *Relational autonomy: Feminist perspectives on autonomy, agency and the social self.* New York: OUP; 2000. pp. 213–235.

26. Meyers DT. *Self, society and personal choice.* New York: Columbia University Press; 1989.

27. Nuffield Council on Bioethics. *Dementia: Ethical issues.* London: Nuffield Council on Bioethics; 2009.

28. Herring J. *Relational autonomy and family law.* Cham: Springer; 2014. pp. 11–25.

29. MacKenzie and Stoljar, 2000, *op. cit.*

30. Hardwig J. What about the family? *Hastings Center Report.* 1990; 20: 5–10.

31. Friedman Ross, 1998, *op. cit.*, p. 45ff.

32. Donchin A. Autonomy and interdependence: Quandaries in genetic decision making. In: Mackenzie C, Stoljar N, editors. *Relational autonomy: Feminist perspectives on autonomy, agency and the social self.* New York: OUP; 2000. pp. 236–258.

33. Shatzman M. *Soul murder: Persecution in the family.* London: Allen Lane; 1973.

34. Granek M, Weingarten MA. The third-party in general practice consultations. *Scandinavian Journal of Primary Health Care.* 1996; 14: 66–70.

35. Balint M. *The doctor, his patient and the illness.* 2nd ed. London: Churchill Livingstone; 2000.

36. Olson DH. Circumplex model of marital and family systems. In: Walsh F. editor. *Normal family processes.* 3rd ed. New York: Guildford; 2003. pp. 514–544.

37. Gilbar R. Asset or burden? Informed consent and the role of the family: Law and practice. *Legal studies.* 2012; 32: 525–550.

38. Howrey BT, Thompson BL, Borkan J, Kennedy LB, Hughes LS, Johnson BH, Likumahuwa S, Westfall JM, Davis A, Degruy F. Partnering with patients, families and communities. *Family Medicine.* 2015; 47: 604–611.

39. Gaver A, Borkan JM, Weingarten MA. Illness in context and families as teachers: A year-long project for medical students. *Academic Medicine.* 2005; 80: 448–451.

40. Foster C, Herring J, Boyd M. Testing the limits of the 'joint account' model of genetic information: A legal thought experiment. *Journal of Medical Ethics.* 2015; 41: 379–382.

FURTHER READING

Friedman Ross L. *Children families and health care decision making.* Oxford: OUP; 1998.

Lindemann Nelson H, Lindemann Nelson J. *The patient in the family: An ethics of medicine and families.* New York: Routledge; 1995.

Cherry MJ. Re-thinking the role of the family in medical decision-making. *Journal of Medicine and Philosophy.* 2015; 40: 451–472.

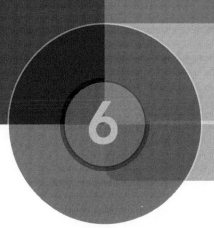

Culture and ethics in healthcare

DAVID MISSELBROOK

Culture and ethics are inextricably bound to each other. Culture provides the moral presuppositions and ethics the normative framework, for our moral choices ... there is also in every culture an admixture of the ethnocentric and the universal.

Edmund Pellegrino[1]

What is truth on one side of the Pyrenees is error on the other.

Blaise Pascal[2]

INTRODUCTION

Culture and ethics are as closely bound together as matter and energy. It is difficult to disentangle their effects, indeed it often seems difficult to distinguish between them. We mainly notice such issues when we look across cultures. We may fail to see the effects of our own culture just as fish are said to be unaware of water.

Humans are social beings. Not just because we live together, but more importantly because we are defined by what Martin Buber sees as 'I – Thou' relationships.[3] We are capable of recognising others as the same sorts of beings as ourselves, and this creates complex networks of relationships and duties between us. These are fundamentally different from the 'I – It' relationships we have with the rest of the outside world. In relating to others, we ourselves become truly human. Buber states, 'A person makes his appearance by entering into relation with other persons'.

But just as humans come in all shapes, sizes and colours, we also have many ways of living together. The way we live expresses the meaning and relationships that we see in our lives together. Viktor Frankl saw our need for meaning to be even more fundamental than our need for mere survival.[4] Althusser argues that our cultures are the places where individual meanings are produced and experienced; thus, to analyse a culture is to analyse our meaning systems.[5] It is these cultural contexts that determine much of our behaviour.

This chapter examines what we mean by 'ethics' and its relationship with moral theory. Might moral theory apply across cultures? How does the culture of both the doctor and the patient determine the social and behavioural assumptions within which ethical decisions are made? This chapter examines the uneasy symbiosis between culture and ethics.

This chapter looks at cross-cultural ethics, taking western and Islamic ethics as an example. It compares moral theory including notions of autonomy between these cultures.

THE MEDICAL CULTURE

I have argued elsewhere that doctors and patients have their own distinct cultures.[6] Indeed, doctors and patients behave as distinct tribes within our broader cultures. Sinclair describes the social transition from laity to doctor.[7] Ironically, our better understanding of scientific epistemology (an excellent way of managing matter/energy entities within the world) arguably disadvantages us from understanding interpersonal meanings. Doctors risk being clever about things and dumb about people. Ratzan dramatically describes this transition as a process of proving our worthiness to be admitted into a different tribe.[8] Doctors may only realise the cultural distance if they are suddenly swapped into the role of patient. There is an epiphany; it is different there! There are too many accounts of this journey to reference, but classics such as Howard Brody's *Stories of Sickness* would be a good place to start.[9] All such accounts however echo Felicity Reynolds' plaintive cry: 'are ... patients fellow human beings?'[10]

For Michel Foucault, the key dynamic was the power relationship between doctor and patient. Foucault characterises doctor's culture as one of domination, enforcing their worldview on patients via a narrow biomedical gaze.[11] One hopes this may be less the case than when Foucault first wrote this in 1963, but we would be naïve to believe that he is wrong. This then is the picture of doctor/patient culture that is our starting point. Note that we have not talked about 'different cultures' in the conventional sense. This is one axis of our gaze. To add an ethical analysis is to add a second axis. To then consider different worldwide cultures is to add a further twist.

TROUBLE WITH MORALS

Differentiating between moral demands and the effects of culture is a challenge. Is normativity – how things ought to be – a property of the world itself or is it just constructed by us? Clearly, morals are not physical objects like atoms or apples. But is morality a fundamental ingredient of the human world, like joy and pain and seeing red? Is morality part of what Bertrand Russell refers to as 'the furniture of the world', a human given?[12] Or, is morality nothing more than a formalisation of social convention, as suggested by contractarianism? We might be Vikings or vegetarians depending on the date.

Mackie points out that

> Disagreement about moral codes seems to reflect people's adherence to and participation in different ways of life. The causal connection seems to be mainly that way round: it is that people approve of monogamy because they participate in a monogamous way of life rather than that they participate in a monogamous way of life because they approve of monogamy.[13]

It may therefore appear that morality is relative – it is constructed to fit the environment and culture of specific societies. What appears to us as instinct or a matter of conscience is social and cultural programming.[14]

However, this argument is less convincing than it seems. Far from a random mix of moral values between cultures, there is in fact convergence of basic moral principles. One could think of the similarities between the Ten Commandments and the Code of Hammurabi, or the general concordance of both codes with the world's current legal systems. While some cultures *tolerate* torture, is there a culture that sees the practice of torture as a virtue? Who proposed that gratuitous cruelty to children was a virtue? What cultures propose random killing or stealing as virtues? In reality, virtually all cultures hold that there are moral categories of right and wrong, and the major virtues in one culture will never constitute the major vices in another. While the expression of social power and meaning varies between cultures, morality tends overall to take a common form.

The main variances are where common moral principles have a contrasting effect in contingent culturally related behaviours, particularly where these involve disputed facts. For example, both pro- and anti-abortionists may have a strong belief in the value of persons; their argument is about what constitutes a person. Singer points out that many of the apparent differences between moral systems are in fact differences in emphasis, or variations in the relative value put on different common goods, often changing with time according to the historical environment of the culture.[15] Developments in value systems often reflect a development towards higher goods such as love or autonomy, as opposed to the following of basic rules.

This therefore gives a picture of a complex system that is dynamic and developing, and yet, tends towards a commonly held intuition that perceives the moral good. This points towards a morality which is part of the 'furniture of our world', relating to hardwired properties of the human condition. As Singer also points out, those few cultures that do form real exceptions to this rule tend to be dysfunctional societies in the process of decay or self-destruction.

WHAT SORT OF MORAL REALISM?

Realism is the claim that our knowledge to some degree tracks the state of affairs in the world as it is in itself. Anti-realism is the claim that our knowledge merely informs us about the state of affairs as constructed in our minds. However, realism is *not* the claim that we have a comprehensive account of the world itself. Neither is it the claim that *all* of our current representations of the world must be true. Realism does not have to be either exhaustive or infallible. I would advocate a *falibilist realist* epistemology. Falibilist realism sees all models that claim to structure knowledge as provisional hypotheses. Thus, models serve an instrumental function. (This is distinct from any commitment to philosophical instrumentalism.) When we nest individual observations or sense perceptions within interpretive models, then we have systems of knowledge that are capable of engaging with the world and that enable us to manipulate parts of it.

Might moral knowledge be realist in this sense? If we accept the failure of relativism to explain the general convergence of morality across cultures, then we are left with different moral realist options. The enlightenment models of duty-based morality (deontology) and consequence-oriented morality (consequentialism, e.g. utilitarianism) both have obvious downsides. Deontology does not help me when duties conflict, such as triage or the balance between my obligations to my patients, my family and myself. Consequentialism cares little for justice or the interests of minorities. However, to correct for deficiencies in a theory does not give one confidence in one's theory. In recent years, virtue theory, or areteic morality, has returned to the fore.[16] Virtue ethics has been criticised as lacking clear guidance to action; however, many (in the British general practice literature, particularly Peter Toon) have shown that this is a superficial and unfounded criticism.[17]

It is true that virtue ethics tends not to give a *simplistic* guide to action. Instead, it offers us a richness and depth that tracks the complexities of human life within our relationship networks. This model is applicable to ethics embedded within specific cultures as virtue theory manifests itself specifically within the social domain.

Not all of life's decisions involve complexity. The more straightforward guides to action may be analogous to the cognitive shortcuts that psychologists tell us we use when evaluating evidence. For this reason, I favour using both deontology and consequentialism, almost as heuristics, within their proper domains with inclusive virtue ethics as the overarching moral structure.[18] However, two examples show that rules are not enough. Kant would not allow us to lie if an axe murderer knocked on our door and demanded to know whether person X was at home. In my view, Kant was wrong. Bentham regarded it as preferable that an innocent man should be hanged rather than risking a loss of faith in the judiciary by revealing a miscarriage of justice. In my view, Bentham was wrong.

Most real human dilemmas are complex because they occur within actual cultures which determine the form of the question. So, in our own culture, in a world where our evidence base is known to be systematically biased in favour of pharma, to what extent am I obliged to advise treatments favoured by official guidelines if they go against my patients' initial preferences?[19] Should I give my patients medical advice based on relative risk reduction or on number needed to treat, knowing that the framing effect is a major determinant of patient response?[20] Should I do more out-of-hours sessions because they are short-handed, or because I need the money, or should I refuse because my family needs me?

Virtue theory acts within cultures, but it is separated from them. It functions as an overall unifying theory and as a court of appeal when we realise that rules or consequences alone are leading us astray. Virtue theory explains the faculty that we use to correct rules when they are wrong as it relates morality to the 'settled dispositions' of humans who are flourishing with respect to their character and humanity within their particular culture.

CROSS-CULTURAL MORALITY

Let us examine the roles of both medical ethics and culture between the contemporary western world and the Islamic world. Clearly, neither world is a simple homogeneous block; therefore, only the broadest brushstrokes are possible.

After living, studying and working in multicultural London for 40 years, I felt I knew plenty about other cultures. Having now lived in Bahrain for 2 years, I realise that being immersed in a different culture is a far more overwhelming, complex and subtle experience. Everything is different. At first glance, I have encountered blatant failures to keep the most basic promises and obligations. 'X is on order for you', but it never arrives. 'I will be there at 2 pm', but you will be lucky to see them by 2.30. One turns up to an advertised event to find nothing there. And conciliatory talk to smooth out disagreement is seen as weakness to be trampled all over. So clearly, the Arab culture must be wrong and the west is right?

Perhaps not. I have come to realise that our list of virtues and duties is pretty much the same. The difference is how we rank them and how we make meaning within our culture in ways that enable us to live together. In the West, keeping promises is a key marker of my integrity. In the East, my behaviour with my family and close friends is the key marker of my integrity. In the West, I will arrive when I have promised. In the East, I will arrive when my nearer obligations (e.g. to my family) are fulfilled. In the West, I can criticise your views directly within a frank discussion. In the East, direct criticism is an affront to my honour and my standing with my peers; it is an insult. So, in the East, one's critique must be elliptic so that you give me the chance to learn from feedback without losing face. In the West, if X is not possible I will say so. In the East, I have no wish to appear unfriendly, so I will say yes but at the same time give you subtle indications that this means no.

We would do well to learn how one another's cultures work and pursue human excellence respectfully within whatever culture we find ourselves to be. In the West, reliability trumps relationships, in the East the reverse. In the West, candour trumps appearance, in the East the reverse. In both cultures, our virtues are broadly the same, but are ranked differently.

FROM THEORY TO PRACTICE: AUTONOMY, DUTY AND CONSEQUENCE IN EAST AND WEST

1. In the West, a very high status is put on individual autonomy. As the nineteenth century British philosopher John Stewart Mill said, 'over himself, over his body and mind, the individual is sovereign'.[21] However, our autonomy is limited by a reciprocal concern for the interests of others. In traditional Islamic cultures, autonomy is also valued but the limits are more clearly defined. In Islam, all acts relate to God's purposes for humans, understood via *Fiqh*, analysis of Islamic law.[22] However, within this framework, every adult has competence to take *Mubah* (permissible) decisions relating to their own life, unless there are genuine reasons otherwise.[23] In Islamic cultures, this is held in balance with the interest of the family or group.[24,25] Thus, the final locus of autonomy is less in the individual and more in the group, usually the family. Choices are therefore made within the context of family and friendship networks. (Interestingly, this shares some features with a feminist ethic in the West.) Therefore, there are cultural differences in the degree of individualism that is acceptable.

2. Deontology seeks to judge actions themselves as wrong (contrary to our duties) or right (according to our duties), typically coming up with a simple duality. Islam nuances this with a graded spectrum from acts that are forbidden (*Haram*) through acts that are generally undesirable (*Makrouh*), to a broad class of acts that are permissible (*Mubah*) to acts that are preferred (*Mustahab*), better (*Wajib*) or obligatory (*Fardh*) (Figure 6.1).[26]

3. Consequentialism seeks to judge actions according to their consequences and then has difficulty in determining the relevant evaluative frameworks for such outcomes, for example, pleasure, preference or welfare. Islam also judges actions according to consequences, but there are well-defined goals for action[27]:
   a. Preservation of life
   b. Preservation of faith
   c. Preservation of the mind and intellect
   d. Preservation of property
   e. Preservation of children and family line.

In the West, we then argue as to whether duty or consequence should take precedence. Islam has a long history of casuistry that can synthesise the nature and consequences of actions

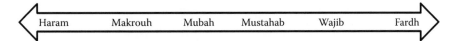

Figure 6.1 Categorisation of forbidden, permissible and obligatory actions.

within a dynamic and flexible framework. Thus, our moral concerns are held in common, but are worked out within different cultural contexts that determine their expression.

CONCLUSIONS

Doctors and patients each live in their own tribes, each with their own culture. This is just as great a gulf as any geographical or ethnic divide. East and West use similar methods of moral reasoning that usually express the same underlying human values and human excellences or virtues. We do this despite different epistemological frameworks, derived from different world views.

In both doctor/patient tribal boundaries and ethnic tribal boundaries, we tend to assume that our culture is right and the other wrong, but this is usually a product of confirmation bias, not of sound reasoning.

When we encounter issues relating to ethical differences between cultures, take five adaptive steps (PETRA), which are as follows:

- *Pause*. Do not rush to judgement because 'they' differ from 'us'.
- *Explore*. Analyse how social meaning is expressed and moral values ranked in both cultures.
- *Think*. Reflect on the strengths and weaknesses of both cultures in question.
- *Respect*. Respect the cultures of others (unless, rarely, they truly represent Singer's unstable or self-destructive society).
- *Adapt*. Learn how to live peaceably with other cultures.

We all share a common humanity that transcends culture and that normally causes our morality to converge. A healthy culture and a flourishing life both need mutual understanding and respect.

REFERENCES

1. Pellegrino E, Mazzarella P and Corsi P, eds., *Transcultural Dimensions in Medical Ethics*. Frederick, MD: University Publishing Group Inc.; 1992, p. 13.
2. Pascal B. Quoted in Berger P and Luckmann T. *The Social Construction of Reality*. London: Penguin Books; 1967, p. 17.
3. Buber M. *I and Thou*. First published in Germany 1923. Smith RG, trans. New York, NY: Scribner; 2000.
4. Frankl V. *Man's Search for Meaning. An Introduction to Logotherapy*. Reprinted: Boston, MA; Beacon Press; 2006.
5. Althusser L. Ideology and ideological state apparatuses. In: *Essays in Ideology*. London: Verso; Eds., Sharma A and Gupta A. 1984.
6. Misselbrook M. *Thinking about Patients*. Oxford: Radcliffe Press; 2001, Chapters 3 and 4.
7. Sinclair S. *Making Doctors*. Oxford: Berg; 1997.
8. Ratzan R. Winged words and chief complaints: Medical case histories and the Parry-Lord oral-formulaic tradition. *Literature and Medicine*. 1992; 11: 94–114.
9. Brody H. *Stories of Sickness*. Oxford: Oxford University Press. 2nd edition; 2002.
10. Reynolds F. Are hospital patients fellow human beings? Personal view. *BMJ*. 1996; 312: 982–3.

11. Foucault M. *The Birth of the Clinic.* London: Routledge; 1989, Ch. 6. (First published as *Naisssance de la Clinique.* France: Presses Universitaires de France; 1963.)
12. Russell B. *Introduction to Mathematical Philosophy.* London: G. Allen & Unwin; 1919.
13. Mackie J. *Ethics, Inventing Right and Wrong.* London: Penguin; 1977, p. 36.
14. Berger P and Luckmann T. *The Social Construction of Reality.* London: Penguin Books; 1967, p. 167.
15. Singer P, Ed. *A Companion to Ethics.* Oxford: Basil Blackwell; 1991, pp. 553–4.
16. MacIntyre A. *After Virtue.* London: Duckworth Press; 1981.
17. Toon P. *A Flourishing Practice.* London: RCGP; 2014.
18. Misselbrook D. Virtue ethics – An old answer to a new dilemma? (A two-part paper.) Part 1. Problems with contemporary medical ethics. *Journal of the Royal Society of Medicine.* 2015; 108(2): 53–6. Part 2. The case for inclusive virtue ethics. *Journal of the Royal Society of Medicine.* 2015; 108(3): 89–92.
19. Goldacre B. *Bad Pharma.* London: Fourth Estate; 2012.
20. Misselbrook D and Armstrong D. Patients' responses to risk information about the benefits of treating hypertension. *British Journal of General Practice.* 2001; 51: 276–9.
21. Mill JS. *On Liberty.* 1859. Reprinted, London: Penguin Classics; 2006, p. 13.
22. Sachedina A. *Islamic Biomedical Ethics, Principles and Application.* Oxford: Oxford University Press; 2009, p. 8.
23. Kamali M. *Principles of Islamic Jurisprudence.* Cambridge: Islamic Texts Society; 2005, pp. 405, 411, 419ff, 428ff.
24. Sachedina, 2009, *op. cit.,* 17.
25. Kamali, 2005, *op. cit.,* 430.
26. Hussein G. 2015. Module 2 – Principles of Western and Islamic Approaches to Bioethics. In: Ware, J. (ed.) *Professionalism and Ethics Handbook for Residents.* Riyadh, Saudi Arabia: Saudi Commission for Health Specialties; 2014, pp. 31–44.
27. Sachedina, 2009, *op. cit.,* 50.

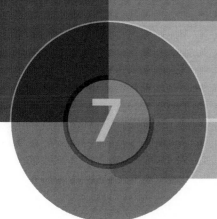

The ethics of complementary and alternative medicine (CAM)

NEVIN MEHMET AND CHRISTINE STACEY

INTRODUCTION

Complementary and alternative medicine (CAM) is a contentious subject within healthcare, mostly surrounding disputes regarding the quality of evidence, versus the efficacy and fervently claimed beneficial effects by CAM practitioners. There is no universally agreed definition of complementary, or CAM,[1,2] although common within much of the literature is the notion that *complementary* pertains to a therapeutic intervention that can be used alongside conventional medicine, whereas *alternative* is an intervention that is used instead of conventional medicine.[3] Baum[4] discusses the use and abuse of language, citing that words such as 'complementary', 'holistic' and 'alternative' used in conjunction with health have been hijacked by a pseudo-culture that applied transient meanings to health. For instance, proponents of disciplines such as homeopathy include traditionalists who require patients to stop all and any conventional treatments/medications and argue that reductionist medical care interferes with the bodies' innate ability to heal itself – with just a little help. Such a perspective is now largely discredited.[5,6] This raises several ethical concerns surrounding potential, emotional and physical harm on vulnerable individuals who seek out CAM at a time when they may feel distrust of conventional medicine or face serious illness and then follow homeopaths (or other therapists) due to fervent unsubstantiated claims.

Healthcare in the past two decades has increasingly focused on well-being, with patients taking responsibility for their own lifestyle choices as opposed to the previous paternalistic doctrine.[7] Patient's autonomous choices are therefore considered to be at the forefront of any healthcare intervention; however, whether CAM is considered an autonomous choice through the lens of healthcare is often disputed.[8] Although CAM has been readily available for many years, there is a dichotomy between appropriate research and efficacy and benefits. Baum[9] states that in the current period of financial austerity, there is no significant research of the requisite standard available in order to make it acceptable for CAM to be funded as a core component of current healthcare provision.

Ethical issues surrounding CAM are steadily moving into the domain of public health ethics as that discipline carries responsibility for the health of the community, with the central concerns of social justice and equity. At its core, public health ethics is centred on not just prolonging but also enhancing life by acknowledging that public autonomy is respected alongside the obligation to prevent harm.[10]

A primary concern in the UK is what appears to be almost total lack of regulation for both CAM practitioners and therapies.[10,11] Furthermore, the continuing trend for accessing CAM reinforces individuals' autonomous choices. If this is conflicting with the potential risk of harm to individuals, that moves CAM into the centrality of the argument of public safety. Nissen emphasises that respect for autonomy, fairness and justice are the most significant issues within the call for research into CAM, as individual choice to engage with CAM does not appear to be diminishing.[12] Often, individuals seeking CAM support are presented with a wealth of information via the internet, which with no effective policing of content of the web makes any ability to make an informed decision to use CAM rendered inadequate.[13] Therefore, regardless of popularity, this lack of evidence substantiating the use of CAM as a direct healing agent, alongside unregulated practitioners leads to concern not only in relation to harm but also in relation to the degree of autonomous choice.

This chapter will deal only with the ethics surrounding therapies considered to be 'complementary' as there is very little ethical support for denying conventional medicine and seeking 'alternative' therapies.

EDUCATION, TRAINING AND RESEARCH

Increasing interest and utilisation of complementary medicine (CM) by the public fuelled the UK medical establishment to call for an investigation into the phenomenon, resulting in the Department of Health (DH) recognising that there appeared to be some value in the management of symptoms of certain illnesses where conventional medicine had little or nothing to offer for complete resolution.[8] The report identified certain therapies, which had a degree of evidence to support their use, others some potential and a few none, also highlighting concerns that included lack of regulation and established education. As a result, many general practice (GP) surgeries sought to establish CM within their own practice[9,14] and a synergistic relationship gradually began to emerge. An example would be the Culm Valley Integrated Centre for Health, which was one of the first NHS GPs to offer its patients a range of CM alongside traditional medical care. Dixon et al.[15] pointed out that the government at that time stated that they wanted to develop a more flexible NHS able to respond to the needs and wishes of patients, allowing them to be more involved in managing their health conditions by giving them more choice, which included access to therapies not considered part of mainstream medicine.

The juxtaposition between CM and research was tenuous as it was based predominantly on lower-order research such as case studies,[16] which were used as justification for use[17]. In order to develop knowledge, quality research undertaken by appropriately trained professionals is required.[18] Therefore, from the 1990s until 2006, CM worked to develop an evidence base, with several universities validating undergraduate and postgraduate degree programmes intending to seek the canon knowledge required to establish CM as a core component of modern healthcare by providing an evidence base.[19] With academically trained CM practitioners, a scientific approach to research began to emerge, although the quantitative versus qualitative argument continued unabated.[16]

Currently, there are no BSc Hons Programmes (undergraduate or postgraduate) cited in the University and Colleges Admission Service (UCAS), although there are foundation and Bachelor of Arts (BA) degree programmes available. The change occurred following Emeritus Professor Michael Baum in 2006,[19] heading a group of 13 eminent names in medicine, by writing to 476 acute and primary care trusts, the *Lancet* and the *Times* denouncing any form of CAM, citing that these were being funded at the cost of life-saving drugs and treatments. This criticism was primarily a response to HRH the Prince of Wales addressing the World Health Organisation as support for other approaches to medicine.[20] The repercussion resulted in the majority of universities who provided BSc degree-level programmes in CM either abandoning or downgrading to BA programmes. Thus, the emerging structure seeking an evidence base for CM almost completely ceased. The ethical, constructive and scientific approach should have demanded clinical research into CM instead of driving it back into the hinterland of care. Searching the Cochrane database for CM reveals numerous trials involving one or more aspects of CM including massage for sleep in intensive care units[21] and acupuncture for insomnia.[22] However, one commonality in these studies was a lack of rigour alongside numbers of participants in the trials. This highlights another significant issue regarding evidence for CM; unless researchers with the knowledge and skills to undertake such research systematically study CM, and such research is adequately funded then, the envious relationship between the disciplines will remain[18] and any benefits to both patients and state-funded healthcare as a whole will be lost. The evidential trail is the key moral driver in that to support CM, evidence from robust research studies must determine availability as without such evidence regulation is impotent and therefore public safety is at risk.

A further issue identified within the HoL (2000) report[3] was the profound lack of regulation of either practitioners or therapies. The King's Fund was tasked by the DH to explore establishing a regulating body that came to fruition with the inauguration of the Council for Natural and Holistic Therapies (CNHC). This council would be equivalent to other health professional regulatory bodies with one exception: it was to be voluntary as opposed to statutory. The CNHC was tasked with developing core curricula for therapeutic disciplines alongside the provision of a register of therapists who had reached a standard of education and training in a recognised establishment.[23] This would give both conventional practitioners and the public a source of therapists who could be relied on to practice professionally and therefore ethically.[16] Similar to the General Medical Council (GMC) and the Nursing & Midwifery Council (NMC), the code of ethics and performance provides all registered practitioners' detailed guidance on ethical practice, with the central focus on ensuring that all practitioners not only practise within the realms of their own therapy, knowledge and expertise but also ensure that informed consent is always obtained, ensuring respect for autonomy.

Although voluntary regulation may go to some lengths to ensure the aims of statutory professional regulation are met, as Stone and Matthews argue, this is not ideal, as when an individual sources a CM practitioner invariably, he or she may be unaware of the CNHC[24]. Furthermore, if dissatisfied or harmed, for example, if a therapist has made a claim that cannot be substantiated, a patient may complain to their usual doctor, who may also be unaware of the CNHC. At the time of writing, the current situation is that the National Institute for Health and Care Excellence intend to remove CM from their current guidance.[25] While obviously a severe setback for proponents of CM, without evidence and regulation, little support may be garnered for its inclusion in a rationed state-funded healthcare system.

Irrespective of whether statutory or voluntary regulation, if a patient is unaware of how or where to obtain a registered and regulated (voluntary) CM practitioner, he or she may be exposed to some degree of harm by a rogue practitioner. The degree of harm may be physical through, for example, toxicity of herbs or essential oils, indeed emotional via vulnerability and claims of 'cure', or financial via continued treatments with very little benefit.[26]

Therefore, an open dialogue between patient and doctor is crucial, or as Stone and Matthews[24] argue, the risk for patients can be a result of the limited knowledge of CM providers or the limited knowledge of conventional doctors on CM that can increase the potentiality of harm for patients accessing CM.

AUTONOMY AND INFORMED CONSENT

Well-being, happiness and living a good life are expectations of modern society with a basic premise dating back to Aristotle.[7] Well-being is subjective, and Moreno-Leguizamon[27] cites Graham[28] and Diener[29] that well-being is about an individual's belief that something in his or her life is desirable, and the increasing popularity of individual well-being has seen an increase in the use of CM to promote general well-being or address symptoms of a range of short- or long-term conditions.[7,8,22,30] Systematic reviews identified that between 2000 and 2013, average use in paediatrics was 46%,[31] and in adults 41%[32] although there has been little change since 2000.[33] Although CM is currently available on the NHS via NICE guidelines on palliative care and back pain, these guidelines are in the process of being rewritten with CM excluded. As a consequence, CM will only be available within the private sector to those with economic means, resulting in unequal access of CM, perhaps going against the ethical principle of social equity. This may result in individuals who previously accessed CM via the NHS seeking out private, 'alternative' and cheaper options, exacerbating existing public safety concerns.

Protagonists of CM probably welcome such limited access, arguing that the fewer people who have access might be in the best interest of individuals. However, this may not apply in all cases, where, for example, within fertility care, it is acknowledged that use of acupuncture may support women undergoing IVF or other fertility treatments by reducing their stress and anxiety.[34–36] This is an excellent example whereby CM can work alongside conventional medicine, rather than causing women to access CM solely due to limited funding opportunities within the NHS, and the potential exploitation of women by CM practitioners working within the private sector claiming to support infertility.

Recent initiatives within the NHS place heavy emphasis on the value of patient choice and patient-centred care, which aims to put individuals at the centre of decision-making around their own treatment options.[16,26,27] The GMC and NMC guidelines require registrants to discuss with patients their treatment and care, and must listen to patients and respect their views about their health.[37–39] Therefore, regard for patients' autonomy and right to self-determination suggests that CM should be available if that is their choice. However, this may not be as simple as one might suggest, as if the efficacy and safety of CM is considered uncertain by doctors, then conflict between, autonomy, beneficence and non-maleficence will ultimately occur. Kerridge and McPhee[40] argue that the central concern is the possibility that conventional medicine practitioners may risk legal liability by ignoring the patient use of and preference for CM. Often, patients are aware that CM is not seen favourably by their usual doctors and this can potentially lead to patients exposed to harm if they choose unregulated 'alternative' practitioners to support their health needs. With the increasing popularity of the need to improve well-being and lifestyle choices along with non-compliance to conventional medication, this may result in detrimental and harmful consequences. Therefore, knowledge and understanding of CM and the differences between 'complementary' and 'alternative' are imperative for primary healthcare.

Recognition of CM would provide opportunity for primary care teams to incorporate broader approaches balancing their own personal values alongside supporting individuals, developing their own models of health and well-being.[25] Owen et al.[41] continue that within the GP 'gate-keeping' role, advising about CM requires some familiarisation of this discipline. Adler and Fosket found that when patients perceived their doctors to be respectful, open minded and willing to listen, they were more likely to reveal use of CM.[42] Patients with cancer tend to be high users of CM outside of oncology units but may fail to disclose such use to their GPs.[25] However, if using herbs or vitamins, there is potential for drug interactions; therefore, open doctor/patient communication about CM is crucial to maintain patient safety and well-being.[30,42,43]

Regardless of disciplinary aspects, informed consent is central to good patient care. Often within CM, consent, as with conventional medicine, can sometimes be assumed in the form of 'tacit consent' and by the nature in which individuals engage with CM, written consent is not often obtained. However, regulatory bodies such as the CNHC require that all registered practitioners must obtain valid informed consent prior to commencing treatment.[44]

Informed consent relies on three fundamental principles: that the individual has capacity, they must be provided with all or at least 'adequate' information prior to consent and provided with time to deliberate the information. (They should also be deciding voluntarily.) Invariably, CM practitioners are practising ethically, by adhering to their regulatory code of conduct. Unfortunately, a paucity of research and an inability to access any valid research result in CM practitioners relying on the limited evidence currently available, invalidating informed consent, even when a written consent form has been acquired.

CONCLUSION

However, there remains a gigantic gap in conventional medicine between patients who would like to discuss CM and primary care teams who do not talk about it with their patients. Dixon and Ham[45] state that the NHS is facing the huge challenge of managing limited resources with an ageing population. They also state that a new model of care is crucial where clinicians work closer together to manage the chronic and complicated medical conditions to meet the needs of these patients. The integrated healthcare discussed in this King's Fund document requires multidimensional working that includes all health and social care directed towards optimal self-care, and prevention of ill health. Therefore, an open dialogue between patients and all the primary healthcare team (PHCT) is key to the future of the NHS. There may even be a dichotomy between GPs and the rest of the PHCT who on the one hand acknowledge the right of patients to make autonomous decisions but vary in the degree to which evidence-based interventions are supported. Therefore, the lack of rigour and evidence of CM immediately makes any discussion including CM into a health and well-being care plan difficult. Regardless of when a patient wishes to include CM into their care plan, the PHCT although they may not be able to condone or offer CM knowledge of the CNHC, would remove many ethical barriers by supporting their autonomous choice, while reducing the possibility of harm. An unwillingness to acknowledge that patients are going to use CM may indirectly place their patient in harm; therefore, the onus is on the GP or other primary care clinician to ensure they are in a position to openly discuss CM even if they do not 'like' it and to direct the patient to where they will most safely find a practitioner. Patients can make poor choices and often look to PHCT for direction, where not knowing is not enough.

REFERENCES

1. National Centre Complementary and Integrated Health. *Complementary, alternative, or integrated health: What's in a name?* MD: NCCIH. 2016; Available at: https://nccih.nih. gov/health/integrative-health [Accessed 25 February 2016].

2. Vickers A, Zollman C. ABC of complementary medicine: What is complementary medicine? *BMJ.* 1999; **7211**: 693–696.

3. House of Lords Select Committee on Science and Technology. *Complementary and alternative medicine 2000.* 6th Report. The Stationary Office. Available at: http://www. publications.parliament.uk/pa/ld199900/ldselect/ldsctech/123/12301.htm CM 5124PDF [Accessed 02 June 2016].

4. Baum M. What is holism? The view of a well-known critic of alternative medicine. *Complementary Therapies in Medicine.* 1998; **6**: 42–44. doi:10.1016/S0965-2299(98)80056-3.

5. Ernst E. The heresy of homoeopathy. *British Homeopathic Journal.* 1998; **87**: 28–32.

6. Ibid.

7. Mehmet N. Ethics and wellbeing. In: McNaught A, Knight A (eds.). *Understanding wellbeing: An introduction for students and practitioners of health and social care.* London: Lantern Press; 2011. pp. 37–49.

8. Shaw A, Thompson EA, Sharp D. Complementary therapy use by patients and parents of children with asthma and the implications for NHS care: A qualitative study. *BMC Health Service Research.* 2006; **6**: 76.

9. Baum M. Complementary and alternative (CAM) medicine and cancer: The ugly face of alternative medicine. Editorial. *International Journal of Surgery.* 2009; **7**: 409–412.

10. Kass NE. Public health ethics: From foundations and frameworks to justice and global public health. *Journal of Law, Medicine and Ethics.* 2004; **32**: 232–242.

11. Ernst E, Cohen MH, Stone J. Ethical problems arising in evidence based complementary and alternative medicine. *Journal of Medical Ethics.* 2004; **30**: 156–159.

12. Nissen N, Weidenhammer W, Schunder-Tatzber S, Johannessen H. Public health ethics for complementary and alternative medicine. *European Journal of Integrative Medicine.* 2013; **5**: 62–67.

13. Fox S. *The social life of health information.* Pew Research Center's Internet & American Life Project; 2011; Available at: https://assets0.flashfunders.com/offering/docu-ment/e670ae83-4b9a-40f0-aac7-41b64dbc7068/PIP_Social_Life_of_Health_Info.pdf [Accessed 02 June 2016].

14. Smallwood C. *The role of complementary and alternative medicine within the NHS: An investigation of the potential contribution of mainstream therapies to healthcare in the UK.* The Stationary Office, London; 2005.

15. Dixon A, Robertson R, Appleby J, Burge P, Devlin N, Magee H. *Patient choice: How patients choose and how providers respond.* 2010. Available at: http://www.kingsfund.org. uk/publications/patient_choice.html [Accessed 02 June 2016].

16. Verhoef MJ, Casebeer AL, Hilsden RJ. Assessing efficacy of complementary medicine: Adding qualitative research methods to the 'gold standard.' *The Journal of Alternative and Complementary Medicine.* 2004; **8**(3): 275–281.

17. Tzu-I Chui. Aromatherapy the challenge for community nurses. *Journal of Community Nursing.* 2010; **24**(1): 18–20.

18. Wardle JL. Involve complementary medicine practitioners in research. *BMJ.* 2008; **337**: 1069–1070.

19. Baum M. An open letter to the Prince of Wales: With respect your highness, you've got it wrong. *BMJ.* 2006; **329**: 118.

20. The Prince of Wales and Duchess of Cornwall. *A speech by HRH Prince of Wales on integrated healthcare at the World Health Assembly.* 2006. Available at: http://www.princeof-wales.gov.uk/media/speeches/speech-hrh-the-prince-of-wales-integrated-healthcare-the-world-health-assembly-geneva [Accessed 06 June 2016].

21. Hu RF. Non-pharmacological interventions for sleep promotion in the intensive care unit. *Cochrane Database of Systematic Reviews.* 2016; **10**. Available at: https://healthmanagement.org/c/icu/news/sleep-in-the-icu-cochrane-review-of-non-drug-interventions [Accessed 06 May 2016].

22. Cheuk DKL, Wing-Fai Y, Chung KF, Wong V. *Acupuncture for insomnia Cochrane common Mental Disorders Group.* 2016; **9**. Available at: http://hub.hku.hk/bitstream/10722/198790/1/Content.pdf?accept=1 [Accessed 06 June 2016].

23. CNHC. *Code of conduct, performance and ethics for registrants.* 2016. Available at: http://www.cnhc.org.uk/pages/index.cfm?page_id=33 [Accessed 07 March 2011].

24. Stone J, Matthews J. *Complementary medicine and the law.* Oxford: University Press; 1996.

25. National Institute of Clinical Excellence. *Supportive and palliative care: Service delivery guideline.* London: NICE; 2015.

26. Hunt K. The regulation of CAM practice in the UK: Can it achieve its aim in safeguarding the public? *Focus on Alternative and Complementary Therapies.* 2010; **14**(3): 160–170.

27. Moreno-Leguizamon CJ. Wellbeing in economic, psychology and health: A contested category. In: Knight A, LaPlaca V, McNaught A (eds.). *Wellbeing policy and practice.* Banbury: Lantern Publishing Limited; 2014. pp. 7–17.

28. Graham C. *The pursuit of happiness: An economy of wellbeing.* Washington: The Brookings Institution Press; 2011 in Knight A, La Placa V, McNaught A. *Wellbeing policy and practice.* Banbury: Lantern Publishing Limited; 2014.

29. Diener E. *The science of wellbeing: The collected words of Ed Diener.* New York: Springer Dordrecht; 2009 in Knight A, LaPlaca V, McNaught A. *Wellbeing policy and practice.* Banbury: Lantern Publishing Limited; 2014.

30. Van Haselen RA, Reiber U, Nickel I, Jakob A, Fisher PAG. Providing complementary and alternative medicine in primary care: The primary care workers perspective. *Complementary Therapies in Medicine.* 2004; **12**: 6–16.

31. Posadzki P, Watson L, Alotaibi A, Ernst E. Prevalence of complementary and alternative medicine (CAM) use in paediatric patients; A systematic review of surveys. *Complementary Therapies in Medicine.* 2013; **21**(3): 224–231.

32. Posadzki P, Watson L, Alotaibi A, Ernst E. Prevalence of complementary and alternative medicine (CAM) use by the general population: A systematic review and update. *Clinical Medicine.* 2013; **13**(2): 126–131. http://dx.doi.org/10.7861/clinmedicine

33. Harris PE, Cooper KL, Relton C, Thomas KJ. Prevalence of complementary and alternative medicine (CAM) use by the general population: A systematic review and update. *International Journal of Clinical Practice.* 2012; **66**(10): 924–939.

34. Cheong YC, Dix S, Hung Yu Ng E, Ledger WL, Farquhar C. Acupuncture and assisted reproductive technology. *The Cochrane Database of Systematic Reviews.* 2013; **7**: 1–74.

35. Manheimer E, Zhang G, Haramati A, Langenber P, Berman BM, Bouter LM. Effects of acupuncture on rates of pregnancy and live birth among women undergoing in vitro fertilisation: Systematic review and meta-analysis. *BMJ.* 2008; **336**: 1–8.

36. Huang DM, Huang GY, Lu FE, Stefan D, Andreas N, Robert G. Acupuncture for infertility: Is it an effective therapy? *Chinese Journal of Integrative Medicine.* 2011; **17**(5): 386–395.

37. Nuffield Trust. *An overview of integrated care in the NHS. What is integrated care?* London: Nuffield Trust; 2011.

38. GMC. *Communication with patients.* 2016. Available at: http://www.gmc-uk.org/guidance/good_medical_practice/communication_partnership_teamwork.aspce/good_medical_practice/communication_partnership_teamwork.asp [Accessed 10 June 2016].

39. NMC. *Code on-line. Put patients first section 2.* 2015. Available at: https://www.nmc.org.uk/standards/code/read-the-code-online/ [Accessed 10 June 2016].

40. Kerridge IH, McPhee JR. Ethical and legal issues at the interface of complementary and conventional medicine. *Medical Journal of Australia.* 2004; **181**(3): 164–166.

41. Owen DK, Lewith G, Stephens CR. Can doctors respond to patients increasing interest in complementary and alternative medicine. *BMJ.* 2000; **322**(7279): 154–158.

42. Adler SR, Fosket JR. Disclosing complementary and alternative medicine use in the medical encounter: A qualitative study in women with breast cancer. *Journal of Family Practice.* 1999; **48**(6): 453–458.

43. Davis EL, Oh B, Butow PN, Mullan BA, Clarke S. Cancer Patient disclosure and patient doctor communication of complementary and alternative medicine use: A systematic review. *The Oncologist.* 2012; **17**(11): 1475–1481.

44. CNHC. *Code of practice informed consent section B4.* 2016, p. 14. Available at: http://www.cnhc.org.uk/assets/pdf/1-058.pdf [Accessed 10 June 2016].

45. Dixon A, Ham C. *Liberating the NHS: The right prescription in a cold climate?* London: The King's Fund; 2010.

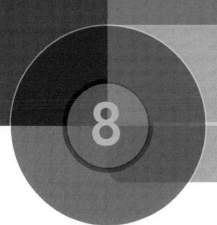

The oughts of omnipractice

8

JOHN SPICER

INTRODUCTION

In a book on the ethics of primary care, we should consider what it is to be a generalist, or to be a clinician involved in generalist practice. This is partially an ontological review of the nature of those who practise in a generalist manner, but is also a utilitarian assessment of why we should have generalists in clinical practice. I will offer some analysis of the word 'generalist' as it is interpreted in various ways within the United Kingdom, and around the world. I ask, therefore, what generalists are and what they do; and perhaps what they should be, given the disparity of esteem with which they are often held.

This area has been the subject of a remarkable flowering of literature in the last few years, where in 2007, several Australasian authors were calling for a 'clear mapping of the generalism as a philosophy of practice'.[1] Writers such as Reeve, concentrating on the interpretive role of the generalist[2]; Gunn et al.,[3] who consider the conceptual basis of generalism; or Heath and Sweeney,[4] who provide a taxonomy of generalism, are all leaders in the field, and would offer the enquiring reader marvellous reviews of this arena in more detail. In this chapter, I will be concentrating on the moral aspects of this and other related material, and attempting to answer the question: 'ought we to have generalists?'

The generalist/specialist divide permeates clinical practice and has deep roots. It is not confined to primary care, the practice of medicine or indeed clinical care more generally. Simplistically, it can be represented schematically thus: at the top of the cone lie the generalists, dealing with a larger number of diverse issues in (usually but not exclusively) less depth than the specialists who lie at the bottom. These latter of necessity deal in rather less diversity of patients' suffering (Figure 8.1).

So, the question to be answered, in a little more detail, could be phrased as an enquiry as to whether those offering care, and thus a response to the human suffering presented to clinicians ought to be delivered by those covering a wide range of expertise, or those with a narrow, though deeper, range of expertise. As ever, the answer is both empirical, or evidential, and normative.

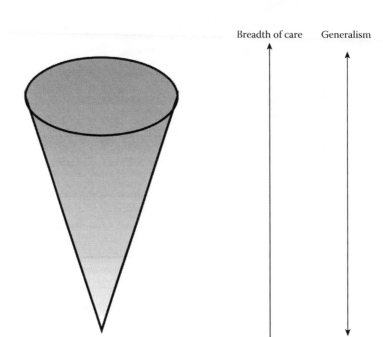

Breadth of care   Generalism

Depth of care   Specialism

Figure 8.1 A cone of care representing 'suffering' of patients.

GENERALISM AND PRIMARY CARE

It seems that the descriptor 'primary care' dates from the 1920s in the United Kingdom.[5] It is not synonymous with UK general practice, US family medicine or the care delivered by a French *omnipracticien[ne]* though the terms are often used interchangeably. However, a broad description of primary care indicates a point of first patient contact, of care delivered within the context of the patient, of being part of the community. Just in themselves, these aspects are of enormous importance; removal of patient to an institution of whatever type might imply a (albeit temporary) loss of connectedness or even self-governance. Implicit, therefore, in defining these terms is a need to define a domain of care, or professional expertise, along with formulating a specific ethics that might lie alongside.[6]

For reference, more modern descriptors of primary care are given by the World Health Organisation (WHO): elaborating patient partnership, enduring patient/clinician relationships, person-centredness and a community responsibility on the part of the clinician.[7] However, interestingly, the WHO also, in a teleological bent, defined goals that primary [health] care should aspire to – mainly in a public health framework.[8] For the WHO, the extra word between primary and care above delineates the wider health promotion context.

If point of first contact matters, then arguably, generalist practice is well-served to confront and deal with the clinical content underlying that first contact. By its nature, it calls for a clinician who can cover a lot of ground: an 'omni-practitioner' as it has been termed in the French style.

In a manner of speaking, the picture of a clinician situated in her community responding to her ill patients of various types, and offering an intervention which is designed to relieve that human suffering is an attractive ethical model. Whether that clinician is medically trained or not may well not matter to the delivery of the aims above, as long as they are delivered. By any measure, to take one of the descriptors above, person-centredness in the clinical interaction is morally good whether the ethical reasoning is utilitarian (a better outcome usually ensues), deontological (as it is consistent with respect for persons) or virtue-based (as good character traits are revealed).[9]

SCOPE

In one view, the distinction between generalist and specialist practice is merely comparative; paediatricians and geriatricians could reasonably describe themselves as generalists, given that they care for patients with a broad range of conditions. However, these professional groups only care for children and older people, respectively. That said, a trend away from super-specialisation is currently detectable in UK secondary care circles, back towards perhaps the 'general medical' hospital practitioner[10] in the aim of better secondary care overall. Perhaps also relevant is the tacit notion that the more 'super' a specialist is, the more expensive to train and more difficult to re-tool him or her also is. (Of late, for example the need for cardiothoracic surgeons has diminished as less invasive therapies have supplanted their work.) However, the 'complete' generalist would cover patients of any age, and has historically done so. Primary care nurses, where their roles are so defined, would have a similar scope of practice, and ideally work in multi-disciplinary teams with their medical colleagues. Such definitional issues are not merely an abstraction, as they seem to have real value for patients. For example, the notion of first contact being with a clinician who is known, whatever the nature of the presenting issue, is something patients prefer, whether or not specialist care needs to be invoked.[11–13]

Allied to this notion of first contact is the potentially undifferentiated nature of the people and problems that present themselves to generalists' 'front doors'. However, in generalist terms, the wide scope of presenting issues is the essence of the job, an essence which generalists ought to embrace. To deal with a smaller number of medical problems may be more comfortable for the practitioner, and the magnification of view is more impressive but it inevitably excludes what surrounds the magnifier's field.[14]

CONTINUITY

Similarly, after first contact, patients prefer to deal with clinicians who know them, or better, where they know each other. This has implications for the quality of care, the value of the relationship and clinical outcome in increasingly fragmented health systems.[15,16] At first sight, the value of continuity may be assumed to be more relevant in the care of serious or long-term conditions, but doctors at least hold that value in minor problems too.[17] What these notions have begun to illustrate in recent years is that there is a body of practice, theoretically and practically, that has been described as relationship-based medicine, building on the relational continuity between clinician and patient.[18] As such, this personal aspect to continuity of care should be differentiated from the continuity illustrated organisationally or in virtue of the information held about a patient by that organisation.[19] In any event, there is increasing evidence that continuity of care is associated with better clinical outcomes, perhaps mediated through accumulated knowledge (of the patient, by the clinician) over time.[20] In an idealised version, what is engendered in this long-term continuity is a species of trust[21] between clinician and patient. Idealised perhaps because like any long-term relationship, that between primary care clinician and patient is not invulnerable, and subject to stress, or even rupture. Where there is a difference of view that cannot be rationalised, or a refusal of treatment held to be implausible or non-indicated, it may break down.[22] That it does not more often is perhaps surprising.

CONTEXT

Generalist clinical practice, in the terms of an omnipractitioner, necessarily describes care of patients in their own contexts, a descriptor which can be drawn widely. Often, care is delivered at the home, meaning a residence, a residential facility or other similar situations. Generally, care is delivered in these community facilities rather than the highly technical environment of the hospital. Essentially these are geographical sites, but of more importance is the social context within which care is delivered: and of crucial import is the family. As mentioned above, some countries refer to their primary care as family medicine for this reason – the same clinician or team of clinicians deliver care to the whole family, whether nuclear, extended or fragmented.[23,24] It might be thought rather archaic to define a mode of clinical practice by reference to those small groups to whom it is targeted. However, human society is still mostly lived in small aggregates of individuals, with whom we may even subsume some of our decision-making, so it does appear logical to deliver primary care on that basis. Readers may note the slightly messy descriptors of site and function here: *community*, *primary*, *family* and *general*, all overlapping in interpretation and meaning. This imprecision represents the real world of care delivery and context and perhaps should be celebrated rather than eschewed? Certainly, a good primary care clinician should have knowledge of the health and well-being factors appropriate to other members of the presenting patient's family if only to understand more of his story. Thus equipped, he or she may be better able to deliver good care.

ROLE

There are aspects of generalist practice that mark it out from specialist practice, not exclusively present, but common enough to describe. Generalists often are unable to make traditionally specific diagnoses, but are nonetheless able to deliver safe care in this uncertain context. It implies a need to be able to tolerate uncertainty and communicate that fact competently to the patient in question.[25] This is often in a clinical context of multimorbidity, where inevitably the care of the patient is more complex than single illness presentations. In addition, the modern primary care clinician will need to have skills in health promotion, rehabilitation and population medicine as well as the patient-directed 'curative' activities described hitherto. Reeve, one of the greatest thinkers in the field, uses the term 'interpretive medicine' to describe a skill founded on individual judgements made by generalist doctors in applying evidence from single condition trials to the multi-morbid patient in question. (It is similar, though not identical, to Toon's description of the interpretative role articulated in 1999.[26]) It is a version of handling the uncertainty in interpreting population-based research to the individual, and a key generalist skill.[27,28] It may even represent an intuitive approach rather than a formal, declarative approach.[29] So, what begins to emerge is a kind of professional identity specific to generalist practice; an identity forged not simply on what the clinician does but also on what he or she is. As such, he or she may even develop traits analogous to virtues in the discharge of generalist practice – and by example, the toleration of uncertainty and the embracing of complexity. Various other authors have contributed to this area over the years, almost too numerous to elaborate, although Balint, Heath and Misselbrook all merit further exploration.[30–32]

A CASE EXAMPLE

> Doris is 70 years old. She lost her husband to a stroke 3 years ago. Her doctor suspected a cerebro-vascular haemorrhage soon after starting anticoagulant treatment for atrial fibrillation (AF). Now Doris has AF and they are discussing therapeutic options. The haematologist is recommending similar treatment on an evidential basis. Doris is not persuaded and would rather take some aspirin.

It is easy to understand Doris' reluctance, given the possibility of her late husband's experience. In the end, the better decision is that founded on her autonomous thinking, informed as it should be by her own assessment of her best interests. A purely evidential account would say that she should take anticoagulants, but that may be inconsistent with her view, even if it is seen as unusual. She may have a predominantly emotional response to the decision founded on her recent bereavement and fellow feelings to her husband's experience.

So, the role of the GP is to mediate all of this, and it is a role with which all generalists are familiar. Is Doris harmed by her non acceptance of an evidence-based treatment? Clearly, she might be so harmed, though it is in a more nuanced research context than may be thought at first; in a recent review, 1 in 25 were helped (strokes prevented) and 1 in 25 harmed (by bleeding) but 1 in 384 seriously harmed (by intracranial bleeding). Each of these figures needs careful translation to the patient, and careful interpretation thereafter. Each of these latter processes might be considered in a highly objective manner by Doris and her clinician, but the end result cannot be but subjective: it is Doris' cardiovascular system and thus she has dominion over any pharmaceutical modification thereof. It may be that the clinician's view is different to Doris', dramatically so perhaps, and the role of her trust in her clinician could be very important. Braunack-Mayer describes this aspect perceptively as '... a vehicle for the exploration of fears and concerns that otherwise might go unvoiced'.[33] As previously noted, that trust relationship is something matured over time, and difficult to establish in the early stages of a clinician–patient relationship. Trust thereby neatly mirrors an aspect of decision-making described by Brody and others, as a process not given as a point in time but something that evolves as the patient perspective matures too, and thus more representative of a fully founded view. It is essentially collaborative and in a case like Doris' that need is self-evident.[34] The collaboration is yet more graphically illustrated by consideration of the uncertainty of the potential benefit. Doris and her clinician cannot know if she would fall into the group harmed or helped by the putative intervention; in an ideal world perhaps her decision-making would be assisted if she knew which would happen, given the treatment as it is. Perhaps, genomics will give her the answer in a few years' time. However, the point as issue here is the sharing and support her clinician can give her in the management of the uncertainty of her possible options. In this and other similar clinical contexts, the generalist must be at least comfortable to practice.

Such dilemmas are amplified even more where the potential intervention is as a result of screening, as opposed to therapeutics. For example, primary care teams – usually doctors and nurses but potentially many other members – could contribute significantly to the prevention of the adverse consequences of hypertension, and already do. In the UK work could reap even greater preventative rewards if it mirrored, for example, the detection and treatment levels achieved in Canada,[35,36] where hypertension control has increased from about 13% to 65% between 1992 and 2002. To achieve this is a laudable population health outcome, of a utilitarian stripe, that hinges on the sum of the individual detection, diagnosis and treatment efforts between clinician and patient, where symptoms are absent.

CONCLUSION: A FEW SALIENT 'OUGHTS'

Firstly, we should consider further the nature of the trust relationship between clinician and patient. It is axiomatic that trust should exist in order for a productive outcome to occur, and where there is a long-term relationship trust might be further engendered than where it is not present. Over time, a patient may see many specialists for many isolated conditions, in a time-limited way, but eventually will return to his or her generalist for continuing care. To do so implies a positive use of trust; it confers a responsibility on the generalist and a reliance on his or her integrity or ability. Such trust might also extend the benefit of generalist care to prevention too. Preventative work is a core function of primary care, even if is not discretely part of the 'cone' above.[37] However, to argue that trust is augmented by long-term relationships is to imply that trust is earned over time – perhaps by the demonstration of benefit or satisfaction for patient. And as O'Neill reminds us, trust is properly co-located with respect to the autonomous decisions of patients, in a modern conception of clinician–patient relationships.[38]

It could also be said that a trusting relationship is fostered by the care of patients in many differing clinical circumstances, neatly summarised as crossing social, physical and psychological boundaries. Lest this statement be taken merely as an assertion, the issues can be researched empirically, difficult as it may seem. We know, for example, that 'being taken seriously' and involvement in decision-making enhance confidence and trust in a primary care clinician.[39] This would seem entirely consistent with generally accepted constructions of autonomy in medicine, where the clear transmission and sharing of information is held to be of great importance to the delivery of ethically sound care. In the elaboration of that patient autonomy, a long-term trusting relationship implies that the generalist will be an advocate for his or her patient in all the various specialist encounters that may occur. Such advocacy may not be comfortable ground to hold in the face of specialists working at the apex of the 'cone of care' but it is a well-described and valuable function.

Secondly, there is an important, if uncomfortable, issue around the status of the generalist. Traditionally, more value has been attached to the work and role of the specialist *vis-a-vis* the generalist. This is not unique to doctors or other healthcare professionals[40] and was also described in UK civil servants in 1968. From a similar era, Lord Moran famously characterised UK general practitioners as those who had fallen off a ladder to the heights of specialism.[41,42] It is not immediately clear why this status differential should have come about, though there is little doubt that it is there and may diminish with increasing experience.[43] One possible explanation originates in the way that undergraduate schools prize specialised knowledge and care over all others, stimulating lifelong attitudes about professional identity. What can be argued forcefully is that interprofessional turf wars of this sort do not do patients any good, and collaborative approaches do.[44] So that where relationships between generalists and specialists sharing care exists are good, better patient outcomes can be assumed.[45,46]

This brings the discussion on to the third aspect we should consider: that of benefit, or its converse, harm. It is axiomatic that clinicians should bring about benefit to their patients, or as it has been put more demotically above, to do them some good. Most medical research is about the benefit various treatments may or may not bring about. We have already seen how one role of the generalist is to interpret research usually of a population-based nature, to the individual patient. Clearly, such an interpretation implies a set of communication skills, of an almost translational type. That the generalist should be skilled not only as a fixer of problems but also as an interpreter, a witness to suffering and bridge between the technical and the personal world is a sentiment argued powerfully in recent years. It is a role applicable to all clinicians to a lesser degree, but certainly to those whose work lies within the parameters of this chapter.[47,48]

Finally, moving from a consideration of the individual patient and his or her interactions with the primary care clinician to the larger issues of the generalist's responsibility to the community, it seems from epidemiological work that a health system that integrates generalist care well improves everyone's health. Such a claim is predicated on assumed improvements in health equity, cost efficiency and public health. Given a generally agreed perspective[49] on the empirical evidence in this area, this is no small claim for the support and continuation of primary care as the vital part of any healthcare system. What is most appealing ethically is the apparent direct connection between the descriptors of primary care as listed above (first access, care co-ordination and person-centred care) and the larger-scale population health outcomes.

To summarise, there ought to be generalists, whose natural home is primary care, for all the evidential and normative reasons explored all too briefly above, and healthcare systems ought to support the development of generalist care similarly. Whilst the largest literature on the subject concerns doctors, the same arguments would support non-medical generalists. This latter fact has been observed in the more isolated parts of, for example, the United States for many years, and not more and more recognised in Europe too.

The ought should therefore be an is, before too long.

REFERENCES

1. Palmer VJ, Naccarella L and Gunn JM. 2007. Are you the generalist or the specialist of my care? *New Zealand Family Physician* 34(6): 394–397. [Now *Journal of Primary Health Care*]
2. Reeve J. 2010. *Interpretive medicine: Supporting generalism in a changing primary care world*. Occasional Paper 88. RCGP. London.
3. Gunn J, et al. 2007. *What is the place of generalism in the 2020 primary care team*. Australian Primary Health Care Research Institute. Canberra, ACT.
4. Sweeney K and Heath I. 2006. A taxonomy of general practice. *British Journal of General Practice* 65(527): 462.
5. Starfield B, Shi L and Macinko J. 2005. Contribution of primary care to health systems and health. *The Milbank Quarterly* 83(3): 457–502.
6. Martin R. 2004. Rethinking primary health care ethics: Ethics in contemporary primary health care in the United Kingdom. *Primary Health Care Research and Development* 5(4): 317–332.
7. World Health Organisation. 2008. *The World Health Report 2008 – Primary health care (Now more than ever)*.
8. World Health Organisation. See http://www.who.int/topics/primary_health_care/en/ [Accessed 10 December 2015].
9. Duggan PS, Geller G, Cooper LA and Beach CM. 2006. The moral nature of patient-centeredness: Is it 'just the right thing to do'? *Patient Education and Counselling* 62(2): 271–276.
10. GMC. 2014. *Securing the future of excellent patient care [The Shape of Training report under Prof D. Greenway]*. http://www.shapeoftraining.co.uk/reviewsofar/1788.asp (accessed June 21, 2017).

11. Waibel S, et al. 2012. What do we know about patients' perceptions of continuity of care? A meta-synthesis of qualitative studies. *International Journal for Quality in Health Care* 24(1): 39–48. DOI: http://dx.doi.org/10.1093/intqhc/mzr068 39-48.

12. Freeman and Hughes J. 2010. *Continuity of care and the patient experience: An inquiry into the quality of general practice in England.* London: The King's Fund.

13. Stein HF. 2006. Family medicine's identity: Being generalists in a specialists' culture. *The Annals of Family Medicine* 4: 455–459. DOI: http://dx.doi.org/10.1370/afm.556.

14. Willis J. 1995. *The paradox of progress.* Abingdon: Radcliffe Medical Press.

15. Stange K, Burge F and Haggerty J. 2014. RCGP continuity of care toolkit: Promoting relational continuity. *British Journal of General Practice* 64(623): 274–275.

16. Maarsingh OR, et al. 2016. Continuity of care in primary care and association with survival in older people. *British Journal of General Practice* 66: 407–408.

17. Schers H, Bor H, van den Bosch and Grol R. GPs' attitudes to personal continuity: findings from everyday practice differ from postal surveys. *British Journal of General Practice* 56: 536–538.

18. Suchman AL. 2006. A new theoretical foundation for relationship based care. *Journal of General Internal Medicine* 21: s40–44.

19. Freeman and Hughes, 2010, *op. cit.*

20. Bayliss EA, et al. 2015. Effect of continuity of care on hospital utilization for seniors with multiple medical conditions in an integrated health care system. *Annals Family Medicine* 13: 123–129.

21. Lings P, et al. 2003. The doctor–patient relationship in US primary care. *Journal of Royal Society of Medicine* 96: 180–184.

22. Doyal L, Doyal L and Sokol D. 2009. General practitioners face ethico-legal problems too! *Postgraduate Medical Journal* 85: 393–394. DOI: http://dx.doi.org/10.1136/pgmj.2008.076604.

23. Dunn EV. 1990. Ethics and family practice: Some modern dilemmas. *Canadian Family Physician* 36: 1785–1787.

24. CFPC Committee on Ethics. 2012. *Ethics in family medicine – Faculty handbook.* http://www.cfpc.ca/ProjectAssets/Templates/Resource.aspx?id=5145#sthash.hj6KViA2.dpuf

25. Trevena L. 2014. Assessing, communicating and managing risk in general practice. *British Journal of General Practice* 64 (621): 166–167.

26. Toon PD. 1999. *Towards a philosophy of general practice: A study of the virtuous practitioner.* Occasional Paper *78.* Exeter: RCGP

27. Reeve J. 2010. Protecting generalism: Moving on from evidence-based medicine? *British Journal of General Practice* 60: 521–523.

28. Reeve, 2010, *op. cit.*

29. Brawn J. 2003. The formal and the intuitive in science and medicine. in *The intuitive practitioner,* Atkinson T and Claxton G (eds.). London: Open University Press.

30. Balint M. 1957. *The doctor, his patient and the illness.* London: Churchill Livingstone.

31. Heath I. 1995. *The mystery of general practice.* Nuffield Trust, London. http://www.nuffieldtrust.org.uk/sites/files/nuffield/publication/The_Mystery_of_General_Practice.pdf [accessed 1 November 2016].

32. Misselbrook D. 2001. *Thinking about patients.* Newbury: Petroc Press.

33. Braunack-Mayer A. 2007. The ethics of primary health care. in *Principles of health care ethics,* Ashcroft RE, Dawson A, Draper H and McMillan JR (eds.). Wiley.

34. Quill, TE and Brody H. 1996. Physician recommendations and patient autonomy: Finding a balance between physician power and patient choice. *Annals of Internal Medicine* 125(9): 763–769.

35. Daskalopoulou S, et al. 2015. The 2015 Canadian Hypertension Education Program recommendations for blood pressure measurement, diagnosis, assessment of risk, prevention, and treatment of hypertension. *Canadian Journal of Cardiology* 31(5): 549–692.

36. McAlister FA, et al. 2011. Changes in the rates of awareness, treatment and control of hypertension in Canada over the past two decades. *CMAJ* 183(9): 1007–1013. DOI: http://dx.doi.org/10.1503/cmaj.101767.

37. Parchman ML and Burge SK. 2003. The patient-physician relationship, primary care attributes, and preventive services. *Family Medicine* 36(1): 22–27.

38. O'Neill O. 2002. *Autonomy and trust in bioethics.* Cambridge, UK: CUP, p. 18.

39. Croker JE, et al. 2013. Factors affecting patients' trust and confidence in GPs: Evidence from the English national GP patient survey. *BMJ Open* 3: e002762. DOI: http://dx.doi.org/10.1136/bmjopen-2013-002762.

40. Subramaniam V. 1968. The relative status of specialists and generalists: An attempt at a comparative historical explanation. *Public Administration* 46(3): 331–340.

41. Loudon I, Horder J and Webster C (eds.). Allegedly made by Lord Moran to the Royal Commission on Doctors and Dentists Remuneration 1958. *Reported in General practice in the National Health Service 1948–77.* Clarendon Press, Oxford.

42. Reeve J, Irving G and Freeman G. 2013. Dismantling Lord Moran's ladder: The primary care expert generalist. *British Journal of General Practice* 63(606): 34–35.

43. Berendsen AJ, Benneker WHGM, Meyboom-de Jong B, Klazinga NS and Schuling J. 2007. Motives and preferences of general practitioners for new collaboration models with medical specialists: A qualitative study. *BMC Health Services Research* 7: 4. DOI: http://dx.doi.org/10.1186/1472-6963-7-4.

44. Rodriguez C, et al. The influence of academic discourses on medical students' identification with the discipline of family medicine. *Academic Medicine* 90(5): 660–670. DOI: http://dx.doi.org/10.1097/ACM.

45. Manca DP, Breault L and Wishart P. 2011. A tale of two cultures: Specialists and generalists sharing the load. *Canadian Family Physician* 57(5): 576–584.

46. King A. 2007. Interprofessional teamworking: A moral endeavour. in *Primary care ethics*, Bowman D and Spicer J (eds.). Radcliffe Publishing.

47. Misselbrook D. 2015. Aristotle Hume and the goals of medicine. *Journal of Evaluation in Clinical Practice* 22(4): 544–549. DOI: htttp://dx.doi.org/10.1111/jep.12371.

48. Owens J. 2012. Creating a patient led NHS: Some ethical and epistemological challenges. *London Journal of Primary Care* 4: 138–143.

49. Starfield B. 2012. Primary care: An increasingly important contributor to effectiveness, equity, and efficiency of health services. SESPAS report 2012. *Gaceta Sanitaria* 26(Suppl. 1): 20–26.

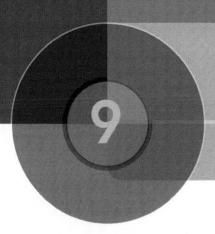

Micro-ethics of the general practice consultation

ROGER NEIGHBOUR

Crucial ethical decisions (arise) in those clinical decisions which at first sight appear to be the simplest and most straightforward.

Paul Komesaroff[1]

One's philosophy is not best expressed in words; it is expressed in the choices one makes … and the choices we make are ultimately our responsibility.

Eleanor Roosevelt[2]

Let me at the outset declare a personal position. I come to this topic not as a professional ethicist, nor even a particularly keen amateur one. My career-long fascination has been with the process of the doctor–patient consultation: its minutiae and subtleties; the way it straddles the concrete and the ineffable; and the extent to which it is a microcosm of the wider world of human relationships. I am also at a time of life when I am no longer afraid to sneak up behind the orthodox ethical establishment and shout a disrespectful 'Boo!' in its ears.

Underlying this chapter is a perennial question: 'Is the devising of a code of medical ethics a top-down or a bottom-up process?' Are general ethical principles pre-determined like statutory laws, thereafter to be uncompromisingly imposed on specific situations? Or is the general, as in case law, to be inferred from multiple examples of the particular? As with most either-or questions, the answer is 'neither; and both'.

Hippocrates, as revealed in the famous oath (see Appendix), which was an early attempt to codify the rights and wrongs of professional practice, was clearly a bottom-up man.

"will teach medical students for free", subscribers to his oath are required to promise, and,
  "I'll support my own teacher, including financially, in his old age". (I like that part.)
  "I will not perform abortions or euthanasia". (Some of us may wish to renegotiate those clauses.)
  "Lithotomy I gladly leave to the surgeons. And when I make house calls, I won't seduce the servants."

Only two of Hippocrates' bullet points are generalisations

"I will treat patients to the best of my ability and to their benefit"

and

"I will maintain patient confidentiality".

The hope has long been cherished that the complexities of the human condition might prove reducible to a convenient handful of universal principles, the 'doctrine of the four humours' being an early example in the history of medicine.* Traditional medical ethical teaching to this day is encapsulated in the four well-known precepts articulated by Thomas Beauchamp and James Childress, and popularised in the United Kingdom by Raanan Gillon: autonomy, beneficence, non-maleficence and justice.[3,4] So fond are we nowadays of the rule and the guideline that the average doctor, challenged as to whether his or her practice is underpinned by any ethical framework, seldom looks any further than this 'motherhood and apple pie' tetrad, which actually amounts to little more than 'Do as you would be done by'. However, just as the doctrine of humours became unsustainable in the face of observation and experience, so too, I suggest, do the shortcomings of the ethical 'big four' become apparent when tested in the fast-moving and unpredictable arena of the consulting room. It is my contention here that ethics on the 'micro' scale of the individual consultation, the torrent of moral choices thrown up by the ebb and flow of dialectic between doctor and patient, obliges us to ponder and challenge some of our personal values at a level below the resolution of conventional 'macro' ethics.

There are important differences between ethical issues on the macro and micro scales, summarised in Table 9.1.

Table 9.1 Comparison of macro- and micro-ethical issues

Macro-ethical issues	Micro-ethical issues
Weighty questions of public interest and lasting general application	More mundane, usually of only local, personal or temporary significance
High stakes, high impact	Lower stakes, low impact
Reflect dilemmas in values of society at large	Reflect alternatives in personal values or attitudes
Often slow to present, and can be anticipated from known developments or trends	Arise in 'here and now' time, in response to immediate and unpredictable circumstances
Slow-moving; can afford to be resolved at leisure, by debate and consensus, in public	Fast-moving; have to be resolved immediately, in private, by the individuals concerned
Resolution clarifies 'what is right in principle'	Resolution suggests 'what is best under the circumstances'
Consistent across cases	Case- and context-specific
High persistence, extensive legacy	Low persistence, local legacy

---

* 'Doctrine of humours' – the belief, dating from Hippocratic times and persisting at least into the eighteen th century, that health required a balance between four bodily fluids: blood, black bile, yellow bile and phlegm.

AN EXAMPLE OF MACRO-ETHICS

As I write (October 2015), world attention has been drawn to the case of 'C', a 10-year-old girl irretrievably brain-damaged from birth. C's loving parents have arranged for her growth to be permanently attenuated with hormonal treatment, in order to keep her small enough for them to be able, as they age, to continue caring for her into her adult life. Media pundits have been largely critical of the parents' decision, and of the doctors who implemented it, invoking the familiar four ethical principles. C's treatment, they maintain, breaches her autonomy, in that she did not consent to it, and her consent may not be assumed. Benevolence and non-maleficence, according to the critics, require that C not be submitted to treatment that distorts her normal development simply for the convenience of others. The principle of justice, they argue, alerts us to the danger that the precedent set by C's case jeopardises the future care of other patients with similar, or indeed lesser, degrees of handicap.

Yet, the same four principles could support an equally cogent case for the opposite point of view. Since C is incapable of understanding her situation, consent can only be given by those legally responsible for her and best placed to construe her best interests, namely, her parents. Normal growth would not add to her happiness, and would in time impair the ability of her parents to manifest their love for her. Other family members also have their wishes, needs and rights; and justice requires these, too, to be factored into any decision.

C's case well illustrates the macro-ethical issues shown in the left-hand column of Table 9.1. It encapsulates a high stakes and increasingly common moral dilemma. Because it resonates with the predicaments of other patients in persistent vegetative state, its implications need to be considered thoughtfully and in depth by a wide range of stakeholders. However, we have to conclude that macro-ethics, while furnishing a useful framework for discussion, does not itself lead to any incontrovertible decision about what is right or wrong, either in principle or in C's particular case. The ethical big four, for all their good intentions, offer C's family little help in their personal agony.

MICRO-ETHICS IN PRACTICE

As an example calling for the nimbleness of a micro-ethical approach, an apparently unremarkable consultation in general practice will serve. Jane D, aged 55, whom you, as her GP, have treated a few times for minor illnesses, comes to see you. She enters the room timidly, looking depressed and anxious, unlike the cheerful person you remember from previous occasions. At virtually every turn, your conversation releases a cascade of micro-ethical dilemmas – rapid-fire, small-scale, low-impact moral choices that have to be made immediately, in real time, by you and you alone, and relevant only to you and your present patient.

Let us eavesdrop on this consultation, and reflect on some of the micro-ethical issues (MEIs) as they occur. Jane D begins:

Patient: *'Good morning, Doctor'.*

MEIs: Will you respond with 'Good morning, Mrs D' or 'Good morning, Jane'? Your choice of a formal or a more intimate greeting imposes your own expectations of the nature of the doctor–patient relationship: business-like and emotionally neutral, or parent–child, or friend-to-friend. The patient's interpretation of these signals may induce a mind-set in which some parts of her agenda (as yet unknown) could be facilitated or inhibited. The 'autonomy' issue of who controls the agenda is heightened by your choice of follow-up: 'How can I help?' or 'What seems to be the problem?'

Patient: *'I, er ... I'm getting these headaches'.*

MEIs: You could (under the rubric of 'non-maleficence' and to avoid missing serious physical pathology) choose to coerce this presentation into the medical model with a closed question such as 'In what part of your head do you feel them?' Or you could allow the patient the autonomy of directing her own narrative with an open question such as 'Tell me more about the headaches'. Alternatively, under a 'beneficence' flag of truth-telling and truth-exploring, you might opt to follow your intuition by saying 'I think you look rather sad'. This latter may ultimately prove more fruitful; but do you have the right to say in effect 'I know better than you what you need to talk about'?

A little later:

You: *'Would you like to tell me why you feel so sad?'*

Patient: *'No, I don't want to talk about it'.*

MEIs: Is the customer always right? The patient's right to privacy and non-disclosure is at odds with your professional experience that talking about an emotional problem is usually helpful. 'First do no harm', we are told. But which is the greater harm: to push the patient into an area of temporary discomfort or to deny her the benefits your clinical acumen may lead to? For you to collude in ignoring cues to hidden agenda may result in inappropriate and possibly damaging investigations and treatment, in somatic fixation, and in the wasting of precious health service resources. It may be possible – and indeed, a tribute to your consulting skills – for you to persuade her to change her mind and consent to some psychological exploration. But would it be ethically right for you to do so? Would this not just be manipulation of a kind usually associated with the used-car salesman?

Unbeknownst to Jane D, her daughter has written to you 'in confidence', telling you that Jane's husband is a violent alcoholic. Husband and daughter are also patients of yours.

MEIs: How far are you bound by the daughter's expectation of confidentiality, if the only way of raising such an important issue with today's patient is by breaching it? Does your duty of care to Jane override your duty of confidentiality to the daughter? What are the husband's rights? What if you suspect there might be criminal domestic violence, or children at risk?

A few minutes later:

Patient: *'You're right, doctor, I am depressed. Do you think some vitamins would help me?'*

MEIs: On the face of it, this is a simple question, to be answered with a truthful and evidence-based 'No; vitamins don't cure depression'. However, the placebo effect, aligned with Jane's expectations and amplified by the authority endowed by your professional status, might be no less effective, and considerably safer, than a pharmacologically active alternative. Is truth-telling more important than beneficence and non-maleficence in this case? Prescribing a conventional antidepressant itself raises ethical issues. How, and how much, will you explain about risks and benefits? Should you prescribe generically or by brand? To whom do you owe the greater loyalty, the treasury or the pharmaceutical company who funded a drug's development? If there is a local prescribing policy, how far are you, an independent professional, bound by it?

Patient: *'And could you sign me off work for a couple of weeks? Only, could you put it down to my bad back, not depression? I don't want them thinking I'm a mental case'.*

MEIs: Your immediate reaction might be a slightly sanctimonious 'I won't tell an untruth on an official document'. But what *is* the truth here? That Jane D doesn't have a bad back (though she could easily say she did)? Or that your patient's interests are best served by a period of respite without the stigma she, probably correctly, anticipates if you put the demands of your own conscience above her right to manage the way her colleagues perceive her? Would there be a victim, apart from the national disease statistics, if you colluded with her in a beneficent white lie?

You notice your computer is reminding you to check Jane D's blood pressure and smoking status for QOF purposes.*

MEIs: Are you justified in imposing this agenda of your own onto the consultation, conflicting as it does with the patient's own priorities? Non-maleficence says you should not; the principle of justice, on the other hand, requires all doctors in the practice to contribute equally to meeting performance targets, for the financial benefit of all.

Patient: *'By the way, when I saw your partner last week I thought he smelled of whisky'.*

And so on. I don't suggest that this ethical soap opera is typical of every consultation, thank goodness. However, it is plausible enough to show how even the most humdrum consultation unfolds moment by moment within a complex and ever-shifting moral landscape. The image I have is of the doctor as a small interplanetary body, like an asteroid, on a meandering path through ethical space, and periodically coming within the gravitational field of one or other of the ethical 'giant planets' like justice or truthfulness or autonomy, which alter the consultation's trajectory as it hurtles on its way without ever bringing it into a stable orbit (see Figure 9.1).

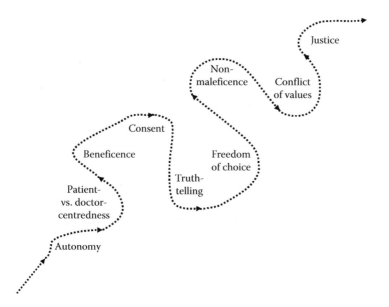

Figure 9.1 The consultation's path through ethical space.

---

* QOF – Quality and Outcomes Framework, part of the United Kingdom's general medical services contract introduced in 2004, linking elements of GPs' remuneration to their performance as measured against a range of clinical and administrative targets.

Micro-ethical issues arise, and have to be resolved, on a more parochial scale than their macro counterparts, below the radar of public attention (see the right-hand column of Table 9.1). They are never going to make headlines, unfolding as they usually do in private between an individual doctor and an individual patient. Although of immediate real-time importance to both parties during the 10 or so minutes of the consultation, their implications rarely impact on other doctors, or other patients. They are so fleeting and fast-moving that, practically, they can often only be identified and considered in hindsight. Yet, the cumulative effect of micro-ethics on the doctor–patient relationship, the mutual trust within which all good medicine needs to be practised, may be profound.

ETHICS IN FUZZY-LAND

Comparing macro- and micro-ethics, it seems to me that there is a parallel with the differences between how specialists and primary care generalists approach their clinical decision-making. Specialists like to deal in certainties; specialist practice is the rigorous pursuit of a definitive diagnosis, on the basis of which a clear-cut, evidence-based management decision can be made. We generalists, on the other hand, live most of our professional lives in 'fuzzy-land'. The problems we deal with are characterised by:

- *Uncertainty:* We may have to make decisions on the basis of incomplete or unreliable information.
- *Atypicality:* The individual patient's problem is seldom an exact fit with the textbook example.
- *Co-morbidity:* Patients often have multiple problems, whose ideal solutions may conflict with each other.
- *Complexity:* The patient's physical condition is affected by multiple psychosocial and cultural factors, not all of which we can identify, let alone control.
- *Indeterminacy:* Problems in primary care are often 'fuzzy', that is, they are hard to analyse, and respond unpredictably to intervention.

These are the hallmarks not just of our clinical world but also of its micro-ethics as well. Most of the ethical questions running through our consultations display:

- *Uncertainty:* There is not enough time fully to explore their implications.
- *Atypicality:* They seldom reduce to a clear-cut example of an established ethical principle.
- *Co-morbidity:* They usually have several ethical components, often conflicting.
- *Complexity:* Their origins and ramifications can be obscure, often involving inaccessible parts of the doctor's or patient's background.
- *Indeterminacy:* They are hard to articulate, often going unrecognised or unexpressed, and their consequences are hard to predict.

There are further parallels between the specialist and the generalist approaches to clinical and ethical decision-making. Traditional medical education teaches us the 'medical model', whereby the patient's presentation of symptoms is followed by history-taking (specific and general), examination and investigations, leading to a diagnosis and hence to treatment. Conventional macro-ethics, based on its four cardinal principles, is similarly methodical in its pursuit of moral certainty – systematic, rule-based, painstaking and time-consuming. However, in the fuzzy-land of general practice we have learned, in the face of time pressure and clinical uncertainty, to do things differently. While the full medical model remains a fall-back 'strategy of last resort', in order to function in real time in the everyday world, we use other, quicker diagnostic strategies such as:

- Pattern recognition
- Hypothesis testing ('try it and see')
- Probabilistic thinking
- Heuristics (hunches, rules of thumb)
- Phronesis (the acumen that comes with experience).*

Within the time constraints of a single consultation, our ethical decision-making of necessity takes similar shortcuts. Over time, we evolve a personal consulting style, unique to us not only in its clinical and communication aspects but also in its ethical underpinning. We build up a repertoire of familiar responses we habitually make to the ethical nuances of the consultation. We learn to perceive and interpret ethical cues subliminally, without always realising that they *are* cues to ethical issues; and for much of the time we respond to them on moral auto-pilot. Our assumptions about how 'autonomy' and 'beneficence' apply to the particular patient in front of us derive largely from our previous experience of that patient, as well as from more questionable cues to the patient's ethical competence such as their social status, cultural background, educational level or language ability. We may subtly influence the patient's right to choose by how we present the available options, particularly if the patient looks likely to choose the 'wrong' one. 'Justice' and 'equity' can take on different meanings according to our position on the political spectrum. Our concept of what constitutes 'truth-telling' is progressively honed by the success or otherwise of our previous attempts at openness.

In short, we do what we usually do for no better reason than that we have grown accustomed to doing it. I'll not claim that this 'on the hoof' approach is the right, or even an acceptable, basis for ethical practice. However, I believe it reflects reality as experienced in over a million GP consultations every day in the United Kingdom.

PRINCIPLISM OR CONSEQUENTIALISM?

Conventional ethical wisdom distinguishes 'principlism' – the pursuit of moral clarity based on axiomatic *a priori* moral principles – from 'consequentialism', which assesses the moral rectitude of an action according to the overall good or harm it leads to. T S Eliot showed himself a principlist when he proclaimed it

… the greatest treason:
to do the right deed for the wrong reason.[5]

Micro-ethicists, on the other hand, are firmly in the consequentialist camp. As Truog and his colleagues point out, the individuals involved in an ethically ambivalent consultation view it in terms of conflicting responsibilities and priorities rather than moral imperatives.[6] In the consulting room, the particular trumps the general.

The distinction between what we might call 'public' macro-ethics and 'private' micro-ethics extends to the different language we use in each context. On the larger stage, where big issues are at stake, we tend to talk of ethical 'questions' (which term implies the existence of answers) or 'dilemmas' (which suggests that moral issues are binary either-or matters of right or wrong,

---

* For a full account of this topic, including heuristics and phronesis, see Ref. 7.

black or white, with no intermediate shades of grey). When speaking of the more intimate setting of the consultation, however, we use softer and more consequentialist language, and talk instead about 'personal values', 'judgement' and 'choice'. If macro-ethics is the pursuit of what is definitely right, micro-ethics will be satisfied if it can feel its cautious way towards what is probably the best thing to do under the circumstances.

Principlism has its four universal pillars – autonomy, beneficence, non-maleficence and justice – on which the moral weight of macro-ethics securely rests. Micro-ethics – the ethics of the one-to-one and the here-and-now – has only the moral code of the individual doctor to rely on. It would be convenient if the latter were constant and consistent for *all* doctors; if every patient could be sure that the value system of every doctor had been quality assured; if the multitude of ethical nuances that influence the course and outcome of every consultation could be documented and scrutinised like a temperature chart. This, of course, is impossible. Every doctor has his or her own unique set of values, attitudes, beliefs, assumptions and predispositions, many of which originate and operate below the threshold of conscious awareness. For the most part, they only reveal themselves moment by moment in the fine detail of the thoughts, words and behaviour that emerge once the consultation is under way.

It is in the detail of individual variation between doctors that both the strength and the weakness of the micro-ethical approach lie. It is a strength that patients can select from a range of approaches until they light upon one that suits their own preference. Just as patients like to be treated as individuals, so too do they appreciate their doctors' freedom, within limits, to express their individuality through idiosyncrasies of consulting style. However, the same freedom that allows creative ethical variation also allows the possibility that an occasional rogue doctor's values will be at serious odds with one or other of the accepted cardinal moral principles. To take an extreme example, the price of ethical pragmatism is an occasional – a *very* occasional – Harold Shipman.*

The freedom to be ethically self-sufficient at the micro level lays upon doctors a responsibility to ensure that their personal values are reliably compatible with patients' well-being. As we have seen, micro-ethical issues cannot be explored or resolved in real time. They are only open to examination before or after they have been expressed in real-life consultations with distinctly non-hypothetical patients. So how is this to be done? I cannot add to the established educational methodologies of case discussion, feedback and reflection. However, I hope that awareness of the micro-ethical dimension in the consultation will emphasise how important this strand is in the education of doctors at every career stage. In primary care, clinical practice teaches us to be humble in the face of human complexity and human frailty, and that's not a bad lesson for ethicists as well.

APPENDIX: THE HIPPOCRATIC OATH[8]

I swear, by Apollo the Physician, and Aesculapius, and Hygeia, and Panaceia, and all the gods and goddesses, making them my witnesses, that to the best of my ability and judgement I will keep this oath and covenant.

To reckon him who taught me this art as dear to me as my own parents; to share my own belongings with him; if he is in need of money, to give him a share of mine; to look upon his

---

* Harold 'Fred' Shipman (1946–2004) was a GP who murdered at least 250 of his patients over a 23-year period whilst preserving the appearance of a devoted family doctor. Four years into an indeterminate life sentence, Shipman hanged himself in Wakefield prison.

offspring as if they were my own brothers, and to teach them this art, if they so wish, without fee; by precept, lecture and every means of instruction I will teach the art to my own sons, and those of my teachers, and to other pupils who have agreed to be bound by the laws of medicine, but to no one else.

I will apply such therapeutic measures as, to the best of my ability and judgement, I consider to be for the benefit of my patients, and to abstain from anything that is harmful or mischievous.

I will neither administer a deadly drug to anyone who asks for it, nor will I make a suggestion to this effect. Similarly, I will not give a woman a pessary to induce abortion. In purity and holiness I will live my life and practise my art.

I will not cut any person for the stone, but will leave this to be done by men who are practitioners of this work.

Whatever houses I visit I will enter for the benefit of the sick, and will abstain from every intentional act of mischief and corruption, including the seduction of any woman or man, be they free person or slave.

Whatever I may see or hear touching on people's lives, whether or not in the course of my professional service, which ought not to be made public, I will not divulge, reckoning that such matters should be kept secret.

As long as I keep this oath inviolate, may it be granted to me to enjoy life and the practice of my art, and to be respected by all men at all times. But if I transgress and break this oath, may the opposite be my fate.

REFERENCES

1. Komesaroff PA. From bioethics to microethics. In *Troubled Bodies: Critical Perspectives on Postmodernism, Medical Ethics, and the Body*, Komesaroff PA (ed.). Durham, NC: Duke University Press; 1995.
2. Roosevelt E. *You Learn by Living*. New York: Harper Collins; 1960.
3. Beauchamp TL, Childress JF. *Principles of Biomedical Ethics*. 7th ed. New York: Oxford University Press; 2013.
4. Gillon R. *Philosophical Medical Ethics*. Chichester: Wiley; 1986 (derived from a 26-part series in *Br Med J* from 1985;290:1117 to 1986;292:543–545).
5. Eliot TS. *Murder in the Cathedral*. 1935.
6. Truog DR, Brown SD, Browning D, et al. *Microethics: The ethics of everyday clinical practice*. John Wiley & Sons, Hoboken, New Jersey. Hastings Center Report 45, no. 1. 2015.
7. Neighbour R. *The Inner Physician*. London: RCGP; 2016.
8. Hippocrates, The oath. In *Hippocratic Writings*, Lloyd GER, Chadwick J, & Mann WN (translators). Harmondsworth: Penguin; 1978, p. 67.

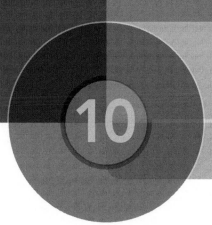

Analysing an *ordinary* consultation

RAFIK TAIBJEE

> John, 45 years old, presents feeling tired. It is likely to be due to working 13 hours a day and stress at home. He also has symptoms of depression. You decide to arrange full blood count (FBC) and renal and thyroid blood tests as there is a slim possibility of anaemia or hypothyroidism, and he does not come in to the clinic very often. You say: 'I'd suggest you get these blood tests if that's OK and then we see you to follow this up ...' John seems content with the plan and arranges to return two weeks later.

This chapter will focus on the concept of informed consent in what is an everyday situation which we may not give much thought to; should a healthcare professional (HCP) explain all the risks and benefits of the tests, and gain specific and explicit consent from John to having them done? I will focus more on the ethical and pragmatic solutions and less on the law, in part as the law offers few answers, because such an unremarkable situation is yet to be legally contested. I will not consider capacity as John is assumed to be an adult who is fully able to consent, being able to receive the information, retain it long enough to make a decision, and weigh it up and communicate his decision.

With increased medical knowledge comes a responsibility to use this judiciously and ensure the patient wants to go on a journey of discovery with the HCP. I come across elderly patients who see death as an inevitable thing and who would rather remain ignorant of any impending suffering or death. They may want to remain positive and would find it difficult if their loved ones expressed anxiety and fear for them. There are many tomes on what to say or do when it comes to resuscitation, or life support machines, or consent to research trials, but these are rarer events. I hope to convince the reader that there is an 'ethics of the ordinary' we need to consider. Much has been written about whether HIV testing requires special consent procedures, but this was rather more in the 1980s when the condition had very different implications. So what of a more everyday investigation, the simple full blood count (FBC)?

OFFICIAL GUIDANCE

To begin, it is instructive to look at UK consent guidance from the medical regulator, an extract of which is reproduced in Appendix. The General Medical Council (GMC) guidance, interestingly entitled 'making decisions together', appears to be more based on virtue ethics. Indeed, most doctors are struck off for dishonesty or integrity issues rather than for clinical incompetence.[1] Broadly speaking, the guidance spells out that patients must be afforded information but the exact way and amount will depend on circumstances. So in some sense, the guidance stipulates a necessity but not the means to know how to do this.

In modern law, the *Bolam* test, being what a reasonable doctor ought to do, has been superseded.[2] The tide started to change in 2004 after the case of Carole Chester who was paralysed after surgery, where Lord Justice Bingham stated in his *obiter dictum* that 'medical paternalism no longer rules and a patient has a prima facie right to be informed by a surgeon of a small, but well-established, risk of serious injury as a result of surgery'.[3]

In March 2015, the UK Supreme Court ruled on the case of *Montgomery*, involving a baby born with cerebral palsy, from shoulder dystocia. There was increased risk due to maternal diabetes, but his mother was not offered a caesarean section. The Supreme Court stated that 'The test of materiality is whether, in the circumstances of the particular case, a reasonable person in the patient's position would be likely to attach significance to it'.[4] This would involve the 'material risks of treatment and of any reasonable alternative'. This significance test from a patient perspective seems set until the next 'reasonable body' of Law Lords redefines the law again. Consent case law has generally involved surgery, so it is unknown how far existing law would extend to blood tests and their consequences.

I will turn to a more instructive ethical approach to the problem. I could adopt an Aristotelean virtue ethics approach, basing the discussion on what a good doctor might do in this situation or any number of other approaches. However, given the dominance in British medical ethics teaching, I have opted to use an approach promoted widely in the UK by Raanan Gillon: the 'Big Four' ethical principles of justice, beneficence, non-maleficence and autonomy.[5] As I hope to demonstrate there is no easy answer, but the way healthcare is set up can make things easier.

JUSTICE

The commonest argument for getting on and arranging the test without more discussion is fair use of resource, and the opportunity cost of clinicians' time being spent explaining the tests rather than on other people or things. This is important if one adopts a utilitarian view of using the limited time to maximise benefit. Doctors cite this reason as a reason for taking shortcuts in gaining consent but this is on a 'dubious ethical basis' as such shortcuts may be more motivated by indolence.[6]

Research has shown that shared decision-making is more valued by younger women and among those with higher educational attainment or more chronic problems. Hence, there may be built-in inequality. This may relate to the time we afford people responding to questions in our consultations, meaning they get more time with the HCP.[7]

An Aristotelian ideal of justice as equity is where those who are equal are treated equally, but those who are unequal are treated unequally. Handling patients differently is legitimate only on the basis of morally relevant differences. Yet, it seems we treat people differently all the time. More educated people with questions often get more time to deal with their information needs, and we know general practitioners (GPs) are not necessarily consistent, ordering more tests for people from higher social classes,[8] or through a perceived need to reassure patients.[9]

BENEFICENCE (AND NON-MALEFICENCE)

Whilst not the purpose of this chapter, we might pause to question why doctors do blood tests in the first place. In this case, the chances of missing anaemia are slim. Did one request the test to help manage uncertainty or perhaps avoid litigation? In other words, for whose benefit?[10] Similarly, Childress states that 'beneficence really masks self-interest', when doctors 'cut corners in explanations'.[11]

But what of beneficence? Some people go as far to say that the confidence an HCP exudes affects overall outcome for the patient, perhaps through some 'Placebo Effect'. There is even some evidence for swifter symptom resolution after a more positive directive style of consultation.[12] These arguments are not very robust and are very situational. A counterargument is that beneficence is marked out though the satisfaction of personal desires and hence is served through autonomy itself.[13]

In terms of non-maleficence, do we do harm by 'torturing patients with possibilities'?[14] GPs commonly do tests when there is no clear diagnosis. Here, John is fatigued and the chance of finding serious physical pathology is low, and the risk of false-positive test results is relatively high. Follow-on tests lead to unfavourable effects such as patient anxiety, high healthcare costs, somatisation and morbidity.[15] Undoubtedly, we try to involve patients more when decisions are less clear-cut, but in so doing, we force them to make a decision when we ourselves may be ambivalent. This results in a patient making a decision armed with less medical knowledge than we possess. Is this morally fair? A lot depends on why they are seeing us as HCPs: for decision making or for information (more on this later).

Informed consent conversations may be in themselves beneficial, as when we finally come upon a diagnosis, it does not come as a complete shock to the patient. In having the conversation, we can also discover that a patient has cognitive impairment, and the conversation can strengthen the doctor–patient relationship making them less 'moral strangers' to each other.[16]

There are perils in the HCP determining beneficence and acting in best interests ahead of getting informed consent. For example, drug testing has led to patients feeling betrayed when they learn that they were tested for substance abuse without their knowledge.[17] However, it is doubtful this would extrapolate to an FBC with fewer social patient consequences or stigma.

Perhaps the strongest argument against beneficence is that we need to know what John would himself consider to be a 'good' outcome. With reduced continuity of care, described as the 'assembly line of medicine',[18] we may not know whether John wants to know he is anaemic, taking into account that it might result in more cancer tests and worry for him. As one would expect, a simple explanation is known to reduce patient anxiety around inguinal hernia surgery, but this situation is more complex.[19] Medical training indoctrinates HCPs into holding normative views about health and illness, and so we develop a strong sense of what is right for the patient.[20] Improving medical outcomes often overrides other values,[21] and even if it does so legitimately, is the universal 'good' extending life expectancy or quality of life?[22]

One solution to this issue is to invoke proportionality. Childress suggests two factors to evaluate: the amount of a loss or gain, and the probability of that outcome.[23] The problem with this is it is not value-free: quantifying harm will depend on an individual's viewpoint. It therefore seems irrational to just 'trust the doctor' and this leads us on to autonomy.[24]

AUTONOMY

Autonomy is loosely translated from Greek as 'self-rule'.[25] Kant believed the 'Categorical Imperative' was the ability to reason and make decision for oneself as the foundation of morality.[26] Strong paternalism has a bad reputation nowadays, but until 1960s beneficence triumphed over autonomy.[27] People believe that the growth of human rights throughout the twentieth century has discouraged passivity and has 'redressed power imbalances'.[28] Moreover, consequentialists argue that patients can participate more if given autonomy.[29] In this case, John might more readily remember to mention an important family history of blood disorders, when the doctor explains the FBC test.

We might endeavour to respect autonomy by becoming 'patient-centred' and find out John's values and acting accordingly. However, autonomy requires decisional authority: having opportunity to make all important choices, not simply giving John the choice over what values to share with us as HCPs.[30] In order to make decisions, John must have the confidence and competence to understand the information we present, otherwise it may provoke stress rather than providing comfort.[31]

Some people argue that patients often waive their right to directly consent on an issue.[32] Indeed, we frequently offer them the choice of being informed as much or as little as they want. However, I would contend that one cannot waive one's involvement in the *decision* without knowing the *specific facts* being considered. In other words, even if we as HCPs offer choices and act as the agent of the patient, the patient needs core information in order to decide to leave it up to us to make the decision in question.[33]

One can read critiques of this stating that 'even sick doctors can ironically prefer paternalism to personal autonomy'.[34] The word 'prefer' being critical here. In other words, autonomy is separate to acting independently, although the two are often fallaciously conflated.

Some argue that it is easier to impart technical information, than to gain all the information relevant to the patient and make the decision as the HCP. After all, with Johari's Window of 'unconscious incompetence' one does not know what one does not know.[35]

HOW MUCH INFORMATION TO GIVE?

The original meaning of doctor was that of 'teacher'. Our role as HCPs is to enhance patient understanding perhaps.[36] Legally, the information provided needs to cover material risks. But, these will differ according to each patient. A one in a thousand risk of blindness in one eye may seem small to one individual, but huge to someone already blind in the other eye. So this does not give an unequivocal, practical answer.

White believes autonomy dictates that decision-makers be given *all* the facts.[37] However, it is not realistic to expect even the best HCP to provide, with no notice, a detailed list of facts. Moreover, I would contend that there is an overemphasis on material risks, spurred on by the law, rather than the benefits. For example, when we initiate medication, we are quick to explain side effects and often slower to know the benefits, often resorting to 'the guidelines say …'. We may in fact be inducing the nocebo effect in our patients: with negative thoughts and pessimism making them experience more ill health.[38]

Is it pointless providing information to John when neither myself, nor John himself, spontaneously thought it necessary?[39] Or, do we have a duty to warn?[40] Indeed, doctors have been shown to typically underestimate patients' desire to be informed and overestimate their desire to be involved in decision-making.[41] Faden found that over 93% of their patient sample felt they personally benefited from the information provided, though their decisions were based on factors external to the information in 88% of cases.[42]

We sometimes know a better treatment exists but is not funded or yet available in our country, like a more expensive variant of a drug. I am not sure whether I always tell the patient this, for fear of losing the placebo effect from the cheaper drug and fearing confrontation. As one research subject said, 'you choose data to help the patient make the decision you think they ought to'.[43] I would also contend that a double-standard exists in that we, as HCPs, discuss and agree to run tests to differing degrees depending on whether it is the patient, or we ourselves, who feel the test might help. I would certainly have spent more time explaining to John why he doesn't need the brain MRI he thinks he does compared with why in fact he did need an FBC test.

TRUST

HCPs value trust as without it our job would be virtually impossible.[44] With increased accountability, trust may diminish. However, less trust may be positive if it aids patient awareness of medical limitations, and makes them take more control of their own illnesses.[45]

Patients may need to trust their HCPs over and above needing information. In a study of breast cancer patients, researchers found that patients' desire for information primarily related to 'maintaining trust and hope', as opposed to empowering them to be decision-makers. Trust was diminished when patients felt misinformed, but trust was augmented when the doctor was adjudged to be open. For this subset of patients, 'what patients sought diverged from the current emphasis on providing information. It was a function not of amount of information but of the nature of information and manner of presentation'.[46] Thus, rather than weighing up technical information, patients make 'second-order judgments of the reliability and trustworthiness of those who offer medical treatment'.[47]

DIVERSE TESTS

Some argue that we have actually started imposing choice on patients. O'Neill feels it should depend on the level of risk involved.[48] A few years ago, HIV testing needed a full discussion and documented consent before being undertaken, but this has changed, perhaps through changes in stigma and treatability. On the contrary, prostate-specific antigen testing for prostate cancer generally is thought to require proper discussion. Some US states like New York have decided to stipulate which tests require written consent, such as for specific genetic conditions.[49]

I believe this is due to the harms and benefits of testing being nearer to each other in magnitude. Therefore, as the benefits could be so great here, such anaemia being curable with dietary change, or being able to stop an antidepressant causing unwarranted side effects being endured, do we need to worry about consent? Extending this further, is an FBC test very different to auscultating the chest and discovering the patient has a pleural effusion which might be due to cancer, or wheeze that might indicate asthma, or a blood pressure indicative of hypertension? Yet, we do not usually gain specific informed consent for these examinations, and rely instead on implied consent or acquiescence.

SEEKING CONSENT

If autonomy is only one amongst the principles, 'perhaps informed consent is not always important'?[50] Indeed, informed consent may simply be a more fundamental entity, providing assurance that a patient has not been deceived or coerced.[51]

Pragmatism might have to rule. In Braddock's research of 81 consultations, each contained at least one decision, with an average of 3.20 clinical decisions per visit (range 1–8, 95% confidence interval 2.85–3.54). Fifteen per cent of the visits involved decision about undertaking diagnostic laboratory tests.[52] Therefore, it seems it might be impossible to gain consent for every decision reached if we attempt to gain consent universally. But then, if HCPs had to decide when to seek consent and when not to, it would leave us confused and uncertain.[53]

Further haziness is caused if one debates whether the consent process requires conscious signposting to the patient. I believe I have learnt, as Elwyn postulates, to ask very specific questions to patients, so that the patient cannot then legitimately say that they were not asked.[54] It is also part of passing clinical examinations, so the examiner can tick off that consent has been gained. Lidz discusses how consent is actually a process that evolves through a conversation, which indeed does seem more natural and less stilted but is harder to record in the medical record.[55]

Finally, I would make the point that providing information does not necessarily mean the patient has understood it, and there is case law to suggest it is the comprehension that matters.[56] If John were to say he understands the FBC test, I would not know if he was simply saying this to be accommodating.[57] We know common medical terms are frequently misunderstood, even 'constipated', 'arthritis' and 'jaundice'.[58] Also, I can inadvertently underplay risks by using descriptors such as 'only' or 'less than', while overplay them using terms such as 'more than' or 'as many as'.[59]

A SOLUTION?

So, up to this point, I suspect the reader, like myself, has found it hard to navigate a clear way through this ethical marshland with multiple conflicting arguments, especially between autonomy and beneficence having dominance.

To my mind, shared decision-making is false. Most often, the HCP makes only one clear plan as an agent, or offers choice from a limited picking list. Informed consent is a 'modern ritual of trust', giving the illusion of challenging authority.[60] Cynics go as far as to say that the skill of the HCP is in making the patient *feel* they were given choices.[61]

A doctor's role is still to give information, and I do not agree that we should be primarily 'information navigators' as Bowman contends.[62] This information, and the way it is delivered, helps patients feel confidence in doctors and move forward in mutualistic relationships, although the nature of these relationships and the reduction in continuity of care are real problems.

In this case, I decided that I wanted to perform a test on John, but really I could have attempted to explain my thought processes to him, being mindful of both the risks: of opening up further uncertainty and worry; and the benefit of treating an uncovered anaemia. So as Brody wrote, I believe disclosure is adequate 'when the physician's basic thinking has been rendered transparent to the patient'.[63] In this case, I did not truly respect his autonomy, but could have at least shown it some regard and possibly gained John's confidence in me, in a pragmatic way through a summarised evaluation.

After all, as Clemenceau purportedly said:

War is too important to leave to the generals.[64]

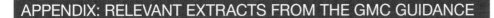

APPENDIX: RELEVANT EXTRACTS FROM THE GMC GUIDANCE

CONSENT: PATIENTS AND DOCTORS MAKING DECISIONS TOGETHER (GMC 2008)

'In deciding how much information to share with your patients you should take account of their wishes. The information you share should be in proportion to the nature of their condition, the complexity of the proposed investigation or treatment and the seriousness of any potential side effects, complications or other risks'.

PARA 4

No single approach to discussions about treatment or care will suit every patient, or apply in all circumstances. Individual patients may want more or less information or involvement in making decisions depending on their circumstances or wishes.

PARA 5

The doctor explains the options to the patient, setting out the potential benefits, risks, burdens and side effects of each option, including the option to have no treatment.

PARA 7

The exchange of information between doctor and patient is central to good decision-making. How much information you share with patients will vary, depending on their individual circumstances. You should tailor your approach to discussions with patients according to:

1. their needs, wishes and priorities
2. their level of knowledge about, and understanding of, their condition, prognosis and the treatment options
3. the nature of their condition
4. the complexity of the treatment, and
5. the nature and level of risk associated with the investigation or treatment.

PARA 8

The doctor should not make assumptions about:

1. the information a patient might want or need
2. the clinical or other factors a patient might consider significant, or
3. a patient's level of knowledge or understanding of what is proposed.

PARA 9

You must give patients the information they want or need about:

1. the diagnosis and prognosis
2. any uncertainties about the diagnosis or prognosis, including options for further investigations

3. options for treating or managing the condition, including the option not to treat

4. the purpose of any proposed investigation or treatment and what it will involve.

PARA 10

If, after discussion, a patient still does not want to know in detail about their condition or the treatment, you should respect their wishes, as far as possible. But you must still give them the information they need in order to give their consent to a proposed investigation or treatment. This is likely to include what the investigation or treatment aims to achieve.

REFERENCES

1. Sokol, D and Bergson, G. *Medical Ethics and Law.* London: Trauma Publishing, 2005.
2. Mason, JK and Laurie GT. *Law and Medical Ethics.* 9th ed. Oxford: OUP, 2013.
3. *Chester v Ashfar* [2004] 4 All E.R. 587.
4. *Montgomery v Lanarkshire Health Board* [2015] UKSC 11.
5. Gillon, R. *Philosophical Medical Ethics.* Chichester: Wiley, 1986 as based on Childress, B et al., *Principles of Biomedical Ethics.* 5th ed. Oxford: OUP, 2001.
6. Orne-smith, A and Spicer, J. *Ethics in General Practice.* Abingdon: Radcliffe, 2001.
7. Edwards, A and Elwyn, G. *Shared Decision-Making in Health Care.* 2nd ed. Oxford: OUP, 2009.
8. Hartley, RM et al. Influence of patient characteristics on test ordering in general practice. *BMJ* 1984; 289: 735–8.
9. van der Weijden, T. et al. Understanding laboratory testing in diagnostic uncertainty: A qualitative study in general practice. *BJGP* 2002; 52: 974–80.
10. DeKay, ML and Asch, DA. Is the defensive use of diagnostic tests good for patients, or bad? *Med Decis Making* 1998; 18(1): 19–28.
11. Childress, JF. *Who Should Decide? Paternalism in Healthcare.* New York: Oxford University Press, 1982.
12. Savage, R and Armstrong, D. Effect of a general practitioner's consulting style on patients' satisfaction: A controlled study. *BMJ* 1990; 301: 968–70.
13. White, BC. *Competence to Consent.* Washington, DC: Georgetown University Press, 1994.
14. Wear, S. *Informed Consent: Patient Autonomy and Physician Beneficence within Clinical Medicine.* Dordrecht, The Netherlands: Kluwer Academic Publishers, 1993.
15. van Bokhoven, MA et al. Blood test ordering for unexplained complaints in general practice: The VAMPIRE randomised clinical trial protocol. *BMC Fam Pract* 2006; 7: 20.
16. Wear, 1993, *op. cit.*
17. Warner, EA et al. Should informed consent be required for laboratory testing for drugs of abuse in medical settings? *Am J Med* 2003; 115(1): 54–8.
18. Wear, 1993, *op. cit.*
19. Kerrigan, DD et al. Who's afraid of informed consent? *BMJ* 1993; 206: 298–300.
20. Rogers, WA and Braunack-Mayer AJ. *Practical Ethics for General Practice.* 2nd. Oxford: OUP, 2009.
21. Pellegrino, ED and Thomasma, DC. The conflict between autonomy and beneficence in medical ethics: Proposal for a resolution. *J Contemp Health Law Policy* 1987; 3(23): 23–46.
22. White, 1994, *op. cit.*
23. Childress, 1982, *op. cit.*
24. Bowman, D and Spicer, J. *Primary Care Ethics.* Abingdon: Radcliffe Publishing, 2007.

25. White, 1994, *op. cit.*

26. White, 1994, *op. cit.*

27. Sokol and Bergson, 2005, *op. cit.*

28. McLean, AM. *Autonomy, Consent and the Law.* Abingdon: Routledge, 2010.

29. Wear, 1993, *op. cit.*

30. White, 1994, *op. cit.*

31. Waller, BN. The psychological structure of patient autonomy. *Camb Q Healthc Ethics* 2002; 11: 257–65.

32. Meisel, A. The exceptions to the informed consent doctrine: striking a balance between competing values in medical decision-making. *Wisconsin Law Rev* 1979; 79(2): 479.

33. Edwards and Elwyn, 2009, *op. cit.*

34. Stirrat, GM and Gill, R. Autonomy in medical ethics after O'Neill. *J Med Ethics* 2005; 31: 127–30.

35. Handy, C. *21 Ideas for Managers.* San Francisco, CA: Jossey-Bass, 2000.

36. Orne-smith and Spicer, 2001, *op. cit.*

37. White, 1994, *op. cit.*

38. Hauser, W, et al. Nocebo phenomena in medicine: Their relevance in everyday clinical practice. *Deutches Arzteblatt Int* 2012; 109(26): 459–65.

39. Wear, 1993, *op. cit.*

40. Maybery, M. *Consent in Clinical Practice.* Abingdon: Radcliffe Medical Press, 2003.

41. Brody, H. *Transparency: Informed Consent in Primary Care.* New York: The Hastings Center, 1989.

42. Faden, RR and Beauchamp, TL. Decision-making and informed consent: A study of the impact of disclosed information. *Soc Indicators Res* 1980; 7: 313–36.

43. Elwyn, G. *Shared Decision Making: Patient Involvement in Clinical Practice.* Nijmegen, The Netherlands: WOK, 2001.

44. Faulder, C. *Whose Body is It? The Troubling Issue of Informed Consent.* London: Virago Press, 1985.

45. Bowman and Spicer, 2007, *op. cit.*

46. Wright, EB et al. Doctors' communication of trust, care, and respect in breast cancer. *BMJ* 2004; 328: 864.

47. Manson, NC and O'Neill O. *Rethinking Informed Consent in Bioethics.* Cambridge: CUP, 2007.

48. O'Neill, O. Some limits of informed consent. *J Med Ethics* 2003; 29: 1–5.

49. Mayo. *New York State Informed Consent Test List.* 2015. Available at: http://www.mayo-medicallaboratories.com/test-catalog/appendix/nys-informed-consent.html (accessed 25 March 2015).

50. Manson and O'Neill, 2007, *op. cit.*

51. O'Neill, 2003, *op. cit.*

52. Braddock, CH. How doctors and patients discuss routine clinical decisions: Informed decision making in the outpatient setting. *J Gen Intern Med* 1997; 12: 339–45.

53. White, 1994, *op. cit.*

54. Elwyn, 2001, *op. cit.*

55. Lidz, CW et al. Two models of implementing informed consent. *Arch Intern Med* 1988; 148: 1385–9.

56. Mason and Laurie, 2013, *op. cit.*

57. Brody, 1989, *op. cit.*

58. Boyle, CM. Differences between patients and doctors. Interpretation of some common medical terms. *BMJ* 1970; 2: 286–9.

59. MacLean, A. *Autonomy, Informed Consent and Medical Law: A Relational Challenge.* Cambridge: Cambridge University Press, 2013.

60. O'Neill, O. *Autonomy and Trust in Bioethics.* Cambridge: Cambridge University Press, 2002.

61. Edwards and Elwyn, 2009, *op. cit.*

62. Bowman and Spicer, 2007, *op. cit.*

63. Brody, 1989, *op. cit.*

64. Jackson, JH. *Clemenceau and the Third Republic.* New York: Macmillan, 1948.

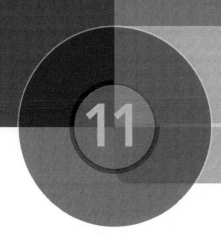

The voice of the patient

11

ROSAMUND SNOW

I hear a lot of stories of patient/clinician interactions from both sides; I suspect you would be surprised which ones make me uncomfortable.

I'm not talking about the extremes at either end of the spectrum – the practices that everyone would agree are very good or very bad. The uncomfortable stories, for me, are those in the area where patient and clinician perspectives clash.

When I listen to the health professionals talking I often hear something like this:

I saw a patient the other day who presented with [*list of biomedical symptoms*]. I thought there might be something else going on, so I probed for more. The patient began to cry and it turned out that she had [*fears, concerns, or a background story beyond the medical symptoms*]. If I hadn't asked, I'd never have found out that information.

Why does that worry me? Are these not the best kinds of doctors and nurses, those who know that we are more than the sum of our body parts, that we have a life outside the surgery? It worries me because, actually, this approach seems to treat the patient's narrative in a similar way to the patient's physical symptoms. It feels as if things have moved from the old model of taking a history to diagnose disease X (treated with a prescription) to the new model where they take a different kind of history to diagnose emotion Y (perhaps treated with something else). It chills me when the stories end with 'and then I found out she was worried about Y' because it seems as if finding out Y was an end in itself, like solving a crossword clue.

There is also an assumption that clinicians have a right to ask us those questions, even if we were not expecting to tell our story or voice our fears.

How did medicine get to this point? Were patients involved in the discussions? If you are a clinician, were patients were involved in setting the curriculum for your education? When you learnt about the ethics and values of probing patients in this way? If not, how can you be sure that this is the right thing to do?

The more discussions I have with patients, the more I hear about healthcare professionals' perspectives on what those patients want to teach, the more I see that there are areas of 'best practice' taken for granted by doctors and nurses with which many patients simply do not agree. Getting patients' stories – or 'eliciting patient narratives', in the academic and educational literature[1,2] – is one of those grey areas. I am not suggesting that all patients agree with this view, or that all patients hate telling their stories all of the time. Of course there are plenty of occasions when we are glad to have had the chance to voice fear, process what has happened to us, or describe the context of life with disease. Of course it is not always a bad thing to talk about patients' emotional lives or elicit their narratives. But at the same time, it is not *necessarily* a good thing; and above all, you do not have the automatic right to ask for our stories.

This becomes a particular issue when our stories cause us pain, when we do not see their relevance to what we are asking you for, or when we are not yet sure how you might judge us or whether you will listen and act. What may seem clear and empathetic to you may be confusing and challenging to us.

As the patient researcher Dariusz Galasiński explains, questions asking things like 'what matters to you?' are not always received in the way you might intend:

> I really wish you, my doctor, stopped thinking of me as a book which simply opens at your say-so. [...] What really (like, really) matters to me, I am not prepared to share publicly. In fact, I am not prepared to share most of what really matters to me with my GP, whom I like and respect. It's none of his business.[3]

You may notice a similar theme in some of these extracts from *What Your Patient Is Thinking*, a series designed with the aim of getting patients of all kinds to contribute to doctors' education:[4]

> I don't want to share too much about my past... If I have come for help with a health problem, please only ask about things that are relevant to that specific problem, and explain why you are asking those questions.
>
> **Kolbassia Haoussou**
> *What Your Patient Is Thinking (November 2016)*

> I don't always [want to] have to refer to my history of abuse or repeatedly tell someone that I don't know, and don't care, about my birth family's medical history. ... As a doctor, you could help me to realise that you are trustworthy by clearly explaining the reasons why you want me to do something.
>
> **Áine Kelly**
> *What Your Patient Is Thinking (March 2016)*

Alarm bells ring in my head when clinicians and academics demand things from patients without explaining to them why the information is needed, or what invisible limits there are for what I am expected to share. 'Ask open questions,' the communications manuals urge, in healthcare professionals' education and in advice for researchers. However, when you are at the other end of those questions, it can feel confusing, trapping and even frightening.

As someone who has struggled with a very demanding chronic condition for more than a quarter of a century, I've interacted with a lot of healthcare professionals. As someone who gets care from a teaching hospital in a university town, I have been asked a lot of questions by educators and researchers too. I am very wary nowadays of taking part in research, because I don't know what will happen to my personal story when it gets to that academic or clinical conference. Will I be positioned as non-compliant or difficult? Or, far worse, will my life story get interpreted with pity? And yet, at the same time, I want stories of people like me to be heard.

Meanwhile, on the clinical side, although my life was probably saved by a doctor who asked me how I was feeling when I was struggling to be brave about a relatively new diagnosis, when I come to the surgery with a specific problem and a short time to get answers, I feel huge resentment at being asked about my emotional life with my condition.

So I change the way I feel about it over time, depending on the circumstances, and I'm just one patient. Clinicians will see multiple patients in a day, all with their own preferences. How on earth are they meant to negotiate this ethical minefield?

Perhaps the answer lies in the quotes above. Whoever you are, reflect on why you are asking a question, consider whether it really needs to be asked, make sure you explain why you need the answer. Offer the option of not replying, or ask permission to ask about things you think might be important, but that we have not brought up ourselves.

I know, from talking to healthcare professionals who just want to do the right thing, that this is a challenging message to hear. But consider this. I give so much information to strangers already – my blood and my blood pressure, my urine, my weight, my height, my nerve function, my eye function, my life style choices – I have spent more than half of my life opening myself like a book to the gaze of doctors and nurses. Some of these pieces of information I want for myself too, because they help me self-manage; but I am not allowed to have them without sharing them, even though they feel like very private parts of my life. I cannot avoid giving doctors these things because I rely on them every single day to prescribe me the medicine that keeps me alive. Unlike Áine or Kolbassia in the quotes above, I have not experienced abuse or torture, but it is still difficult for me to say no to clinicians' questions – doctors have had the power of life and death over me since I was a teenager. Their judgement of my self-management has impact on the work I am allowed to do, my chance of being able to drive and my opportunity to get a mortgage. If they probe for the parts of me I have not volunteered, I feel as if they want to own every bit of me, body and soul. If their questions made me cry, I have to walk back out past the eyes in the reception area, I have to get myself under control so I can go back to work, I have to live with the feelings unleashed in those last few minutes of the short consultation. If I'm not ready for that, then I don't want you, the questioner, to make it your business.

So, if you were taught that a good healthcare professional elicits patient narratives, treats the whole patient, bears witness to the patient's suffering or simply asks for the patient's ideas, concerns and expectations, bear in mind that not all of us actually want that all of the time. Some of us find it confusing, irrelevant and intrusive. If you are developing tools or research or guidelines, think about the assumptions you are making. Remember that so much of healthcare 'good practice' has been developed with very little patient input, bringing in that critical reflection to bear on everything you learn.

You could even apply that principle to this book. Ask yourself as you read: who is speaking here? Do they include the direct patient voice, the increasing amount of information online and in print where we are telling you what we like and dislike? Do you really know what your patient is thinking? Have you even earned the right to know?

REFERENCES

1. Tate P, Tate L. What you need to achieve in a patient encounter or consultation. In: *The doctor's communication handbook*. 7th ed. Abingdon: Radcliffe; 2014. p. 60–81.
2. Washer P. Recognising and responding to cues. In: Washer P, editor. *Clinical communication skills*. Oxford: Oxford; 2009. p. 24.
3. Galasinski D. What Matters to you? 2016. [cited October 20, 2016]. Available from: http://dariuszgalasinski.com/2016/08/09/what-matters-to-you/
4. Various authors. What your patient is thinking series. London: The BMJ; 2015 [cited October 20, 2016]. Available from: http://www.bmj.com/specialties/what-your-patient-thinking

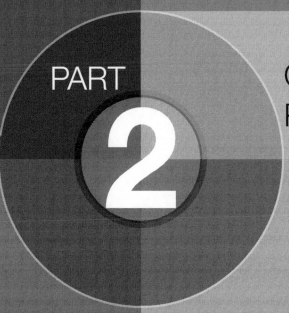

PART 2

ON VULNERABLE PATIENTS

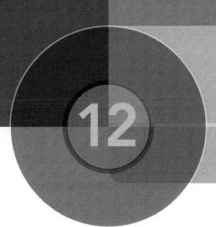

Children and the ethics of primary care

PEKKA LOUHIALA

The ethics of everyday life, the morality of the ordinary, is the 'place' in which medical ethics is enacted. The routine interaction between doctor and patient, not the dramatic life-and-death decision making that dominates the thinking of bioethicists, defines the 'space' of relationship, where the quiet, ongoing administration of care is most characteristically enacted.[1]

INTRODUCTION

Children are not small adults. From a purely physiological point of view, preterm newborns, term newborns, infants and older children are in many senses *qualitatively* different from adults. Their disease processes are different and effects of medical interventions may differ from that seen in adults.

Psychological differences between different age groups of children and adults are obvious too.

It follows from these physiological and psychological differences that also moral questions related to the healthcare of children are different or at least the weight of certain values is different from that in the case of adult patients.

The focus of academic medical ethics (or bioethics) is almost exclusively on situations and cases that are extreme or unusual, at least from the point of view of primary care. This applies also to ethics education, which 'may fall short of capturing the full spectrum of ethical considerations encountered in clinical care'.[2] Many clinical decisions of everyday practice seem simple and straightforward, but contain value judgments that are there whether the physician is aware of them or not.[3] Truog et al.[2] have characterised the latter approach as 'microethics' or 'view from the inside', while the traditional approach in bioethics has been a 'view from the outside'. These views are, of course, complementary rather than contradictory.

The aim of this chapter is to demonstrate the wide variety of ethical decisions that are present in everyday primary practice with children. I begin with an example that demonstrates the multitude of small ethical decisions made in a very common and often uncontroversial case in primary care.[4] I then continue with two cases from primary care and discuss issues related to autonomy in the light of them.

PHILOSOPHY MEETS THE MIDDLE EAR

CASE 1

Harry is 18 months old and has had symptoms of common cold for 3 days. He was better and already feverless but wakes up in the middle of the night, complaining of pain in his ears. His temperature is rising again[4].

All primary care physicians and most parents recognise the story and the first diagnosis that comes to their mind is acute otitis media (AOM), one of the most common diseases in childhood.

Sometimes the diagnosis of AOM is simple, but sometimes it is not. Most cases resolve spontaneously but it is difficult or impossible to predict the value of antibiotics in individual cases. From the point of view of the physician, the questions seem to be:

1. Does this child have AOM?
2. Do antibiotics help him or her?
3. What other treatment does the child need?
4. How should the follow-up be organised?

In an era of (so-called) evidence-based medicine and with thousands of clinical studies addressing AOM, one would think that there are straightforward answers to these questions. Unfortunately, there are not, and even in the case of clear results, one has to remember that science provides only mechanisms and probabilities. *Somebody* has to interpret what these probabilities mean for *this* particular patient in *this* particular context.

Clinical practice guidelines have been developed to help practitioners in their daily decision-making. They summarise the available scientific data concerning a specific clinical question. Usually, a guideline provides first a definition of a disease and then presents data on various strategies for treatment and prophylaxis.

1. *Does this child have AOM?*

   The first small ethical decision may have to be made even before the full diagnostic process is complete. Visualising the tympanic membrane is essential for the diagnosis but very often there is earwax preventing this and sometimes the removal of it is far from easy. Does full visibility of the tympanic membrane outweigh the discomfort caused in the child when trying to remove the wax? As many clinicians, children and parents know, this discomfort is sometimes not minor.

   The diagnostic process is not made easier by the lack of an unequivocal definition of AOM. The abstract of the American guideline[5] promises to provide a 'specific, stringent definition of AOM', but in the main text it is noted that 'there is no gold standard for the diagnosis of AOM'. Further on it is noted that 'AOM has a spectrum of signs as the disease develops' and that 'criteria were chosen to achieve high specificity recognizing that the resulting decreased sensitivity may exclude less severe presentations of AOM'. The Finnish guideline[6] provides a definition, which is first circular: 'Acute otitis media means acute-onset, short-lasting and clinically verifiable inflammation of the middle ear'. This is then clarified by the following:

   > There are signs of inflammation in the tympanic membrane and there is secretion in the middle ear. In addition, at least one of the following symptoms or signs can be

found: upper respiratory symptoms (rhinitis, cough, fever, throat pain, ear pain), poor hearing and crying.

In the light of these guidelines, it is obvious that there is a grey zone in which it is not easy to determine whether the child has AOM or not.

2. *Do antibiotics help him or her?*

Decisions about treatment involve more value judgements. In many cases, the diagnosis is obvious, and the next question seems to be whether the child needs antibiotics or not. Again, the guidelines differ, and it is not obvious that the circumstances in different countries explain the variation.

In Finland, the recommendation is to prescribe antibiotics as a rule if the diagnosis is 'certain enough'. The guideline allows, however, a possibility for follow-up without antibiotics, if the parents agree. In Australia, the first suggestion for a mildly unwell child over 12 months is no antibiotics for the first 24–48 hours. According to the Scottish guideline, 'Children diagnosed with acute otitis media should not routinely be prescribed antibiotics as the initial treatment'.

Another way to evaluate the need for antibiotics is the *number needed to treat* (NNT), which in this case means the number of children needed to have a course of antibiotics for one child to benefit. According to one analysis, the NNT is 17.[7] Again, the interpretation of this figure in the clinical context is a value judgment. NNT figures as such are not small or large but must be interpreted in a context, depending on the seriousness of the condition and the potential harms of the treatment.

The guidelines agree largely on the choice of antibiotics and suggest amoxicillin as a first choice if the child is not allergic to penicillin. The length of the course varies, however, and there may still be complex questions that need an answer – and a value judgment. What if the child has had a course of amoxicillin before and has developed a rash in the same context? It is widely known that most suspected allergic reactions to antibiotics are false alarms but how much weight should be given to this possible complication? Parents may also have preferences for the choice of a drug. If every single dose means a fight between the child and her parents, and the parents suggest a single daily dose of azithromycin for 3 days instead of a dose of amoxicillin twice a day for 5 days, what kind of a role should these kinds of preferences have in the decision-making?

From the point of view of a single patient, broad spectrum but generally safe antibiotics like amoxicillin are a better choice than narrow-spectrum antibiotics like penicillin V. However, from the point of view of *future* patients, narrow spectrum would be a better choice.

3. *What other treatment does the child need?*

Since pain is often the major symptom of AOM, all guidelines emphasise its treatment. There are several alternatives available but – somewhat surprisingly – the supporting evidence is weak. Only one randomised placebo-controlled study has addressed the effect of paracetamol, one of the oldest and most widely used analgesics, in the treatment of otalgia in AOM.[8] The dose of paracetamol in that study was small, and the differences between the treatment groups were not large. My guess is, however, that practically all practitioners treating children with AOM would consider it unethical *not* to give these children pain medication. Correspondingly, they would probably not agree to participate in a new study comparing paracetamol with placebo and in the treatment of pain associated to AOM. These are strong and interesting value judgments that prefer common experience to scientific evidence.

The guidelines do not mention non-pharmacological treatments of AOM at all. Many parents and practically all clinicians are aware of the effect of sleeping position on the symptoms of AOM. There are no randomised trials on this, but a raised sleeping position for these children is often recommended. This advice is based on *common sense*.

4. *How should the follow-up be organised?*

There are still value judgments to be made after the initial decisions concerning treatment. These judgments concern, for example, follow-up and possible advice on lifestyle issues.

There is no evidence for or against routine re-examination of symptomless children. However, the Finnish guideline recommends a routine re-examination within 3–4 weeks. The Australian guideline does not mention follow-up at all. The Scottish guideline suggests re-examination only for children who originally had a discharging ear. The American guideline leaves it to the clinician to decide on possible reassessment of some patients like young children with severe symptoms.

Day care for large groups of children and parental smoking are two well-known and significant risk factors for AOM. Should the clinician ask questions about these or give advice to the parents about these risk factors? These are further value judgments that have to be considered related to the care of the acute illness.

SO WHAT?

In sum, this clinical example of an extremely common childhood disease demonstrates the multitude of values and value judgments that are present at all levels of clinical decision-making.

If there is evidence for or against something, it is, of course, important to consider, but evidence as such is blind. Numbers do not dictate, they only advise. Sometimes even ethicists don't see this:

> Either the evidence is valid, in which case you must attend to it; or it is not, in which case you have to act based on some sort of reason; or you just do not know, but need to decide on a course of action nonetheless. 'Art' will not help you here – neither hunches, guesses nor intuition.[9]

This statement resembles the *naturalistic fallacy*[10] and seems to derive 'an ought from an is'. Although Goodman argues otherwise, there is no compelling reason for the clinician to act in one direction or another, *whatever* the evidence is. Clinical evidence is expressed in the form of probabilities and a treatment decision calls for a value judgement in any case.

The central role of values does not imply, however, that value conflicts are common. On the contrary, in the vast majority of cases, the value worlds of physicians and patients overlap quite sufficiently, and no conflicts arise.[11]

WHOSE AUTONOMY?

> The pendulum has swung from rather crass paternalism practised 50 or 60 years ago to an obsession with autonomy which allows patients with questionable autonomy to come to harm.[12]

CASE 2

There is an outbreak of measles in the community. Four-year-old John has not been vaccinated in the routine vaccination programme because his parents were afraid of serious harmful effects of the MMR vaccine. Now the parents are, however, worried and turned to their GP/GPN for advice.

Autonomy is one of the central values in patient care, and it is certainly true that the expansion of its role has made the doctor–patient relationship 'more open, more adult, more transparent and more attentive to the patient's values and wishes'.[13] At the same time, it has been forgotten that a 'radically independent, autonomous person is at best an idealised portrait of a fictional character, part of an elaborate ideological cartoon of Western culture'.[1] We all are, after all, essentially dependent beings.[14]

The psychological growth of children varies considerably and exact age limits for the ability to decide about personal health issues would not do justice to all children. The Finnish Act on the status and rights of patients,[15] for example, does not specify age limits but states, instead, that 'the opinion of a minor patient on a treatment measure has to be assessed if it is possible with regard to his/her age or level of development'.

When the child grows, his or her role in the decision-making process also grows. This is obvious in long-term relationships, when, for example, a child with diabetes takes more responsibility of his or her own care. Even a small child can participate *somehow* in the process and find it important and meaningful.

Disagreement about necessary investigations or treatment is not uncommon and it may take place between the family and the healthcare personnel or within the family. Often, however, the basic problem is more about communication than about medical matters.

In the case of a seriously ill young child, the situation is clear. According to the tradition in medical ethics and legal practice in Western Europe, parents do not have a right to deny a potentially life-saving treatment to their child. In less severe cases, however, it is thought that the parents in a way represent the future autonomous person the child will one day be.

In case 2, the child is healthy. There is, however, a small but real chance for the development of a life-threatening condition. If he is vaccinated, there is a small but real chance for adverse effect due to the vaccine (although *not* the effect the parents are afraid of).

The ethical challenge in case 2 is to find the acceptable degree of persuasion in this particular family. The decision takes place on a continuum, where the parents and the clinician reach a decision together.[16] One end of the continuum represents classical paternalism where treatment would be provided without discussion. This would be appropriate in life-threatening conditions but not in this case. At the other end of the continuum, the GP would present factual information only and the parents would then decide.

Most cases in real life fall somewhere in the grey area between the extremes. The GP may try to persuade the parents to allow vaccination but voluntariness has to be preserved. Using rational arguments and presenting scientific evidence are compatible with parental autonomy, but it should be remembered that fully neutral communication is not possible. Facts presented to the patient or family are always a subset of all available facts, and the views of the professional are present in the communication act, however neutral he or she tries to be.

Refusal of childhood immunisations is in many cases based on biased information, nowadays often found on the Internet. However, it is thought that very few families use complementary or alternative therapies only. The parents in case 2 seem to trust their GP because they turn to her for advice. This is not surprising because there is evidence that parents, in general, trust doctors more than they trust other sources of health information.[17] Discussing another case concerning refusal of immunisation, paediatrician-ethicist John Lantos suggests that we 'should encourage parents to question our recommendations, just as we encourage students to do, and welcome the opportunity to explain why we recommend the treatments that we recommend'.[16]

CASE 3

Sarah is a 6-year-old girl who presents with fever and sore throat. She is not critically ill or dehydrated and she is cooperative in the beginning. However, she refuses to open her mouth for a throat swab test. The parents try their best and the GP tries her best but nothing helps.

In case 3, the child does not seem to have a serious disease. Again, there is a small but real chance for the development of a life-threatening condition. Without a strep A test, it is not possible to know whether she needs antibiotics or not.

Whatever the experience and communication skills of the GP, sometimes they are not enough. In her vivid essay *Illness Not as Metaphor* paediatrician Perri Klass[18] describes

the demon child from hell … the child, who was already feeling sick, was now emotionally distressed and unwilling to cooperate with the insertion of a cotton swab into the back of her oropharynx. She signified this unwillingness by keeping her teeth absolutely clenched, against all the best efforts of her mother, the intern, and me. And she was successful.[18]

Klass was the senior clinician and she made the final decision to surrender. The point in her essay was elsewhere and she did not discuss the scenario further. This case illustrates, however, a common situation in primary care paediatrics: a GP has to balance the potential gains and harms of two options. One option is to cause significant emotional distress in the child and obtain the test result. The other option is to accept some uncertainty and make a treatment decision without this particular test. The risk–benefit balance is different in each option. In other words, the *best interests* of the child must be considered.

These scenarios are familiar to any physician working with children. Their basic structure is, however, universal in medicine, which is, by definition, an art in which uncertainty is the only certainty. Nowhere in medicine is this truer than in primary care.

REFERENCES

1. Tauber AI. *Patient Autonomy and the Ethics of Responsibility.* Cambridge: MIT Press; 2005.
2. Truog RD, Brown SD, Browning D, et al. Microethics: The ethics of everyday clinical practice. *Hastings Center Report* 2015; 45(1): 11–17.
3. Komesaroff PA. From bioethics to microethics: Ethical debate and clinical medicine. In: Komesaroff PA, editor. *Troubled Bodies: Critical Perspectives on Postmodernism, Medical Ethics, and the Body.* Durham, NC: Duke University Press; 1995. pp. 62–86.
4. Louhiala P. But who can say what's right and wrong? Medicine as a moral enterprise. In: Evans M, Louhiala P, Puustinen R, editors. *Philosophy for Medicine: Applications in a Clinical Context.* Oxford: Radcliffe Medical Press; 2004. pp. 135–41.
5. Lieberthal AS, Carroll AE, Chonmaitree T, et al. The Diagnosis and Management of Acute Otitis Media. *Pediatrics* 2013;131:e964–e999. http://pediatrics.aappublications.org/content/pediatrics/early/2013/02/20/peds.2012-3488.full.pdf [Accessed 29 May 2016].

6. Acute otitis media (online). Current Care Guidelines. Working group set up by the Finnish Medical Society Duodecim. Helsinki: The Finnish Medical Society Duodecim, 2010. Available at: http://www.kaypahoito.fi/web/kh/suositukset/suositus?id=hoi31050 [Accessed 3 July 2017].

7. Glasziou PP, Del Mar CB, Sanders SL, Hayem M. Antibiotics for acute otitis media in children (Cochrane Review). In: *The Cochrane Library*. Issue 2. Oxford: Update Software; 2002.

8. Bertin L, Pons G, díAthis P, et al. A randomized, double-blind, multicentre controlled trial of ibuprofen versus acetaminophen and placebo for symptoms of acute otitis media in children. *Fundam Clin Pharmacol* 1996; 10: 387–92.

9. Goodman J. *Ethics and Evidence-Based Medicine*. Cambridge: Cambridge University Press; 2003.

10. Ridge M. Moral Non-Naturalism. In: Zalta EN, editor. The Stanford Encyclopedia of Philosophy (Fall 2014 Edition). Available at: https://plato.stanford.edu/archives/fall2014/entries/moral-non-naturalism/. [Accessed 3 July 2017].

11. Louhiala P. Deciding on treatment. In: Louhiala P, Heath I, Saunders J, editors. *The Medical Humanities Companion Volume Three: Treatment*. Oxford: Radcliffe; 2014. pp. 47–50.

12. Loewy E. In defense of paternalism. *Theor Med Bioeth* 2005;26: 445–68.

13. Pellegrino E. Physician integrity: Why it is inviolable. *In: Connecting American Values with Health Reform*. Hastings Center; 2009, pp. 18–20. Available at http://www.thehastings-center.org/Publications/Detail.aspx?id=3528 [Accessed 15 December 2015].

14. Nys T, Denier Y, Vandevelde T. Introduction. In: Nys T, Denier Y, Vandevelde T, editors. *Autonomy & Paternalism. Reflections on the Theory and Practice of Health Care*. Leeuven: Peeters; 2007, pp. 1–22.

15. Ministry of Social Affairs and Health, Finland. No. 785/1992. Act on the Status and Rights of Patients (unofficial translation). Available at: http://www.finlex.fi/en/laki/kaan-nokset/1992/en19920785 [Accessed 3 July 2017].

16. Weddle M, Empey A, Crossen E, et al. Are pediatricians complicit in vitamin K deficiency bleeding? *Pediatrics* 2015; 136: 753–57.

17. Freed GL, Clark SJ, Butchart AT, Singer DC, Davis MM. Sources and perceived credibility of vaccine-safety information for parents. *Pediatrics* 2011; 127(Suppl 1): S107–12.

18. Klass P. Illness not as metaphor. *N Engl J Med* 2014; 371: 2057–59.

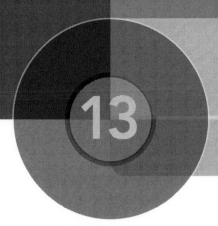

On frailty and ethics: Negotiating narratives

13

DEBORAH BOWMAN

The sixth age shifts
Into the lean and slipper'd pantaloon,
With spectacles on nose and pouch on side,
His youthful hose, well saved, a world too wide
For his shrunk shank; and his big manly voice,
Turning again toward childish treble, pipes
And whistles in his sound. Last scene of all,
That ends this strange eventful history,
Is second childishness and mere oblivion,
Sans teeth, sans eyes, sans taste, sans everything.

(As You Like It, Act 2, Scene 7)

INTRODUCTION

In his speech on the seven ages of man, Jacques offers a narrative of age and diminution that continues to resonate. Its description of an ageing process that is both inevitable and bleak is poignant because we both recognise and fear the account. The shrinking of a human life, both literally and metaphorically, is captured in the term 'frail'. This chapter will explore the ways in which a diagnosis of frailty creates particular ethical questions that are, it is argued, richly elucidated and understood by a narrative approach. It is suggested that there are different types of narratives – societal, cultural, pathographies[1] and individual – each having a role in informing how we think about, and respond to, the concept of frailty.

ON FRAILTY

The British Geriatrics Society describes frailty as 'a distinctive health state related to the ageing process in which multiple body systems gradually lose their in-built reserves'.[2] The predominant narrative of frailty is one of vulnerability, diminution, dependence, deterioration, loss and risk. It is a curiously dualist concept in Western medicine, principally referring to physical weakness and decline. In non-medical contexts, fallibility may be described as indicative of the frailty of human nature, but in relation to health, frailty largely denotes physical decline. This is not an idle observation. The ethical landscape of how we respond to situations is shaped, in the first instance, by the ways in which we conceptualise a problem or a question. What would it mean to your understanding and response to frailty if it were more inclusively described? If it were no longer the preserve of the older person? If it were something that existed without physical representation? The narrative of how we have come to define and understand frailty itself is, of course, integral to our ethical response, yet it is rarely considered or discussed.

The pathographies of the frail are commonly relayed by others: by carers, relatives and health and social care professionals rather than by the individuals experiencing frailty themselves. What it means to be frail is, of course, culturally and socially situated. Narratives about ageing, class, gender, community, connectedness and care all inform the perception and experience of frailty. Within each of those narratives are multiple other stories that twist and turn to render each person's experience unique and significant.

WHY NARRATIVE?

There are, of course, many ways of discerning and considering ethical questions. Narrative is fundamentally an approach that is concerned with ways of knowing. It does not merely acknowledge the value of interpretation and the possibility of multiple meanings, it celebrates that complexity.[3] Moreover, narrative ethics requires attention to the plural voices (and silences) in an account or a situation. It is as concerned with absence as with presence and with the unsaid and with the said.

Narrative may function at multiple levels, allowing us to notice points of commonality and divergence. For example, in considering frailty, a narrative approach will attend not only to the story of the patient but also to those of carers, professionals and policymakers. That is not to suggest that each account is afforded equal weight or influence, but it is to allow for a rich understanding of the ways in which the concept of 'frailty' is created and understood by different parties.

Narrative ethics attends to both the 'telling' and the 'ways of knowing'. It is concerned with both content and form.[4] It has a theoretical foundation[5] but also seeks to foster narrative skills in practitioners to inform work with patients and families. Its premise is the individual and the specific matter in making ethical decisions. It is a counter to the objectivity, reductionism and generalisability of a traditional biomedical approach. It recognises the inherent humanity in healthcare[6] and prioritises relationships.

NARRATIVE AND CASES

Cases and scenarios are common in both medicine and ethics. They offer an authentic way for professionals and students to learn about the application of ethical theory and models in practice. However, narrative ethics offers a challenge to the reliance on, and prevalence of, cases.[7]

Consider, for example, the following case which might be the prompt for discussion of the ethical issues arising in respect of frailty.

Elspeth Mayhew is 86 years old. She is a widow and lives alone in her bungalow. Her daughter, Mary, lives with her family about 2 miles away and visits her mother three times a week. Elspeth also joins Mary's family for Sunday lunch every week. Elspeth's son, John, lives approximately 70 miles away. Elspeth is on a statin, an ace-inhibitor, a diuretic and analgesia for arthritis. She visits her GP, Dr. Mehta, every month. Elseph also has her blood pressure checked regularly by the practice nurse, Lina Rossco.

Mary arrives at Elspeth's bungalow one day to find her mother on the hall floor after a fall. Mary calls an ambulance and Elspeth is taken to A&E where she is found to have a Colles fracture of the wrist. Staff at A&E are concerned about Elspeth who seems a bit disoriented. They also note that she smells of urine and they decide to admit her to a general medical ward. Elspeth does not settle in the ward. She doesn't eat or drink and appears alternately tearful and withdrawn. The ward sister expresses her concerns and asks nursing staff to pay particular attention to Elspeth. Elspeth is visited by a physiotherapist, Marcus, who recommends specific exercises and encourages her to mobilise. Elspeth is polite, but resists telling him 'everything hurts'. The healthcare assistant, Javick, spends most time with Elspeth.

The healthcare team is unsure what to do next. Elspeth does not seem well and Mary is adamant that she should not be discharged. Elspeth says little, but keeps asking when she can go home. John is shocked and alarmed by the change in his mother. He disagrees with Mary about what should happen and suggests to the ward sister that their mother would be much better off in familiar surroundings.

The scenario above is a typical account, capturing the broad biopsychosocial aspects of Elspeth's 'case'. The discussions that might arise from such a description could be rich, but they will necessarily be partial and constrained by both the form and content of the case as presented. Firstly, the act of writing a case is itself a moral and interpretative act.[8] Choices, which are rarely explicit, about language, emphasis, the exclusion or inclusion of information and point of view all inform and shape how an ethical problem is perceived and understood. The author or presenter of such a summary has the power to determine both form and content[9] to inform ethical engagement and analysis. Imagine if the 'case' above were reworked into first person narratives of the *dramatis personae*: Elspeth, Mary, John, Dr. Mehta, Lina, the practice nurse, the unnamed A&E doctor, Javick the healthcare assistant, Marcus, the physiotherapist and the ward staff. The verb 'imagine' is important here; rarely, if ever, will healthcare professionals have the time or scope to explore an individual's narrative in depth, but even limited engagement with unmediated or 'tidied' narratives will yield unique and invaluable insights.

Consider, for example, Elspeth's own story about her fall and the days afterwards.

I love my bungalow. We came here so I didn't have to deal with stairs. I am not as steady as I was – but then I go and do a stupid thing anyway. Stupid. Stupid. I could hear Hugh, in my mind's eye scolding me as I got on that stool to look at the light bulb. 15 years gone, but still with me. It happened in flash. I was lying there like Thora Hird in that piece about the biscuit and the sofa, by – you know – the man – chap with glasses. Northern. I don't know how long I was there. In the hall. I could see the shadows of people outside the glass in the door, but no one was coming my way. I needed the loo and it was cold.

Don't know how long – but Mary eventually came. She does most Tuesdays. Not always – busy lives they all lead. She's got a key and next thing I know, she's fussing over me telling me not to move and to count to ten and all sorts of nonsense she's seen on the TV. It was hurting then and my skirt was rucked up, but I couldn't make myself decent.

I don't remember the drive to the hospital. I spoke to a young doctor but – well, it was just about the arm really. She looked really tired and so young. Not like Dr. Mehta; he's always interested. No matter what, he makes time and he listens, really listens. Mary was on her phone, cancelling plans and telling John to come down. No need. Such a fuss. I was ready to go home after the cast was put on, but they brought me up here. My clothes are in a bag and I am stranded. They keep doing things to me – the cuff on and off – on and off – squeezing, like a vice. When Lina – the nurse who works with Dr. Mehta – takes my blood pressure, she tells me the numbers – the 'scores on the doors', she says – we have a giggle, me and Lina.

Back and forth they come – back and forth – I've been here answering the same questions for days now – new people coming and going – what do they do with the answers? Busy, always busy, I suppose. I asked Javick – he's the assistant who likes music – how can he feel like singing in here. He laughed and starting humming the death march and winked at me. He's the only one whose made me smile in here.

I hate the food – dinner at 5 o'clock – 5 o'clock – and those horrible plastic jugs of squash and water. Like children. All day and night, people are crying and moaning. Those that aren't sleeping round the clock like they're already dead. That young man who wants me to exercise doesn't seem to realise – it is all so painful. They lock us in you know. Locked in. Why? Penned in. Cornered – like the wounded creatures we are, I suppose. I wept when I realised – I can't stop – stop – crying. I just want to – need – to get out of here. My library books are due tomorrow. I can't even read here: too noisy and bright – noise – horrible – all the time. Sorry, I don't usually complain. I just feel so – so well, just – you know – just – sorry.

If we consider content first, the ethical questions and priorities are altered by Elspeth's narrative. The details that matter to her are barely mentioned, if they appear at all, in the 'case study'. We learn of her emotional responses, the priority she affords to dignity, independence, kindness and freedom, her relationships with her family and different members of staff, her perceptions of the care she has received, the significance for her of the sudden shift from independence to dependence and the ways she experiences the monolithic and systemic routines of healthcare. If we were to consider what autonomy and care might mean for Elspeth, we would have a far richer, more nuanced and authentic understanding based on even this short first person account.

When we look at the form of Elspeth's short narrative, we find other significant considerations. Elspeth moves between tenses: past, present and future versions of her life collide in one brief excerpt. She references stories of ageing and vulnerability that she knows, with a sense of fear or at least apprehension. Elspeth's language is broken, altered and incomplete. Sentences trail off. Her words are disrupted. It is not just her wrist that is fractured. Fluency seems to be related to trust: her sentences about Dr. Mehta, Lina and Javick are complete, well crafted and punctuated. The language frequently evokes themes of being trapped, loss and compulsion: for example, the blood pressure cuff is compared with a vice and on discovering the wards are locked, the verbs she uses are 'penned' and 'cornered'. There are comparisons with animals, children and the dead: those without power, freedom and choice. Within the fractured language is a sense of urgent emphasis and bewilderment. It is a narrative that calls for others to attend to a pain that is existential as well as physical.

There is a raw despair in Elspeth's narrative. In a few paragraphs, we are shown the extent of her loss and fear. We do not know what preceded this fall nor do we know, for certain, what will follow. However, the narrative makes it clear that the shockwaves of this fall are far reaching. Whether the fall was a consequence of frailty or leads Elspeth to be described in future as 'frail' may be clinically necessary, but it is not ethically sufficient. To care ethically for Elspeth means engaging with the depth of her loss and what it means for her. Narrative is uniquely suited to the task.

Of course, it is not just Elspeth who has a narrative to share about this incident. Space precludes it, but it would be fascinating to hear, or imagine, the accounts of each of the people named in the vignette. All of those involved, including perhaps some, such as Javick who might not routinely be part of clinical team meetings and care decisions, will have a unique perspective and together they are charged, by working with Elspeth, with finding meaning[10] in this complex situation to negotiate a coherent and supportive response. What might a multidisciplinary team meeting that adopted a narrative approach and used narrative skills yield in terms of rich meaning-making? How might it differ if staff were invited to share their first-person accounts of looking after Elspeth and in explicitly considering how they interpret what it means to 'care' for her?

NARRATIVE SKILLS AND QUESTIONS

There are many ways in which narrative can inform and enhance ethical practice. Whatever the situation, the questions in the box below will provide useful narrative prompts.

- Who is the author?
- From what point of view is the story told?
- What is the difference between an author and a writer or a narrator?
- What role do the characters or people play?
- Who is absent from the account or story?
- What is the language like and how does it influence reading of the story?
- Are metaphors and imagery used in the account?
- What possible meanings and interpretations are there for the text as presented?
- When and how does the plot develop?
- Which 'characters' or people are active and which are silent?
- What is included and what is omitted
- Who is the audience or reader?
- What are the themes, archetypes and subtext of an account?
- What are the relational and communication dimensions of this ethical question or 'problem'?

STORIES OF FRAILTY

It is not only the individual patient or client whose narrative matters. Diseases, groups of people and professions all have their own narratives in which recurrent themes and unarticulated values shape how a condition, patient or professional is understood and interpreted. What then are the themes that imbue the concept of 'frailty' and how might these inform our responses to the 'frail'?

The principal concepts that underpin Western concepts of frailty are, it is suggested, risk, uncertainty, vulnerability, dependency and, perhaps most difficult of all, inevitability. These conceptual cornerstones are difficult for patients, families and professionals alike.[11] There is not much to comfort in a narrative that is preoccupied with increasing risk, heightened vulnerability, unchosen dependency, confusing complexity and unknowable uncertainty. The close association of frailty to age raises further difficult questions. Narratives of ageing and being an older person are too often predicated on incapacity, increasing problems and unavoidable decline.[12] Within those narratives are woven further influential stories,[13] such as those of class, gender[14] and status.

Of course, these themes recur and dominate because they reflect, to some extent, the lived realities of frailty: its unpredictable quality, the loss of independence and the spectre of an uncertain, but probably, deterioration. Healthcare students are, rightly, taught about the risks of frailty and the importance of recognising and responding to it. However, in recognising frailty, one may also be unquestioningly accepting a narrative that obscures, reduces and hinders an ethical response. For if the narrative of frailty implies marginalisation, weakness and deterioration, what might the implications be for agency and choice?[15] If effective 'management' of risk becomes the priority, what is left of imaginative and responsive person-centred care? Indeed, what a challenge it is to find the person amongst the dominant discourse of loss, decline and risk. A narrative response to frailty then must attend not only to the accounts of the individuals involved but also to the narrative of the condition itself.

NARRATIVE AND FRAILTY: CLOSING THOUGHTS

If frailty is an altered state in which agency and identity are at risk, an ethical response that attends to meaning, an individual's sense of self and relational priorities is required. Narrative not only allows for, but also demands, that the subjective, the qualitative and the individual are afforded as much moral weight as the objective, the measurable and the generalisable. To attend to ethics is to attend both to ways of knowing and to ways of being.

Each situation or experience of frailty is unique and cannot be fully captured by universal laws or principles. The clinical encounter is but a small part of someone's story. As such, the transition to 'frailty' arises in the context of a 'life story' and without attention to the same, moral analysis will be partial and inadequate. Much of ethics is concerned with 'problems' and arguing a 'position',[16] but in situations of frailty and long-term relationships, the aim of ethical analysis may not be to 'solve' the problem, but to open up dialogue, share norms and values and to explore tensions between perceptions.

All those who are involved in illness and ethical decision-making contribute to making meaning and interpreting that experience. Narrative ethics provides a framework within which to demonstrate the courage, imagination and wisdom to navigate, both with patients and other professionals, diverse perspectives, contested meanings and multiple interpretations. It is a means by which priorities, and therefore, care can be flexibly negotiated, extending the boundaries of relationships beyond the 'management' of risk to recognise the inherent humanity in health encounters. Moral vision is broadened, understanding deepened and relationships strengthened: what better ballast might there be against both the rhetoric and realities of frailty?

REFERENCES

1. Frank, A. W. *The Wounded Storyteller: Body, Illness and Ethics.* Chicago, IL: The University of Chicago Press, 1995.
2. *Fit for Frailty: Consensus Best Practice Guidance for the Care of Older People Living with Frailty in Community and Outpatient Settings.* British Geriatrics Society, June 2014. http://www.bgs.org.uk/campaigns/fff/fff_full.pdf (accessed 2 March 2016).
3. Charon, R., Montello, M. *Stories Matter: The Role of Narrative in Bioethics.* New York: Routledge USA, 2002.
4. Hudson, A. Narrative in medical ethics. *BMJ* 1999; 318: 253.
5. Lindemann Nelson, H (Ed.). *Stories and Their Limits: Narrative Approaches to Bioethics.* New York: Routledge USA, 1998.
6. Brody, H. *Stories of Sickness.* (2nd Ed.) Oxford: Oxford University Press, 2003.
7. Hurwitz, B. Textual practices in crafting bioethics cases. *Journal of Bioethical Inquiry* 2012; 4(9): 395–401.
8. Hurwitz, B. Form and representation in clinical case reports. *Literature and Medicine* 2006; 25: 216–240.
9. Chambers, T.S. The bioethicist as author: The medical ethics case as a rhetorical device. *Literature and Medicine* 1994; 13(1): 60–78.
10. Brody, H. 'My Story is Broken; Can You Help Me Fix It?': Medical ethics and the joint construction of narrative. *Literature and Medicine* 1994; 31(1): 79–92.
11. Chapman, S. Theorizing about aging well: Constructing a narrative. *Canadian Journal on Aging* 2005; 24(1): 9–18.
12. Feldman, S. Please don't call me dear: Older women's narratives of health care. *Nursing Inquiry* 1999; 6(4): 269–276.
13. Kaufman, S. The social construction of frailty: An anthropological perspective. *Journal of Aging Studies* 1994; 8(1): 45–58.
14. Grenier, A., Hanley, J. Older women and 'frailty': Aged, gendered and embodied resistance. *Current Sociology* 2007; 55(2): 211–228.
15. Gilleard, C., Higgs, P. Frailty, disability and old age: A reappraisal. *Health* 2011; 15(5): 475–490.
16. Bowman, D. What is it to do good medical ethics? Minding the gap(s). *Journal of Medical Ethics* 2015; 41(1): 60–63.

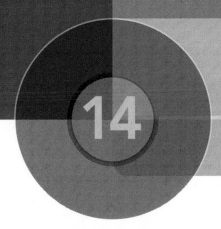

Achieving a good death in primary care: Ethical challenges at the end of life

BENEDICT HAYHOE

14

INTRODUCTION

Providing treatment and care towards the end of life will often involve decisions that are clinically complex and emotionally distressing; and some decisions may involve ethical dilemmas and uncertainties about the law that further complicate the decision making process.

General Medical Council, UK, 2010

Approximately 500,000 deaths occur each year in England, a number predicted to rise by 17% from 2012 to 2030.[1] Most of these people will be likely to have significant contact with primary healthcare, and with numbers of those dying at home approaching 50%,[2] primary care professionals may reasonably anticipate a growing need for their involvement in the care of people at the end of life. end of life care is therefore an increasingly important aspect of primary care, and one acknowledged to be complex, not only clinically but also emotionally, ethically and legally.[3] Nevertheless, still representing a relatively small proportion of overall workload, end of life care may be an area for which many primary care professionals feel ill prepared, particularly in relation to the ethical problems it may entail.[4]

This chapter will provide an overview of some major ethical challenges faced by professionals in this area of healthcare, starting with a brief consideration of what may constitute a 'good death', before discussing key issues such as autonomy, analgesia, life-sustaining treatments and advance care planning (ACP). Viewed largely from the perspective of the UK general practitioner, concepts discussed will also be relevant to other primary care disciplines including nursing, pharmacy and counselling.

GMC guidance[3] refers to patients as 'approaching the end of life', when they are considered likely to die in the next 12 months, and includes not only those whose death is imminent and those with significant life-threatening conditions, but also premature neonates whose prospect of survival is very poor, and patients diagnosed with persistent vegetative state (PVS) for whom a decision to withdraw treatment may lead to death.

Primary care physicians' exposure to the undoubtedly ethically challenging situations of care of premature neonates and patients in PVS is considered likely to be minimal and as such outside the scope of this chapter, which will focus on end of life care of adult patients in the primary care setting. Nevertheless, primary care professionals may find themselves in situations where they need to discuss these difficult cases with families or carers, and it is hoped that the following pages may provide some general principles that are transferrable. In addition, various sources of further information and guidance are available, which readers may find useful.[3,5]

A GOOD END TO LIFE

Palliative care is an approach that improves the quality of life of patients (adults and children) and their families who are facing problems associated with life-threatening illness. It prevents and relieves suffering through the early identification, correct assessment and treatment of pain and other problems, whether physical, psychosocial or spiritual.

WHO, 2015.[6]

Euthanasia, in the uncontroversial sense of a 'gentle and easy death',[7] must be the hope of all patients and the aim of all end of life care services. Philosophical debate has existed for centuries regarding the essential components of such a death,[8] and some acknowledgement of this may be helpful in considering ethical aspects of end of life care.

Whilst various theories on what might constitute a 'good death' exist, it has been argued[9] that 'hedonism', the ethical theory that pleasure should be sought and pain avoided, might be consistent with accepted approaches to palliative care; negative hedonism would require the absence of adverse symptoms such as pain, depression and anxiety, while positive hedonism, as does Christian teaching, focuses on personal growth, awareness, preparedness and acceptance.

Empirical evidence supports hedonism,[1] with factors identified as most important to people at the end of life including having pain and other symptoms effectively managed, being surrounded by loved ones and being treated with dignity. Similarly, consistent with a 'Four principles' perspective, in seeking to do that which is good for patients and avoid harm (beneficence and non-maleficence),[10] good end of life care will consequently aim to address both these areas, providing effective, evidence-based, scientific treatment of medical symptoms, in a holistic approach encompassing careful consideration of emotional and spiritual needs.

Indeed, overall context and holistic care are especially important; end of life cannot be considered in isolation from the rest of life,[9] or indeed from the rest of society, so consideration must be given to patients' previous and current situation in establishing plans and goals for care. Furthermore, simply targeting and conforming to 'objective goods', such as pain control and presence of family, do not automatically result in 'good' subjective experiences for patients;[11] a checklist approach will not guarantee a 'good death'.

Whilst being treated with dignity does not necessarily equate with respect for autonomy, evidence suggests that some degree of control over the circumstances of end of life care is desirable for patients,[12] so respect for autonomy will clearly be an important consideration.

SELF-DETERMINATION AT THE END OF LIFE

Autonomy can be understood as the ability of individuals to exercise self-determination or free will in making decisions. Arising from utilitarian philosophy[13], a right to self-determination in relation to medical treatment has become widely established in law[14,15] and now underpins a number of essential aspects of medical practice, such as confidentiality, consent and capacity, arguably of particular importance in end of life care.

Respect for individual autonomy will also be consistent with deontological (duty-based) ethical approaches, and is a key concept in duty-based professional ethical guidelines such as those provided by the UK General Medical Council.

In the context of end of life care, this leads to a central aim to support patients' autonomy in achieving their own 'good death', offering them, and enabling them to make, choices that make this possible. This aim provides a basis for requirements to respect patients' decision-making capacity, offer them choice in aspects of care and treatment in such a way that they are able to make informed decisions to consent to or refuse them, support them in planning for future care, and be open and honest in disclosing information, whilst keeping their information confidential from others.

However, situations may occur where, for example, patients, families and medical professionals disagree about the best course of action, patients' wishes cannot be supported, or patients lack the capacity to make decisions for themselves, leading to criticism of the value given to autonomy in contemporary ethical medical practice.

In the case of patients who lack capacity, it has been suggested that autonomy fails to provide an appropriate understanding of their experience of life and illness[16], such that reference to autonomy in relation to these patients is 'highly incongruous'[17]. Even where patients have the ability to make their own decisions, too great a focus on autonomy may not be helpful, with conflict between patients' views that 'doctor knows best' and professionals' strong belief in patients' autonomy leading to patients being left to fend for themselves in making decisions, 'abandoned to their own autonomy'[18] by 'inverse paternalism'[19].

For some, therefore, focus on self-determination may arguably offer a temptation to professionals to transfer responsibility for complex and difficult treatment decisions back to patients[20]. Others criticise the importance given to autonomy in the area of end of life care more generally, suggesting that it fails to guide respect for individuals effectively.[21,22]

These arguments support a less rigid, more 'Communitarian' approach to respect for autonomy in end of life care, 'respect for persons'[23], where emphasis is given to the broader context of the individual, encompassing concepts such as dignity and individuality, and including consideration of his or her social situation, relationship with family and carers and emotional and spiritual background.

Perhaps, this may recall an idealised view of the UK GP, known to patient and family over years and available to provide holistic support as well as medical care. While this may no longer be a common reality of primary care, this kind of approach to patients at the end of life would seem an appropriate aim and one which is achievable using a team-based model of care.

ANALGESIA, SEDATION AND THE DOCTRINE OF DOUBLE EFFECT

When caring for patients in end of life situations, it will frequently be necessary for primary healthcare professionals to address troublesome symptoms such as pain, agitation, shortness of breath and excessive respiratory secretions, and indeed, notwithstanding the importance of the holistic approach discussed above, practical management of symptoms at the end of life will often be a major part of the primary care clinician's role.

Clearly, ethical arguments support the need to control these symptoms in order to facilitate experience of a 'good death'. However, provision of treatment to deal with such symptoms has been complicated by concerns about the possibility of adverse effects, particularly the potential for shortening of life.[24]

A concept identified particularly with Catholic theology, but widely referred to in medical ethical practice, the doctrine of double effect distinguishes between actions with intended consequences, and those with consequences that are merely foreseen. Used particularly in justifying not only use of opioids in potentially fatal doses but also in the use of sedation at the end of life,[25] the doctrine was introduced into English law in the case of *R v Adams*,[26] which established that a doctor is 'entitled to do all that is proper and necessary to relieve pain and suffering, even if the measures he takes may incidentally shorten life'.

Despite subsequent judicial approval[27] and wide official acceptance of the doctrine,[28,29] it has been criticised for a number of reasons. Firstly, it is very difficult to distinguish between foresight and intention. Furthermore, for some, this does not matter. Consequentialists argue that consequences determine the moral nature of acts, so any 'killing' is the same, regardless of intention. In a similar way, the doctrine is inconsistent with English law on murder which considers the foresight of virtually certain consequences to amount to intention.[30,31]

However, notwithstanding considerable ongoing debate about the place of the doctrine in English law,[25] dealing with severe pain and distress at the end of life remains a familiar situation in primary care and a practical solution to management is necessary. A sensitive approach may avoid the suggestion that the doctrine of double effect is being used to allow euthanasia, whilst enabling adequate symptom control: careful dosing, following accepted guidelines on escalation until pain is controlled, with clear reference to clinical effect.[9] In fact, it is now recognised that the risk of death as a result of opiate analgesic use is generally only through inappropriate use; where prescribed correctly, there may in fact be no 'double effect' in this situation.[24]

The use of sedation in end of life care has been the subject of even greater controversy, with concern about its distinction from euthanasia as well as a view, likely derived from Christian philosophy, that awareness may be an important element of end of life, allowing individuals to experience death for the purpose of personal growth and reconciliation.[9] A consequence of this has been an impact on treatments in general; it is often considered that patient awareness is key factor in deciding on medications used in end of life care.

While use of 'terminal sedation', or drugs for the purpose of sedation only, would not usually be familiar in end of life care in the primary care context, the use of opiate analgesics and other medications to relieve pain and distress, which may also cause sedation, is commonplace. For some patients, it will be personally important to experience life fully and to its natural end, but for others not doing so may be of positive benefit.[9] As we have seen, controlling pain and suffering is consistent with hedonistic theory as well as duty-based ethical medical practice; avoiding awareness of these symptoms through sedation may be equally valuable.

Open discussion with patients, and judicious prescription, in conformity with accepted practice would seem to be essential here, both legally and in terms of a pragmatic ethical approach.

WITHHOLDING AND WITHDRAWING MEDICAL TREATMENT

In primary care, withholding and withdrawal of life-prolonging medical treatments are most likely to refer to situations such as withdrawal of routine medications, food and fluids, withholding of antibiotics, and decisions not to refer to hospital, call ambulances or perform cardiopulmonary resuscitation.

Conventional medical practice requires a presumption, based on ethical, legal and human rights principles, in favour of prolongation of life wherever possible.[3] However, situations where for reasons including patient choice, effectiveness and burdensomeness of treatment, it is considered acceptable to withhold potentially life-sustaining treatment, or withdraw it once started.

Justifying what appears to contravene the accepted principle of preservation of life, it is argued that withdrawal of life-prolonging treatments that no longer confer benefit is followed by death that is incidental. In the English courts, this has been defended on the basis of a distinction between 'acts' and 'omissions',[27] as well as by reliance on the doctrine of double effect; this accords with Christian philosophy that, while all life has intrinsic worth and dignity, it is not an absolute good to be maintained at all costs.[32]

A complex area of ethical and legal debate, with strong criticism of both the legal situation[27] and professional guidance,[33] the concept of withdrawal or withholding of treatments remains contentious, and most especially if any suggestion exists that this may be less to do with patients' 'best interests' and more with healthcare resources. In the UK this was demonstrated by the recent controversy surrounding the 'Liverpool Care Pathway', a checklist approach designed to facilitate end of life decisions, including the withdrawal of active treatment where appropriate.[34] Great public concern arose from a suspicion that there might be a connection between decisions to withdraw or withhold treatments for patients at the end of life and financial incentives for hospitals to place patients on a pathway of care which might result both in earlier death and cost-saving for healthcare services.

Nevertheless, it seems clear that circumstances do exist where, 'the principle of the sanctity of human life must yield to the principle of self-determination',[27] or, in the case of patients who lack capacity, burdensomeness or futility of treatment makes it no longer ethically desirable to start or continue. An interesting example of a situation of this kind, likely to become a more common occurrence in primary care, is deactivation of implantable cardioverter defibrillator (ICD) devices.[35] Repeated defibrillation at the end of life can cause physical discomfort and emotional distress to the patient, as well as emotional distress to families. While it is argued[36] that there is an acceptance on implanting these devices for a balance between discomfort caused by shocks from the defibrillator and the benefit in prevention of sudden death, changes in the clinical situation may result in significant changes in this balance, such that it represents a trade-off that is no longer acceptable to the patient.

Consequently, the continuing benefit of ICDs in the context of other life-threatening conditions needs to be reviewed and discussed with patients to establish their wishes and ensure understanding; insufficient knowledge amongst ICD recipients may result in stressful and painful end of life situations.[36,37]

This has parallels with decisions not to carry out cardiopulmonary resuscitation, where significant misunderstanding amongst public and professionals of the success rates of community CPR and consequently the futility of its use in many situations leads to unrealistic expectations which have a profound effect on decision-making.

MAKING DECISIONS IN ADVANCE

A process of discussion with patients aiming to establish healthcare preferences in case of future mental incapacity[38] ACP is now established in statute in the UK's *Mental Capacity Act 2005*. Outcomes of such discussions may include advance statements of wishes, advance decisions to refuse treatment, and appointment of lasting powers of attorney. Increasingly promoted in primary care, guidance recommends that ACP should be offered routinely to patients in this setting,[39] especially to those at the end of life.[3]

However, although most GPs have conversations with their patients about end of life care wishes, 25% still say they have never initiated such a discussion,[40] and knowledge and understanding of the process of ACP, as well as experience of its use, may be limited.[41]

While ACP has clear ethical value in terms of respect for persons and particularly for autonomy, and consequently a strong argument can be made for its greater use in end of life care as well as more generally, a number of important criticisms and ethical concerns have been raised.

Perhaps most centrally, ACP has been criticised in terms of its assumption that individuals are able accurately to predict their wishes for future,[42] with evidence suggesting substantial instability in individuals' choices over time[43] and some questioning whether we in fact have the durable identity or 'personhood' relied on by the concept.[44]

A concept centred on respect for autonomy may not be universally applicable culturally, with evidence of a variety of culturally specific beliefs about ACP.[45] Similarly, religious values may have significant influence on people's use of ACP,[46] defining their views on decision-making at the end of life.

Given the substantial decision-making powers afforded to those appointed with the power of attorney, coercion, particularly where financial issues may be involved, is a significant concern in ACP, with family dynamics often difficult for healthcare professionals to judge.[47] At the same time, there must be an awareness of the motivations of professionals and healthcare systems in promoting ACP, with the suggestion that ACP may be used as a means to reduce healthcare costs, which is of particular concern.[48]

Cardiopulmonary resuscitation is commonly discussed as part of ACP, and refusal of this intervention can be made in the form of an advance decision to refuse treatment. Where a clinical decision, as distinct from one as part of an ACP discussion, is made that cardiopulmonary resuscitation should not be attempted, the courts have recently made it clear that it is essential that this should be discussed with the patient, or with the patient's relatives if he lacks capacity, unless there exist strong reasons not to do so.[49,50]

ASSISTED SUICIDE

Suicide in the face of terminal illness may, in giving control over timing and manner of death, and avoiding pain and suffering, seem to meet some requirements of a 'good death',[9] although it would likely fail to allow opportunity for positive experience of continued awareness and personal growth. Nevertheless, apart from contravening a societal acceptance of sanctity of life, and a general moral intuition that 'killing' is wrong, recent parliamentary debate on assisted dying[51] has confirmed what has been indicated in a number of court cases,[52,53] that English law will not support assisted suicide and that there exists no 'right to death' commensurate with the recognised 'right to life'.

However, situations are likely to continue to arise where patients with terminal illness express the wish to end their lives. Where they seek advice on this and related issues, including consideration of the possibility of travelling abroad to facilitate assisted suicide, patients may see their GP as the most obvious professional to approach. With the possibility of a real risk, greater for health professionals where there exists a duty of care, of prosecution in the UK,[54] primary care clinicians will need to exercise caution in avoiding anything that might be interpreted as facilitating suicide.[55] Such patients will clearly be deserving of respect and compassion, and nothing would suggest that doctors should not engage in discussion with them. Indeed, some attempt, if not to dissuade them, at least to clarify misunderstandings where their decision may be based, for example, on false assumptions about the course of illness or expected experience of end of life may be considered the duty of the caring clinician. Emphasis on palliative care will also be key, with palliative care services ideally placed to respond to the symptoms, concerns and fears of patients at the end of life.

RESOURCES AND RATIONING

It has long been recognised that any ethical system of care must have an acknowledgement of distributive justice, giving a means to balance the rights of individuals and respect for their autonomous wishes with the needs of other individuals and of society as a whole. This will be true in end of life care as in any other area of medicine, and indeed may be a particular issue here; the gap between diagnosis with life-threatening illness and receiving palliative care, for example, is often considerable.[40]

Emphasis is placed in palliative care practice on choice, with use of advance decision-making to respect patients' autonomous wishes. However, in reality, the opportunity for patients to exercise autonomy in this way in current healthcare environments may be severely limited by resource constraints, with evidence, for example, that cost and supply are frequently a key determinant of place of death rather than choice.[56]

Given increasing involvement of GPs in decision-making regarding resource allocation, some may be in the difficult position of having responsibility for care of patients at the end of life, whilst at the same time rationing a limited budget.[57] A difficult balance will need to be struck between care of patients at end of life, in accordance with their conception of a 'good death', and availability of resources and consequent impact on and justice to others.

Nevertheless, with openness and planning with patients, this process may become easier; allowing patients the opportunity to avoid burdensome, futile and unwelcome interventions at the end of life may result in decisions which both support their conception of a 'good death' and incidentally save costs for healthcare services.

CONCLUSION

A complex area of clinical practice, end of life care requires primary care professionals to give great consideration to ethical issues, making sensitive balances involving the wishes and needs of patients on a background of a sometimes less than clearly defined legal framework and inadequate resources.

Whilst following accepted clinical guidelines and working within legal boundaries, the key to the ethical care of patients in the end of life situation will be a holistic approach. Here, emphasis will be on the social 'context' of the individual, giving greater consideration to relationships with family, carers and with wider society, with early discussion and future planning, and openness and honesty about realistic goals and outcomes of care.

With its unrivalled opportunities for follow-up and development of a caring relationship over time, primary care is arguably an ideal environment to approach end of life care in this way, with the aim of achieving close alignment with patients' wishes for a 'good death'.

REFERENCES

1. NHS England. Actions for end of life care 2014–16 [Internet]. 2014 [cited 2016 June 19]. Available from: https://www.england.nhs.uk/wp-content/uploads/2014/11/actions-eolc.pdf

2. National End of Life Care Network. Data sources: Place of death [Internet]. [cited 2016 June 17]. Available from: http://www.endoflifecare-intelligence.org.uk/data_sources/place_of_death

3. General Medical Council. *Treatment and care towards the end of life: Good practice in decision making.* London: GMC; 2010.

4. Addicott R. The Kings Fund: End of life care [Internet]. 2010 [cited 2016 June 17]. Available from: http://ejournal.narotama.ac.id/files/End%20of%20LIfe%20Care.pdf

5. British Medical Association. *Withholding and withdrawing life-prolonging medical treatment: Guidance for decision making.* 3rd ed. London: BMA; 2007.

6. World Health Organization. Palliative care: Factsheet No. 402 [Internet]. 2015 [cited 2016 June 19]. Available from: http://www.who.int/mediacentre/factsheets/fs402/en/

7. 'Euthanasia, n' [Internet]. OED online. 2015 [cited 2016 June 19]. Available from: http://www.oed.com/view/Entry/65140

8. Mendelson D. Roman concept of mental capacity to make end of life decisions. *Int J Law Psychiatry.* 2007;30(3):201–12.

9. Woods S. *Death's dominion: Ethics at the end of life.* London: Open University Press; 2006.

10. Beauchamp T, Childress J. *Principles of biomedical ethics.* 6th ed. Oxford: Oxford University Press; 2008.

11. Dworkin R. Liberal community. *Calif Law Rev.* 1989;77(3):479–504.

12. Martin D, Thiel E, Singer P. A new model of advance care planning: Observations from people with HIV. *Arch Intern Med.* 1999;159(1):86–92.

13. Mill J. *On liberty, utilitarianism and other essays.* Oxford: Oxford University Press; 2015.

14. *Schloendorff v Society of New York Hospital* [1914] 211 N.Y. 125, 105 N.E. 92.

15. *Sidaway v Board of Governors of the Bethlem Royal Hospital* [1985] 1 All ER 643, HL.

16. Dresser R. Missing persons: Legal perceptions of incompetent patients. *Rutgers Law Rev.* 1994;46(2):609–719.

17. Gormally L. *The dependent elderly: Autonomy, justice and quality of care.* Cambridge: Cambridge University Press; 1992.

18. Kessel A, Meran J. Advance directives in the UK: Legal, ethical, and practical considerations for doctors. *Br J Gen Pract.* 1998;48(430):1263–6.

19. Malpass A, Kessler D, Sharp D, Shaw A. 'I didn't want her to panic': Unvoiced patient agendas in primary care consultations when consulting about antidepressants. *Br J Gen Pract.* 2011;61(583):63–71.

20. Hilden H-M. End of life decisions: Attitudes of Finnish physicians. *J Med Ethics.* 2004;30(4):362–5.

21. Burt R. The end of autonomy. *Hastings Cent Rep.* 2005;35(6):S9–13.

22. Sullivan M. The illusion of patient choice in end of life decisions. *Am J Geriatr Psychiatry.* 2002;10(4):365–72.

23. Torke A, Alexander G, Lantos J. Substituted judgment: The limitations of autonomy in surrogate decision making. *J Gen Intern Med.* 2008;23(9):1514–17.

24. Notcutt W, Gibbs G. Inadequate pain management: Myth, stigma and professional fear. *Postgrad Med J.* 2010;86:453–8.

25. Huxtable R. Get out of jail free? The doctrine of double effect in English law. *Palliat Med.* 2004;18(1):62–8.

26. *R v Adams* [1957] Crim LR 365.

27. *Airedale NHS Trust v Bland* [1993] 1 All ER 821, HL.

28. House of Lords Select Committee on Medical Ethics. *Report of the select committee on medical ethics.* HL Paper 21-I of 1993–4. London: HMSO.

29. New York State Task Force on Life and the Law. *When death is sought: Assisted suicide and euthanasia in the medical context.* New York: NYSTF; 1994.

30. *R v Woolin* [1999] AC 82.

31. Williams G. *Intention and causation in medical non-killing: The impact of criminal law concepts on euthanasia and assisted suicide.* Abingdon: Routledge-Cavendish; 2007.

32. Clarfield A, Gordon M, Markwell H, Alibhai S. Ethical issues in end of life geriatric care: The approach of three monotheistic religions – Judaism, Catholicism, and Islam. *J Am Geriatr Soc.* 2003;51(8):1149–54.

33. Keown J. *Euthanasia, ethics and public policy: An argument against legislation.* Cambridge: Cambridge University Press; 2002.

34. Neuberger J. More care, less pathway: A review of the Liverpool Care Pathway [Internet]. 2013 [cited 2016 Jun 19]. Available from: https://www.gov.uk/government/uploads/system/uploads/attachment_data/file/212450/Liverpool_Care_Pathway.pdf

35. Beattie J. ICD deactivation at the end of life: Principles and practice [Internet]. British Heart Foundation; 2013 [cited 2016 Jun 17]. Available from: https://bhfweb.preceden-thost.com/~/media/files/publications/hcps/icd-deactivation.pdf

36. Strömberg A, Fluur C, Miller J, Chung M, Moser D, Thylén I. ICD recipients' understanding of ethical issues, ICD function, and practical consequences of withdrawing the ICD in the end of life. *Pacing Clin Electrophysiol.* 2014;37(7):834–42.

37. Groarke J, Beirne A, Buckley U, O'Dwyer E, Sugrue D, Keelan T, et al. Deficiencies in patients' comprehension of implantable cardioverter defibrillator therapy: ICD patient comprehension paper. *Pacing Clin Electrophysiol.* 2012;35(9):1097–102.

38. Hayhoe B, Howe A. Advance care planning under the Mental Capacity Act 2005 in primary care. *Br J Gen Pract.* 2011;61(589):e537–41.

39. Royal College of Physicians of London. *Advance care planning: National guidelines.* London: RCP; 2009.

40. Public Health England. National End of Life Care Intelligence Network: What we know now [Internet]. 2015 [cited 2016 Jun 19]. Available from: http://www.endoflifecare-intelligence.org.uk/view?rid=872

41. Hayhoe B. Advance care planning in primary care in the East of England: A qualitative study [MD Thesis]. University of East Anglia; 2013 [cited 2016 Jun 19]. Available from: https://ueaeprints.uea.ac.uk/48803/1/2013HayhoeBWJMD.pdf

42. Fagerlin A, Schneider C. Enough: The failure of the living will. *Hastings Cent Rep.* 2004;34(2):30–42.

43. Christensen-Szalanski J. Discount functions and the measurement of patients' values. Women's decisions during childbirth. *Int J Soc Med Decis Mak.* 1984;4(1):47–58.

44. Dresser R. Bound to treatment: The Ulysses contract. *Hastings Cent Rep.* 1984;14(3):13–16.

45. Perkins HS, Geppert CMA, Gonzales A, Cortez JD, Hazuda HP. Cross-cultural similarities and differences in attitudes about advance care planning. *J Gen Intern Med.* 2002;17(1):48–57.

46. Johnson K, Elbert-Avila K, Tulsky J. The influence of spiritual beliefs and practices on the treatment preferences of African Americans: A review of the literature. *J Am Geriatr Soc.* 2005;53(4):711–19.

47. Schiff R. Living wills and the Mental Capacity Act: A postal questionnaire survey of UK geriatricians. *Age Ageing.* 2006;35(2):116–21.

48. Hayhoe B, Howe A. Advance care planning: An unsuitable subject for QOF? *Br J Gen Pract J R Coll Gen Pract.* 2014;64(629):649–50.

49. *Winspear v City Hospitals Sunderland NHS Foundation Trust* [2015] MHLO 104.

50. *R (Tracey) v Cambridge NHS Foundation Trust and Ors* [2014] EWCA Civ 822.

51. HC Deb 11 Sep 2015, column 656 [Internet]. 2015 [cited 2016 Jun 19]. Available from: http://www.publications.parliament.uk/pa/cm201516/cmhansrd/cm150911/debt-ext/150911-0001.htm#15091126000003

52. *R (on the application of Pretty) v Director of Public Prosecutions* [2001] UKHL 61.

53. *Ms B v an NHS Hospital Trust* [2002] EWHC 429 (Fam).

54. Crown Prosecution Service. Policy for prosecutors in respect of cases of encouraging or assisting suicide [Internet]. 2010 [cited 2016 Jun 19]. Available from: https://www.cps.gov.uk/publications/prosecution/assisted_suicide_policy.pdf

55. British Medical Association. Responding to patient requests relating to assisted suicide: Guidance for doctor in England, Wales and Northern Ireland [Internet]. 2015 [cited 2016 Jun 19]. Available from: https://www.bma.org.uk/-/media/files/pdfs/practical%20 advice%20at%20work/ethics/20150153%20bma%20guidance%20on%20assisted%20 suicide%20update%202015.pdf?la=en

56. Meier D, Morrison S. Autonomy reconsidered. *N Engl J Med* [Internet]. 2002 [cited 2016 Jun 19];346(14). Available from: http://www.hadassah-med.com/media/2003242/07Auton omyreconsidered.pdf

57. Sheehan M. It's unethical for general practitioners to be commissioners. *BMJ.* 2011;342:d1430.

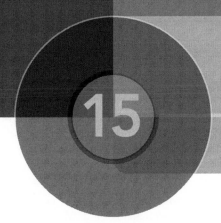

The ethics and challenges in caring for vulnerable migrants in primary care

PAQUITA DE ZULUETA

INTRODUCTION

Migration, and forced migration in particular, caused by war, violence or the threat of starvation and extreme poverty is one of the defining humanitarian and political issues of the day. The mass exodus from war-torn Syria and other countries has led to the highest level of refugees and displaced people since World War II; by 2015, 65.3 million people displaced worldwide, with 12.4 million newly displaced. Over 3700 of the million crossing the Mediterranean to Europe died at sea.[1] However, the staggering numbers tend to conceal from view the tragic loss of life and the human suffering endured by individuals. Compassion, in this context, fades or collapses.[2] Metaphors can and do shape our moral perceptions and predispositions.[3] Words such as 'swarm', 'flood', 'tsunami', 'swamp' and even 'cockroaches' convey the idea of a malignant force that will overwhelm and engulf Western countries, inevitably leading to fear, anger and defensiveness. The threat and reality of terrorism in Europe exacerbates this fear. The asylum seeker becomes the Other, 'not like us', an inferior or dangerous alien, and our sense of connection and common humanity is blunted or attenuated.[4] Even the term 'migrant' has a pejorative ring, and 'illegals' even more so. Not all healthcare professionals are impervious to these emotionally charged political currents that threaten to distort ethical perceptions and therapeutic relationships.

ATTITUDES TO MIGRANTS AND THE RISK OF DEHUMANISATION

There has been a progressive and inexorable hardening of attitudes towards those seeking asylum in the UK as in the rest of Europe. Since 1985, the UK government has introduced a range of measures to prevent or deter new arrivals. Consistently, negative media and harsh political depiction of refugees and asylum seekers fuel public hostility, indirectly leading to further 'massive loss of life'.[5] However, even if there is a human tendency for 'othering', we can move from 'I-it' to 'I-Thou', as advocated by the philosopher Martin Buber.[6] The capacity for expanded compassion can be cultivated by developing our self-awareness and moral imagination, and is highly relevant to how healthcare professionals view and behave towards vulnerable migrants. The sociologist-philosopher Zygmond Bauman, referring to Levinas, proposes that the stance towards asylum seekers as 'security problems' leads to the erasure of 'face' – a metaphoric name for those aspects of the Other that place us in a condition of ethical responsibility and that guide us to ethical action.[7] By erasing the face, we dehumanise individuals, ceasing to consider them as fellow human beings worthy of our care. Individual stories or images often have more power in conveying the horror and suffering of the plight of others.[8] Yet, viewing many such harrowing images can eventually lead to desensitisation, and if the emotions aroused – sadness, empathy and outrage – cannot be translated into helpful action, they risk sliding into apathy and cynicism.[9]

A CALL TO HUMAN VALUES

At its core, our response to forced migration is about our human values: How much do we care about the suffering and loss of dignity of our fellow human beings, and what are we prepared to do about it? This issue is particularly pertinent to healthcare professionals and raises questions for them such as: Do the goals of medicine and professional duties transcend issues of 'entitlement' and nationality? How can we combine justice with compassion? Should healthcare professionals act as agents of the state or should they be prepared to challenge and even disobey state policies and regulations if they believe them to be inhumane and contrary to their Hippocratic commitment to serve all those in clinical need? How far should general practitioners (GPs) act as advocates (rather than gatekeepers) for the vulnerable and marginalised? Healthcare professionals, as responsible and advantaged citizens and as healers dedicated to serving the sick and vulnerable, face ethical dilemmas and challenges in the care of those who have been forced to migrate, including those trafficked in or enslaved in the UK.[10]

PROVISION OF HEALTHCARE FOR THE HEALTH NEEDS OF VULNERABLE MIGRANTS

Vulnerable migrants have a variety of unmet healthcare needs, many brought on by the harsh conditions imposed on them, and an unresponsive healthcare profession.[11] This represents a failure of ethics in its broadest sense. Socio-economic status and migration *per se* account for many of the health discrepancies between vulnerable migrants and non-migrants.[12] Asylum seekers and refugees suffer a disproportionate burden of physical, mental and social morbidities.[13,14] They may suffer severe and intractable mental health problems requiring specialist mental healthcare, often in low supply.[15] Social issues abound such as isolation, poverty, social stigma, difficulties finding adequate housing or schools, unemployment, cultural differences requiring significant adaptation and language barriers. There are problems and challenges to be resolved at all levels: biomedical, psychological, social, cultural, ethical and even spiritual. Additionally, individuals who have suffered trauma, torture and degradation may be very reluctant or even unable to articulate their experiences, and often present with vague symptoms of somatic pain, making communication more challenging. It takes time to establish trust. It also needs the health professional's willingness and openness to listen, and wise discernment to elucidate the real causes for the suffering.[16] It may require specific education and training, which may be lacking.

PERINATAL CARE AND HEALTHCARE FOR CHILDREN

Immigrant women are already disadvantaged and more likely to have adverse obstetric outcomes.[17] Barriers to healthcare for pregnant women can have significant adverse effects on both maternal and child health. The UK government in its policy document *Maternity Matters* highlights the importance of good antenatal care for women and their offspring, and the need to target deprived communities and ensure that their needs are treated with equal importance and respect.[18] Yet, the facts regarding the perinatal care for undocumented pregnant women in the UK are shockingly at odds with these policies and aspirations.[19] Antenatal care is considered 'emergency care' and cannot legally be withheld, but is fully chargeable. Vulnerable immigrant women, often destitute and with no surplus income, are usually unable to pay the substantial charges (around £6000 at the time of writing), leading them to avoid antenatal care and to resort to delivering at home without professional assistance, sometimes with fatal outcomes.[20] The majority of women are unable to access a GP or receive the recommended number of antenatal visits.[21] Pregnant women face additional stressors to those already experienced by vulnerable migrants, such as trafficking for sex work, violence or female genital mutilation (FGM).[22] GPs and midwives are ethically constrained as they cannot refer these women to an affordable system and yet may not be able to provide a safe alternative.

Children, either unaccompanied or of vulnerable parents, also endure hardship and deprivation. The majority escape recommended vaccinations and are turned away by GPs.[19] Despite moral obligations from the *UN Convention on the Rights of the Child*[23] and UK legislation for the protection and provision of care for children, professionals are failing to do so.[24]

In summary, vulnerable migrants potentially represent a substantial workload (and potential economic burden) for busy primary care practitioners. Unsurprisingly, there may be reluctance to take this work on, and this is reflected by the difficulties that migrants encounter when trying to access primary care.[25] However, despite the challenges of working with deprived, marginalised patients, doctors can thrive in this work and there is no correlation between practice area deprivation and GP well-being.[26,27] Working with vulnerable migrants can be rewarding and meaningful work. Various proposals have been suggested and a variety of successful innovations implemented to compensate and support primary care professionals such that they can deliver culturally sensitive, appropriate care for this group of individuals.[12, 28–30]

ELIGIBILITY OF ACCESS AND BARRIERS TO HEALTHCARE

Although the basic human right of access to health services has been enshrined in numerous international and European declarations and legal instruments, one of the most fundamental barriers to migrants in accessing health services is the lack of systems for ensuring that their legal entitlements are known and respected in practice.[12] The UK *Immigration Act* 2016 sets out to make it more difficult for irregular immigrants to access public services or the job market in the UK.[31] Besides the common lack of knowledge and understanding of the healthcare system and their legal entitlement to primary care, asylum seekers and undocumented migrants have to surmount other barriers such as language barriers, obstructive bureaucracy, fear of being reported or arrested and direct or indirect discrimination leading to denial of health coverage.[28,32,33] Asylum applicants and their dependents form only 7% of net migration to the UK and 0.5% of applicants for social benefits,[34] yet they are portrayed as 'freeloaders' sapping the NHS. Most vulnerable migrants do not access healthcare for several years, even if suffering from untreated health conditions.[33] However, even in these cases, errors may be made and the claim may not be 'bogus' but hard to prove within the strict legal criteria.[35,36] Their lives may still be at risk and they may eventually qualify for asylum on humanitarian grounds.[37]

ELIGIBILITY FOR PRIMARY HEALTHCARE

At the time of writing, access to primary care is still free to those who seek asylum, including those whose applications have failed, who are homeless, without documents or who have come to UK shores through unofficial routes – sometimes unhelpfully referred to as 'illegals' – a term that brands them as criminals underserving of treatment. Anyone can register and consult a GP or a practice nurse without charge.[38] A practice nurse can refuse an application but not on discriminatory grounds, and must still offer free emergency care for 14 days. Unfortunately, many of those working in primary care are unaware of this, not helped by complex or misleading guidance.[39] Not all services in primary care are necessarily free; referrals to community services such as physiotherapy, blood tests, X-rays and other tests may be chargeable. This may place primary care professionals in an ethical quandary if inability to pay creates a barrier to optimal care. Evidence suggests that many GP practices do turn away vulnerable migrants, even those with urgent health problems.[39] How can this denial of care be ethically justified?[40]

ELIGIBILITY FOR SECONDARY CARE

The complex changes regarding charges for 'overseas visitors' are listed in government guidance.[38] Services free to vulnerable migrants include: family planning (but not termination of pregnancy), diagnosis and treatment of specific infectious and sexually transmitted diseases (including HIV) and the treatment for a physical or mental condition caused by torture, FGM, domestic violence or sexual violence. Treatment under the *Mental Health Act* is also free to everyone. All accident and emergency (A&E) services, including walk-in and urgent care centres, are free at point of use to all patients, but this does not include services once the patient has been admitted as an inpatient. Healthcare organisations such as hospital trusts have a legal obligation to recover charges for treatment from those ineligible to the NHS. Although clinicians decide on the necessity for treatment, overseas visitor managers have an imperative to show that every effort has been made to obtain payment in the period before the treatment starts. One can readily imagine the potentially ethically fraught and ugly scenarios that may occur in the context of caring for sick, vulnerable migrants. GPs have to refer acutely ill patients for secondary care, in the knowledge that they may be asked to pay and cannot afford to do so or somehow manage if secondary care is aborted and patients in desperation attend GP clinics.[41]

ETHICAL 'LENSES'

The way we treat asylum seekers carries unavoidable ethical dimensions that cannot be elided by referring to bureaucratic diktats.[33] On the everyday level, the ethical issues GPs and primary care practitioners face in relation to vulnerable migrants are broadly the same as for any of their patients, albeit some of the issues, such as justice and human rights, may be more salient. I will use the 'ethical lenses' of rights, duties, virtues and utility for exploring general and specific ethical issues in relation to treating vulnerable migrants, endeavouring to arrive at a multifaceted and rich perspective that is helpful to those working in primary care.

DUTIES AND HUMAN RIGHTS

Much of the discourse in relation to vulnerable migrants accessing healthcare is framed in the language of rights. The *Universal Declaration of Human Rights* (1948) is based on fundamental ideas of universality, equality and non-discrimination and evolved from recognition that denial of human beings' intrinsic worth and dignity can lead to slavery, egregious exploitation and mass murder.[42] The *European Convention on Human Rights* (EHCR), ratified by the UK, sets out individual rights.[43] The introduction of the *Human Rights Act* (1998) in the UK enabled claimants to bring an action in the national courts rather than the EHCR. Its implementation has generated acrimony and political controversy. Article 12 of the *International Covenant on Economic and Social and Cultural Rights* sets out 'The right of everyone to the enjoyment of the highest attainable standard of physical and mental health'.[44] The denial of access to free healthcare for failed asylum seekers (who cannot work and earn legally) violates international law and is inhumane.[35]

Respect for individual rights and individual autonomy has also become a central tenet in contemporary medical ethics. However, even if human rights have been politically legitimated and ratified, this does not provide ethical justification for those rights.[45] O'Neill claims that grounding human rights in a conception of the good (such as Aristotle's concept of human flourishing or *eudaimonia*)[46] is fraught with difficulties in our pluralistic world, and that any right requires its counterpart obligation or has no force. She proposes anchoring human rights in an account of human obligations or duties. She lists five advantages: Firstly, obligations are structurally connected to rights; secondly, the connection to action can be well articulated; thirdly, that obligations can be more readily distinguished and specified than rights and fourthly, that this approach is less individualistic than rights-based approaches. Finally, she submits that obligations can be better justified than rights. Another disadvantage of rights is that they may clash (although the same applies to principles or duties), and it is unclear how to prioritise a right or decide which individual or group takes precedence.

HUMAN NEEDS AND SOLIDARITY

Despite the rigour of her arguments, O'Neill's framework appears to leave out an important dimension in the humane response to the needs of marginalised vulnerable members of our society. Michael Ignatieff eloquently argues for the possibility of a shared understanding of the human good. He proposes that we should base a theory of rights on needs, and that needs create responsibilities that can be mediated by the state (although he expresses caveats regarding state-run impersonal and standardised care for unique individuals). Sharing responsibility for the care of needy strangers helps to create a moral humane society.

> It is this solidarity among strangers, this transformation through the division of labour of needs into rights and rights into care that gives whatever fragile basis we have for saying that we live in a moral community.[47]

Ignatieff suggests that it is essential to agree on the necessary preconditions for human flourishing, even though it can be difficult to reach agreement on the basic necessities that people should be entitled to. Language of rights is unable to articulate the needs we have as social beings, and money cannot buy the human gestures that confer respect. The manner of giving counts, as does the moral basis on which it is given. We can respect people's rights but still demean them as persons. A decent and humane society, therefore, requires a shared language of the good, and a theory of needs is integral to this. Ignatieff also critiques Rawls' theory of justice[48] which focuses on the 'basic goods' required for personal freedom, by pointing out that 'many of the essential requirements for a decent life – love, respect, solidarity with others – cannot be sensibly justified as necessary for personal freedom'. Social isolation and loneliness are potent causes of misery and illness, the fate of many undocumented migrant.[49] The overemphasis on individual freedom and the scepticism towards social justice and solidarity, characteristic of libertarian philosophers such as Robert Nozick, attacks the political philosophy and social ethics underpinning the welfare state, and challenges the very notion of a society as a moral community.[50] Yet, to ask the question whether welfare rights, such as rights to healthcare and education, are more important than civil rights, such as freedom of speech, creates a false dichotomy since they are interdependent; one cannot exercise one's autonomy without physical health and the basic means for survival. Doyal and Gough's theory of needs proposes that objective and universal needs are necessary for successful social participation, and that individuals cannot flourish if deprived of opportunities to do so.[51] They offer two categories of need: firstly, survival and physical health, and secondly, individual autonomy, which involves understanding, absence of disabling mental illness and social opportunity. Vulnerable migrants often have needs in both categories. Doyal and Gough define access to healthcare as a key 'intermediate need', and that those in a position to intervene and meet the need for survival and mental and physical health (i.e. healthcare professionals) have a moral duty to do so. This need also creates a duty to involve vulnerable migrants in research,[52] actively campaign for resources and training and collaborate with others, including community groups, political leaders and non-governmental organisations to improve the conditions for vulnerable migrants.

Although clinicians usually work within a needs-based approach to distributive justice, prioritising care for those in need can be challenging. Distributive justice issues are an everyday issue for GPs, including the vexed question of appointment times for optimal care and fairness. By what criteria do we define 'need' and to what dimensions of a person's illness do we allocate greater time? Selectively excluding vulnerable migrants from accessing healthcare is based on a system of merit, not need, involving the judgement that they are not 'worthy' of care.[53]

In conclusion, a needs-based approach fits within ethical frameworks of both rights and duties. It also underpins Aristotle's theories of justice and of flourishing – treating 'equals equally and unequals unequally'.[46] Access to good healthcare, however, is necessary but not sufficient to promote health and flourishing – social and environmental factors are often more important, and socio-economic inequality in itself has adverse effects.[54] Restricting migrant's access to healthcare undermines social inclusion strategies needed to reduce health inequalities.[55] Arguably, we need to widen the scope to include social justice and social responsibility.[53] Recognition of solidarity as a public good emerges from a needs-based approach, with reciprocal care for everyone's needs and interests, social inclusion and non-discrimination. Solidarity is both an instrumental good – people are objectively better off in solidarity-based societies – and an intrinsic good fostering moral communities.[56] Solidarity acknowledges our shared vulnerability and humanity.[57]

A human rights approach in healthcare, however, may at times have the edge; the language of human rights confers more dignity than needs and can be psychologically empowering when applied to vulnerable and marginalised groups.[58] Involving them in actively taking control of aspects of their health in the community can help to restore self-respect and promote well-being. Health professionals, with their authority and power, are uniquely placed to act as advocates for patients. A human rights perspective endorses them in their advocacy role, and enjoins them to be politically active when rights are violated – resisting policies of exclusion, lobbying policymakers to legislate for policies that are humane and just, speaking up for asylum seekers to have access to the healthcare they need and exposing inhumane and/or inadequate conditions detrimental to patients' health and well-being. In other words, 'giving voice to the voiceless' – sometimes coined 'advocacy ethics'.[59]

PROFESSIONAL DUTIES

Professional ethics is usually expressed as duties and codes of conduct rather than core values. The UK General Medical Council invokes the vaguely defined duty not to 'discriminate unfairly against patients or colleagues'[60] The World Medical Association (WMA) is more prescriptive and creates a positive duty of care for health professionals to act as advocates for patients by promoting the 'fundamental right' for people in clinical need to receive medical care and to speak out against legislation that prevents this.[61]

The UK Royal College of General Practitioners (RCGP) emphasises that all vulnerable migrants have the right to be fully registered with NHS general practice and are entitled to primary medical services without charge. 'General Practitioners should not be expected to police access to healthcare and turn people away when they are at their most vulnerable'. Although this is the crux of the matter, GPs have the *discretion* to refuse registration as long as this is not for discriminatory reasons (in line with the *Equality Act 2010*).[62] The RCGP also points out that practices are not required to check identity or immigration status although there may be 'practical reasons to do so'. Herein lies the difficulty – it is very difficult for a vulnerable person who lacks confidence and knowledge of the system to challenge a hostile practice manager or GP receptionist stating that 'the list is closed' or proof of residence is obligatory. Bureaucracy, prejudice and/or GPs' struggle to cope within a system that is already overloaded and underfunded create barriers to access. Caring for vulnerable migrants in the primary care setting does not represent supererogation or altruism, but simply 'doing one's job' – acting in all patients' best interests.[63]

Professional codes tend to narrowly focus on clinician–patient relationships and not the wider ethical issues or the institutional and societal context within which health professionals function. Conflicting duties emerge in this context between GP's role as gatekeeper (justice) protecting the NHS' resources, and the Hippocratic (healing) role, also framed as the healthcare provider's moral rather than political obligation.[40] Yet, as discussed above, this dichotomy need not exist if we view healthcare professionals' healing and advocacy roles as integral to promoting solidarity, flourishing for all, and a more egalitarian society.[53]

VIRTUE-BASED ETHICS

Professional duties can also be viewed from the lens of virtue ethics (VE). VE offers a way of addressing ethical challenges that can be more helpful and adaptable than rights, rules and principles. Indeed, professional codes are often not followed or perceived as relevant.

As abstract prescriptions, they can fail to connect with the lived experience of practitioners and of their patients.[64] The same may be true for 'principlism'.

> Principles are thought to be too abstract, too removed from the contextual and experiential complexity of clinical decision-making, and too conducive to an overly rationalistic, quasi-legalistic ethics that over-emphasizes quandaries and stifles compassion and moral creativity.[65]

Arguably, 'code ethics' lacks coherence unless placed within a comprehensive and shared tradition of human flourishing (*eudemonia*) and a consensus on what constitutes good practice.[66] Aristotle's VE provides a framework that is not based on rules or prescriptions, but is set in the context of a society within which individuals can live in harmony.[46] VE relies on the intrinsic motivation to develop the virtues needed for a flourishing life and to cultivate the goods internal to practice.[67] Virtues are predictable predispositions leading to good deeds, not just good intentions. They are honed and habituated by constant practice, analogous to learning to play an instrument well ('ethics' is derived from the Greek word *ethos,* 'habit' or 'custom'). VE focuses on the particulars, and does not rely on rules or ready-made formulae, but develops more from the 'bottom up', using the virtues of discernment and practical wisdom to reflect, deliberate and discover the best way forward. Importantly, VE acknowledges the synergistic relationship between emotions and cognitions in moral reasoning, a relationship confirmed by modern day neuroscience.[68] VE, as interpreted by MacIntyre[67] and Toon,[66] emphasises sustainable communities, individual and shared narratives, relationships, collaboration, reciprocity and mutual trust. Even if one takes the view that a shared notion of the good is impossible, Pellegrino proposes that professional ethics can and should be underpinned by virtue-based ethics.[65]

THE VIRTUES OF COMPASSION AND JUSTICE

Among the virtues, Pellegrino lists 'fidelity to trust', fortitude, benevolence, reasonable self-effacement, compassion, justice and prudence or practical wisdom (*phronesis*). To these I would add courage. All of them are relevant in the care of vulnerable migrants but compassion is central to our response to their suffering. It is a complex emotion that includes cognitive, affective and motivational elements. My understanding of compassion is close to that of Gilbert (a psychologist)[69] and Nussbaum (a philosopher),[70] such that it encompasses empathy – both emotional ('feeling with'), and cognitive (being able to adopt the perspective of the other person) – distress tolerance, and, most importantly, the motivation to alleviate the suffering, leading to purposeful, appropriate action, even if this simply means active listening. I have written elsewhere on compassion and the tensions in accommodating it within modern medicine[71] and modern medical ethics.[64] Medicine, at its core, should be based on an ethic of alleviating suffering and promoting healing and flourishing. Compassion does not fit well within a positivist mechanistic paradigm requiring measurable outcomes, or within a market-based, industrialised system of care. With compassion we acknowledge our common humanity and vulnerability, yet profoundly respect the uniqueness and dignity of individuals and their stories. Elisabeth Porter argues that we can expand an ethics of care and compassion to a 'politics of compassion', which 'links the universal and the particular in that it assumes a shared humanity of interconnected, vulnerable people and requires emotions and practical, particular responses to different expressions of vulnerability'.[72] Compassion is not 'soft', but demands strength, wisdom and courage. It may demand 'professional anger' – for health professionals know the pain and suffering endured by their patients and should speak on their behalf, challenging others when they behave unethically, or treat patients in a way that is callous and cruel.[73,74]

PUBLIC HEALTH ETHICS, UTILITARIANISM AND POLITICS

There are robust utilitarian and public health reasons for vulnerable migrants to retain access to primary healthcare. Firstly, limiting access to GP surgeries will lead individuals with untreated illness to present at a later stage to A&E services, costing considerably more to the NHS, using more resources and creating unnecessary suffering.[75] Secondly, primary and secondary prevention of chronic diseases such as diabetes and hypertension is much more cost-effective than treating the late sequelae of the disease.[76] Thirdly, containment and control of communicable diseases would be more difficult and expensive.[77] Concerns have been raised, however, regarding the cost of treating failed asylum seekers in the NHS in the light of pressure on finite NHS budgets.[78] This is a legitimate concern, yet arguments can be made that the UK is a wealthy country and should be able to afford healthcare for the small number of additional people, particularly as this will save money in the long run. Furthermore, the great majority of vulnerable migrants are healthy, well-educated and more than willing to work and participate in society as tax-paying citizens; ignoring this represents a shameful capital and social waste. Public health and primary healthcare are inherently political as they are involved in caring for and educating individuals or communities with potentially competing interests, and are involved in the exercise of power and authority.[59] Aristotle viewed ethics as inseparable from politics. How the *polis*, city or state functions is inextricably bound up with how its citizens can flourish.[47]

AUTONOMY AND CONSENT IN A MULTICULTURAL CONTEXT

Lack of understanding and communication difficulties can vitiate valid adequately informed consent. Good communication is particularly important in the context of intimate examinations or invasive procedures. Patients may come from cultures where individual autonomy is an alien concept and where the head of the household (male) is expected to make the decisions, although this may change with time and adaption to the new culture.[79]

CONFIDENTIALITY AND FGM

Confidentiality demonstrates respect for autonomy and helps to create and maintain trust, facilitating timely and responsive healthcare. Vulnerable migrants live in fear of deportation and may be very reluctant to give much information to healthcare professionals for fear of denunciation. Although primary care is free at the point of access, patient confidentiality is now seriously threatened with non-clinical data sharing between NHS Digital and the Home Office.[80] This threat is significant, particularly as administrators may be more willing to denounce patients they perceive as 'illegal'. Compulsory denunciation or even criminalisation of those providing care to refused asylum seekers is already a reality in some countries.[81]

FGM is a procedure that involves partial or total removal of the female genital organs for cultural reasons, has no health benefits and can cause significant suffering as well as gynaecological and obstetric complications.[82] Health professionals need to be aware that women migrants are likely to have had this procedure if they come from certain countries such as Egypt, Sudan, Eritrea and Somalia. FGM has become a highly topical issue in the UK with extensive media coverage, educational programmes and legislation criminalising those who perform or assist in FGM (*Female Genital Mutilation Act 2003*). FGM also generates specific issues of consent and confidentiality. Doctors have strongly criticised the government-led FGM-enhanced data collection involving mandatory submission of particularly sensitive patient-identifiable medical information to third parties. This disclosure threatens medical confidentiality and the clinician–patient relationship.[83]

INTERPRETERS

The use of professional interpreters has been shown to improve patient care and satisfaction and lower healthcare costs represents a good practice. However, in practice, this may not always be possible and a relative may sometimes act as interpreter, creating ethical pitfalls, particularly with women whose dominant or abusive partners may not be willing to reveal their real stories, or when there are sensitive intimate issues. Gender, cultural, tribal and political issues may arise, creating tensions and mistrust. Consent to the presence of an interpreter must be agreed to. A qualitative study revealed a number of ethical issues, including concerns about confidentiality and accurate transmission of information – a concern that is shared anecdotally by many health professionals. There was also a mismatch between perception of roles with patients expecting advocacy and interpreters neutrality.[32]

CONCLUSION

Denial of healthcare to vulnerable migrants is widespread in the UK (and elsewhere) and cannot be ethically justified whether we adopt the lens of rights, duties, virtues or utility. It also does not make rational or economic sense. Healthcare professionals cannot prevent wars and the gross economic inequalities that create forced migration, but they can show moral leadership and model a humane response to the refugee crisis.[84] They can also fulfil their professional roles by speaking up for the vulnerable and marginalised in clinical need and responding compassionately to their suffering. Their role as healers should not be combined with that of border control agents. This is particularly the case for primary care clinicians in the UK who are often the first port of call, and who are still able to offer free healthcare. Compassion can be combined with justice. Human flourishing, both for ourselves and for our fellow human beings, is a good that primary healthcare professionals should be willing to pursue and defend.

REFERENCES

1. United Nations Refugee Agency. *Global trends: Forced displacement in 2015.* Geneva, Switzerland: UNHCR. http://www.unhcr.org/uk/576408cd7.pdf (accessed July 22, 2016).
2. Cameron CD, Pyne BK. Escaping affect: How motivated emotion regulation creates insensitivity to mass suffering. *J Pers Soc Psychol* 2011;100(1):1–15.
3. Lakoff G, Johnson M. *Metaphors we live by.* Chicago, IL: Chicago University Press, 2003.
4. Humphries B. Supporting asylum seekers: Practical and ethical issues for health and welfare professionals. *Irish J Appl Soc Stud* 2006;7(2):76–86.
5. Stone J. *The Independent. Katie Hopkins' migrant 'cockroaches' column resembles pro-genocide propaganda, says the UN.* www.independent.co.uk/news/uk/katie-hopkins-migrant-cockroaches-column-resembles-pro-genocide-propaganda-says-the-un-10201959.html (accessed January 10, 2016).

6. Buber M. *I and Thou.* London: Bloomsbury 2013 (original translation by Ronald Gregor Smith Edinburgh: T & T Clark 1937).

7. Bauman Z. Strangers are dangers…Are they indeed? In: *Collateral damage. Social inequalities in a global age.* Cambridge: Polity Press, 2011.pp. 1–10.

8. Västfjäll D, Slovic D, Mayorga M, Peters E. Compassion fade: Affect and charity are greatest for a single child in need. *PLoS One* 2014;9(6):e100115. doi:10.1371/journal.pone.0100115.

9. Gallagher A. The ethics of migration and what moves us to care. *Nurs Ethics* 2015;22(7):741–2.

10. The Centre for Social Justice. *It happens here. Equipping the United Kingdom to fight modern slavery.* London: Centre for Social Justice, 2013.

11. Haroon S. *The health needs of asylum seekers. Briefing Statement.* London: UK Faculty of Public Health, 2008.

12. Rechel B, Mladovsky P. Ingleby P, Mackenbach JP, McKee M. Migration and health in an increasingly diverse Europe. *Lancet* 2013;381:1235–45.

13. Burnett A, Peel M. Health needs of asylum seekers and refugees. *BMJ* 2001;322:544–7.

14. Tribe R. Mental health of refugees and asylum seekers. *Adv Psychiatr Treat* 2002;8:240–8.

15. McColl H, Bhui K. Mental healthcare of asylum-seekers and refugees. *Adv Psychiatr Treat* 2008;14:452–9.

16. De Zulueta P. The body tells a story. *BMJ* 2003;326:666.

17. Hayes I, Enohumah K, McCaul C. Care of the migrant obstetric population. *Int J Obstet Anesth* 2011;20:321–9.

18. Department of Health. *maternity matters: Choice, access and continuity of care in a safe service.* London: DoH, 2007.

19. Chauvin P, Simonnot N, Vanbiervliet F, Vicart M, Vuillermoz C. Access to healthcare for people facing multiple health vulnerabilities. Paris: Médecins du Monde Network, 2015.

20. Taylor D. *NHS charges putting pregnant migrant women in danger. The Guardian* 2013. http://www.theguardian.com/society/2013dec27/nhs-charges-pregnant-migrant-women-danger (accessed January 16, 2016).

21. Shortall C. McMorran J, Taylor K, et al. *Experiences of pregnant migrant women receiving ante/peri and postnatal care in the UK: A Doctors of the World Report on the experiences of attendees at their London drop-in clinic.* Doctors of the World, 2015. http://b.3cdn.net/droft heworld/5a507ef4b2316bbb07_5nm6bkfx7.pdf (accessed January 16, 2016).

22. Asif S, Baugh A, Jones W. The obstetric care of asylum seekers and refugee women in the UK. *The Obstet Gynaecol* 2015; 17:223–31.

23. United Nations. *Geneva declaration of the rights of the child.* United Nations, 1924. http://www.un-documents.net/gdrc1924.htm (accessed September 2, 2015).

24. Lancet, Editor. Adapting to migration as a planetary force. *Lancet* 2015;386:1013.

25. Jones D, Gill PS. Refugees and primary care: Tackling the inequalities. *BMJ* 1998;317:1444–6.

26. Stevenson AD, Phillips CB, Anderson KJ. Resilience among doctors who work in challenging areas. A qualitative study. *Br J Gen Pract* July 2011; doi:10.3399/bjgp11X583182. e404–410.

27. Grieve S. Measuring morale—Does practice area deprivation affect doctor's well-being? *Br J Gen Pract* 1997;47(422):547–52.

28. British Red Cross. *Not gone, but forgotten. The urgent need for a more humane asylum system.* London: British Red Cross, 2010.

29. Wind-Cowie M, Wood C. *Do No harm.* London: DEMOS, 2014.

30. Fassil Y, Burnett A. *Commissioning mental health services for vulnerable adult migrants.* London: Mind, 2015. NHS England publication; Gateway ref 03512.

31. Immigration Act 2016 http://www.legislation.gov.uk/ukpga/2016/19/pdfs/ukpga_20160019_en.pdf (accessed 18 July, 2016).

32. O'Donnell CA, Higgins M, Chauhan R, Mullen K. 'They think we're OK and we know we're not'. A qualitative study of asylum seekers' access, knowledge and views to health care in the UK. *BMC Health Serv Res* 2007;7:75.

33. de Zulueta P. Asylum seekers and undocumented migrants must retain access to primary care. *BMJ* 2011;343:d6637.

34. Blinder S. *Migration observatory.* Oxford: Briefings Asylum, 2016.

35. Hall P. Failed asylum seekers and health care. *BMJ* 2006;333:109–110.

36. Vernon G, Feldman R. Refugees and asylum seekers in primary care. From looking after to working together. In: *Working with vulnerable groups. A clinical handbook for GP's. Gill P, Wright N, Brew I (eds.).* London: Royal College of General Practitioners, 2014. pp. 71–87.

37. Reeves M, de Wildt G, Murshali H, et al. Access to health care for people seeking asylum in the UK. *Br J Gen Pract* 2006;56:306–8.

38. NHS Entitlement: Migrant Health Guide. Public Health England Migrant Health Guide July 31st 2014. https://www.gov.uk/guidance/nhs-entitlements-migrant-health-guide (accessed June 28, 2016).

39. Farah W, Hundt A, Qureshi F. *Access to primary care for migrants is a right worth defending.* Migrants Rights Network, 2011. http://www.irr.org.uk/pdf2/Access_to_Health_Care.pdf (accessed September 26, 2013).

40. Taylor K. Asylum seekers, refugees, and the politics of access to health care: A UK perspective. *Br J Gen Pract* 2009;59:765–72

41. de Zulueta P. *Why are the most vulnerable still denied health care? BMJ Blogs* 2013. Available at: http://blogs.bmj.com/blogs/2103/12/20/paquita-de-zulueta-why-are-the-most-vulnerable-still-denied-healthcare/ (accessed December 21, 2013).

42. Universal Declaration of Human Rights. *United Nations General Assembly*, Paris, 1948. http://www.un.org/en/universal-declaration-human-rights/ (accessed July 20, 2016).

43. The European Court for Human Rights. *Council of Europe F-67075 Strasbourg–cedex.* http://www.echr.coe.int/Documents/Convention_ENG.pdf (accessed November 3, 2015).

44. United Nations. *International covenant on economic, social and cultural rights.* New York; United Nations, 1966.

45. O'Neill O. *Autonomy and trust in bioethics.* Cambridge: Cambridge University Press, 2002.

46. Aristotle. *The ethics of Aristotle. The Nichomachean ethics.* (Trans. JAK Thomson). Harmondsworth: Penguin, 1955.

47. Ignatieff M. *The needs of strangers. An essay on privacy, solidarity, and the politics of being human.* New York: Penguin Books, 1984, p.10.

48. Rawls J. *A theory of justice,* 2nd ed. Cambridge, MA: Harvard University Press, 1999.

49. Steptoe A, Shankar A, Demakakos P, Wardle J. Social isolation, loneliness, and all-cause mortality in older men and women. *PNAS* 2013;110(15):5797–801.

50. Nozick R. *Anarchy, state and utopia.* Malden, MA: Basic Books,1974.

51. Doyal L, Gough I. *A theory of human need.* London: Macmillan, 1991.

52. Giving voice to the voiceless. Involving vulnerable migrants in healthcare research. *Br J Gen Pract* 2016;66:284–5.

53. Dwyer J. Illegal immigrants, health care, and social responsibility. *Hastings Center Report* 2004;34:34–41.

54. Marmot Review Team. *Fair society, healthy lives; Strategic review of health inequalities in England post-2010.* 2010. http://www.instituteofhealthequity.org/projects/fair-society-healthy-lives-the-marmot-review/fair-society-healthy-lives-full-report (accessed July 30, 2016).

55. Romero-Ortuño R. Access to health care for illegal immigrants in the EU. Should we be concerned? *Eur J Health Law* 2004;11(3):245–72.

56. Gheaus A. Solidarity, justice and unconditional access to healthcare. *J Med Ethics* 2016;0:1–5.

57. Brainsack B, Buyx A. *Solidarity: Reflections on an emerging concept in bioethics.* London: Nuffield Council, 2011.

58. Ashcroft R. Standing up for the medical rights of asylum seekers. *J Med Ethics* 2005;31:125–6.

59. Callahan D, Jennings B. Ethics and public health: Forging a strong relationship. *Am J Public Health* 2002;92(2):169–76.

60. General Medical Council: *Good medical practice.* London: GMC, 2013.

61. World Medical Association. *WMA council resolution on refugees and migrants.* Adopted by the 203rd WMA Council Session, Buenos Aires, April 2016. https://www.wma.net/policies-post/wma-council-resolution-on-refugees-and-migrants/ (accessed July 23, 2016).

62. Failed Asylum Seekers, Vulnerable Migrants & Access to Primary Care. RCGP Position Statement, Updated January 2013. http://www.rcgp.org.uk/policy/rcgp-policy-areas/asylum-seekers-and-vulnerable-migrants.aspx (accessed July 22, 2016).

63. Downie RS. Supererogation and altruism: A comment. *J Med Ethics* 2002;28:75–6.

64. de Zulueta PC. Suffering, compassion and 'doing good medical ethics'. *J Med Ethics* 2015;41:87–90.

65. Pellegrino ED. Towards a virtue-based normative ethics for the health professions. *Kennedy Inst Ethics J* 1995;5(3):253–77.

66. Toon P. *A flourishing practice?* London: Royal College of General Practitioner, 2014.

67. MacIntyre A. *After virtue.* 2nd ed. Notre Dame, IN: University of Notre Dame, 1984.

68. Damasio AR. *Descartes' error. Emotion, reason and the human brain.* New York: Putnam, 1994.

69. Gilbert P. *The compassionate mind: A new approach to life's challenges.* London: Constable and Robinson, 2009.

70. Nussbaum MC. *Upheavals of thought. The intelligence of the emotions.* New York: Cambridge University Press, 2001.

71. de Zulueta P. Compassion in 21st Century medicine: Is it sustainable? *Clin Ethics* 2013;8(4):119–28.

72. Porter E. Can politics practice compassion? *Hypatia* 2006;21(4):97–123.

73. McNeill PM. Public health ethics: Asylum seekers and the case for political action. *Bioethics* 2003;17:487–502.

74. McCartney M. All asylum seekers should be treated with humanity. *BMJ* 2011;343:d5571.

75. Delamothe T. Migrant healthcare: Public health versus politics. *BMJ* 2012;344:e924.

76. Gulland A. Providing preventive care to migrants saves money, study finds. *BMJ* 2015;351:h4806.

77. Hargreaves S, Holmes A, Friedland JS. Charging failed asylum seekers in the UK. *Lancet* 2005;365:732–3.

78. Newdick C. Treating failed asylum seekers in the NHS. *BMJ* 2009;338:b1614.

79. Fan R. Self-determination vs. family determination: Two incommensurable principles of autonomy. *Bioethics* 1997;11:309–22.

80. Travis A. *NHS hands over patient records to Home Office for immigration crackdown. The Guardian*, January 2017. https://www.theguardian.com/uk-news/2017/jan/24/nhs-hands-over-patient-records-to-home-office-for-immigration-crackdown (accessed January 25, 2017).

81. Vernon G. Denunciation: A new threat to access health care for undocumented migrants. *Br J Gen Pract* 2012. 62(595):98–99 doi: 10.3399/bjgp12X625265.

82. *Information regarding the WHO classification FGM.* http://www.who.int/reproductivehealth/topics/fgm/overview/enFGM and a resource pack is available at http://www.gov.uk/government/publications/female-genital-mutilation-resource-pack (accessed July 30, 2016).

83. Bewley S, Kelly B, Darke K, et al. Mandatory submission of patient identifiable information to third parties: FGM now, what next? *BMJ* 2015;351:h5146.

84. Abbasi K, Patel K, Godlee F. Europe's refugee crisis: An urgent call for moral leadership. *BMJ* 2015;351:h4833.

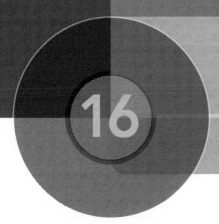

Proximity, power and perspicacity: Ethical issues in primary care research

JONATHAN IVES

INTRODUCTION

The need to be attentive to ethical issues when conducting healthcare research almost goes without saying, but it is always tempting to begin a chapter such as this with an historical account of how and why we have the system of ethical research governance that we do, and explain why it is needed. Tempting, but, given the amount of ink that has already been spilled on the subject, certainly unnecessary. For any reader who is a researcher or a clinician, and is yet to be convinced of the need to pay attention to research ethics, I respectfully suggest you seek a new profession. It is important to note, of course, that one can appreciate the importance of being attentive to ethical issues, whilst still being critical of the current system of ethical governance that is in place, at either an institutional, local or national level, which can be cumbersome, and occasionally as obstructive and burdensome as it can be useful.[1] I would direct an interested lay reader to general and historical texts, such as Annas and Grodin's account of the *Nazi Doctors and the Nuremberg Code*,[2] or Jones' account of the Tuskagee syphilis experiments,[3] which provide vivid and sufficient justification for this kind of chapter being included in a volume such as this. An excellent, and brief, introduction to core principles can be found in articles by Slowther et al.[4] and Shaw et al.[5] on ethical issues and research governance.

This chapter will not provide an account of why research ethics is important, or provide an overview of research ethics in general. Rather, it will highlight particular 'problem areas' that may become prominent when research takes place in primary care specifically. Further reading on research ethics in primary care can be found in Roger Jones' *The Ethics of Research in General Practice*,[6] and the series of articles in *Family Practice* by Ives et al.,[7] Draper et al.[8] and Wilson et al.[9]

The chapter will begin, importantly in the current climate, by providing a brief account of why primary care practitioners and practices (henceforth referred to collectively as 'Primary Care') ought to conduct, or facilitate (henceforth referred to collectively as 'participate in'), research, and outline some thoughts on what factors might be important when making a decision whether or not to participate in a particular project (which is itself an ethical issue that has received scant attention to date). It will then move on to consider some problematic areas for research ethics in primary care, organised around the theme of 'proximity'.

THE OBLIGATION TO RESEARCH IN PRIMARY CARE

The question of whether primary care ought to participate in research may not strike one immediately as an ethical issue but, arguably, it is one of the most important. Another way to understand the question is to ask whether primary care does something *wrong* by failing to participate in research.

In their 2008 paper, Ives et al. argue that there is indeed an obligation for primary care to participate in research, but noted that this obligation might be discharged in myriad ways. Three arguments were offered in support of this claim, summarised below:

1. The argument from fairness

"Free riding occurs when one person benefits from the efforts of others whilst simultaneously and inexcusably avoiding contributing to this effort him/herself. Free riding is wrong because it is unfair. All family doctors benefit from medical research in some way. Family doctors who benefit from research without contributing to the research effort are free riding. Therefore, it is wrong (because it is unfair) for family doctors not to participate in research."[10]

2. The argument from reason (a Kantian argument)

"Medicine, as a legitimate scientific practice, requires ongoing, high quality research to be conducted. If all doctors refused to take part in research, medicine would lose its legitimacy. No family doctor would reasonably wish for medicine to lose its legitimacy. Therefore, no family doctor should refuse to participate in research."[11]

3. The argument from utility (a utilitarian argument)

"We all have an obligation to maximise goods and minimise harms, including family doctors. The aim of medical research is to maximise good and minimise harms. Overall, participating in research will maximise goods and minimise harms. Therefore, family doctors should participate in research."[12]

Whilst there is not space in this chapter to critically assess these arguments, they certainly seem to provide a *prima facie* case for their being, all other things being equal, an obligation to take part in research. We need, therefore, to consider what may make things unequal: what might shift the balance and make non-participation ethical? One such factor may be resource.

RESOURCE AND RESEARCH ETHICS IN PRIMARY CARE

Let us first deal with the easiest question. If we accept the very plausible Kantian trope of 'ought implies can',[13] we can straightforwardly accept that when resource scarcity makes it impossible to take part in research, there cannot be an obligation to do so. This leaves two scenarios:

1. Where resource is abundant.
2. Where resource is available but competed for by other legitimate and required activities.

Dealing with (1) also appears straightforward. Given that there is a *prima facie* obligation to participate in research, if participation is made easy by an abundance of resource, then there is a clear obligation to do so. Furthermore, when primary care does participate in research, it is reasonable, as Draper et al.[8] argue, that it should be reimbursed for associated costs and so does not make a loss.

The more difficult question (2) is essentially a question of prioritisation: To what extent should primary care be obliged to *prioritise* research over other activities? Answering this question will undoubtedly require us to identify, and characterise in a morally meaningful way, the kinds of activities that primary care might engage in. This is certainly beyond the scope of this chapter, but let us assume, for simplicity's sake, that we can distinguish broadly between three core activities, which there is a *prima facie* obligation to perform, but will likely be in resource competition:

1. Life-saving/maintaining services
2. Life-enhancing services
3. Service enhancement.

It would be reasonable to assert that category 1 ought to take priority over categories 2 and 3. The argument over what falls within each category will be lengthy and difficult, and will require complex arguments over the correct conception of health and well-being goods (for a good example of this debate, see Kraut's *What is Good and Why: The Ethics of Well-being*),[14] as well as debates about efficacy; however, for the sake of argument and for illustrative purposes, let us say that this would mean services such as screening, prescribing, blood pressure clinics and such like would be *prima facie* prioritised over fertility services and cosmetic procedures (with the caveat, and moot assumption, than in the majority of cases, whilst certainly impactful, the need for such services does not lead to significant health problems that might place an individual case into category 1). Category 3 would involve a range of activities, which could be directed towards enhancing either category 1 or category 2 activities – and this would include, *inter alia*, all kinds of clinical and service delivery research. It is reasonable to suppose, if thus far the argument is plausible, that category 3 activities that enhance category 1 activities ought to be prioritised over those that enhance category 2 activities. The more difficult question is to what extent category 3 activities that enhance category 1 activities ought be prioritised over category 2 activities themselves; and this is a grey area in which genuine dilemmas gain traction.

The preceding discussion cannot offer an answer to any particular question of whether or not an individual doctor or practice ought to support a particular piece of research, but it does suggest that when primary care is faced with the option of participating in research, it should, at least, consider the following before making a judgement about whether participation is obligatory, supererogatory or impermissible:

1. There is a *prima facie* obligation to participate in research, and research ought to be considered a core activity.
2. Given (1), when refusing, the burden of argument lies with you to show that:
    a. Compliance is impossible (therefore not obligatory).
    b. Compliance is unreasonable (because it would place an unreasonable personal burden on staff in terms of time and effort).
    c. Compliance is ethically impermissible (because it would impact negatively on category 1 or category 2 activities).
3. Some trade-off may be acceptable between a negative impact on a category 1 or 2 activities and research that has a good chance of enhancing those activities.

Having now explored the question of whether primary care ought to take part in research, the remainder of this chapter will use the theme of 'proximity' to explore some particular ethical challenges in primary care research.

PROXIMITY ...

One of the reasons that primary care may be seen as fertile ground for research, and research recruitment, is the proximity of the family doctor to their patient population. Although some might argue that this proximity is being eroded, it is still the case that many family doctors have long-standing relationships with their patients, and families of patients, which engender confidence and trust, and provide the family doctor with a more intimate and contextualised understanding of the patient than secondary or tertiary practitioners might expect to have. To a large extent, research in primary care makes use of (or potentially exploits) this proximity. The remainder of this chapter is organised around the notion of proximity and how it may raise ethical questions in two particular areas: power and perspicacity.

POWER ...

A staple concern of research ethics is that participation in research must be fully informed and voluntary, and this requires all participants to have as full as possible an understanding of the research and to have chosen to participate in the absence of coercive influence (although see Manson and O'Neil's excellent book[15] that challenges standard ways of thinking about informed consent). These are important because they allow a patient to exercise autonomy. Autonomous persons are able to exercise their own judgement about how they live their life, and to act autonomously requires both freedom to make a choice (the absence of coercion) and sufficient information on which to base a choice. Any form of deception (including providing false or incomplete information) or coercion (applying pressure or force) makes a person either less autonomous, or prevents a person from being able to exercise autonomous choice.

In the context of primary care research, the proximity between clinician and patient (often a result of long-term care relationships), an invitation from a clinician to participate in research may be perceived by a patient as something that cannot be refused, either because they feel they owe something to the clinician or because they are concerned about the impact of a refusal on their ongoing care. It is, perhaps, given that if a patient believes that non-participation will have a negative impact on their ongoing care, this is coercive and entirely unethical to exploit. The risk of this happening can be mitigated by carefully constructing information sheets and recruitment processes that stress explicitly that care will not be affected whatever decision is made.

Considering the former case, where a patient consents to participate because he or she feels something is owed to the clinician, challenging questions arise about the nature of, and relationship between, coercion, motivation and autonomy. As Beauchamp and Childress[16] have noted, it is important to recognise a distinction between

> a subjective response in which people comply because they feel threatened ... (and) ... coercion ... because coercion requires that a real, credible and intended threat is brought on a person so that his or her self-directiveness is displaced. (p. 164)

To briefly explore this, let us consider three cases in which a patient consents to participate in research.

1. *A woman consents to complete a questionnaire about her diet and weight loss, even though she does not want to and does not feel she has time, because her doctor has asked her to as favour because responses are low, and she feels she owes her doctor this, given that her doctor has been so understanding and helpful.*

This case seems to be an example of something unacceptable. The reason for this is that the doctor has expressly asked the patient to participate as a favour, and this seems incommensurate with the nature of the professional relationship. The fact that someone might perform such a favour is not itself problematic. In the context of a friendship or spousal relationship, for example, favours may be common currency, and acting against one's desires because one feels one owes a favour is not normally considered to be problematic (as long as the favour is commensurate with what is 'owed'). In this case, the completion of a questionnaire is not at all dangerous or burdensome. The problem here is not that there is coercion; a person may be free to feel that they owe anything to anyone, and that is a matter of personal moral choice. A sense of 'owing' one's doctor is not, arguably, even entirely inappropriate. Many doctors do go above and beyond their professional duties, and a patient wishing to reciprocate and offer something in return is not obviously morally wrong. Rather, the clear wrong here lies in the doctor trying to *exploit* that sense of 'owing' in the patient.

2. *A man consents to undergo experimental surgery to treat prostate cancer, even though he is worried about the risks and would prefer the standard intervention, because his doctor has invited him to and he feels he owes his doctor this, given that his doctor has been so understanding and helpful.*

This case seems almost identical to the case above, except that (1) the intervention is more burdensome and (2) the doctor has not sought to exploit a sense of 'owing' in the patient. Despite the fact that the intervention is more burdensome, this case seems more acceptable than the first. The reason for this lies in the fact that the doctor has not, in any sense, sought to *exploit* a sense of obligation in the patient. The patient has volunteered it. The wrong is arguably in the asking, not in the giving, and if the patient wishes to perform a reciprocal act, and chooses to do it in this way, then arguably there would be a wrong in preventing the patient from doing so. As Wilson et al. have noted:

> It is … not necessarily wrong for a patient to act upon a sense of obligation to their family doctor if that obligation is well placed and is not being exploited. A sense of just reciprocity may indicate a well-adjusted moral person and if a person feels the obligation to reciprocate, participating in research may be an appropriate way of doing so providing it is proportionate.[17]

However, there is something uncomfortable in the fact that the patient is so acting because he feels he owes the doctor, because this again seems to wrongly characterise the relationship between a doctor and a patient. The key ethical question, however, as noted above, seems to be whether this sense of owing is being *exploited* or not – and much of this will depend on how the individual patient experiences and perceives the obligation, suggesting that effective and open communication during recruitment is key to ethical practice.

3. *A man consents to undergo experimental surgery to treat prostate cancer, even though he is worried about the risks and would prefer the standard intervention, because he feels he has gained much from the NHS over the years and he ought to give something back. Helping the next generation of cancer sufferers by taking part in research seems a good way to do this.*

The third case is similar to the second, except that the motivation to act comes not from a sense of owing the doctor anything but a strong moral conviction that one should contribute something back to society. Despite the risks and burden, this case seems more acceptable. The intuitive appropriateness of this, however, seems to come from the generalness of the obligation 'to society' rather than 'to this individual', and it is not clear whether there is any morally relevant difference that would justify treating the two differently.

These examples, and our brief analysis of them, raise two important and vexatious questions. If a patient decided to consent to participate in research out of a sense of moral obligation: (1) To what extent ought that sense of obligation be questioned and/or considered inappropriate or a coercive influence, when we do not consider a sense of moral obligation (generally) to be coercive? and (2) To what extent should it matter who/what the recipient of that sense of obligation is? We are generally free, within the bounds of law, to determine our own sense of moral obligation, and to say that I am permitted to be motivated to take part in research out of a sense of moral obligation to society in general, but not out of a sense of moral obligation to an individual health professional, seems problematic. However, the difficulty in demarcating and isolating a person's motivation, and the risk of slipping into coercive practice, might mean that, overall, ethical practice is better served by drawing a line to avoid any risk of exploitation arising from a patient's sense of owing their doctor (a response based on some form of rule-consequentialism). There is obviously no ethical problem with a patient experiencing a sense of owing their doctor, and it may be entirely morally appropriate; but, there may be a wrong in capitalising on that moral sense, just because of the risk of exploitation. Research in primary care, just because of the proximity between patient and clinician, must be particularly attentive to that risk. It should not assume that a patient's motivation is suspect or inappropriate just because it may include some sense of personal obligation to the clinician; but, it also should not be assumed that a person could not feel coerced simply in light of who is doing the asking.

PERSPICACITY ...

Family doctors may be assumed to have special insight into their patients, derived from their proximity to them, which can be useful for both selecting and targeting putative participants. There are both positives and negatives to this, meaning that perspicacity borne out of proximity may be a double-edged sword.

Firstly, family doctors may be in a relatively unique position of knowing how 'research friendly' their patients are. Family doctors are usually notified if a patient is taking part in a clinical trial, and may also be privy to details about other forms of health-related research participation. As 'gatekeepers', family doctors may potentially use this knowledge in two ways.

Firstly, there is potential for this knowledge to be used to target 'research friendly' patients. This is only likely to be an issue when recruitment and sampling are non-random (e.g. purposive sampling for qualitative research), where patients are approached on the basis of fulfilling certain set criteria. The mandate to efficiently meet recruitment targets may encourage the approachment of patients who are likely to say yes to research. The potential problem here is that 'research friendly' patients may then become overburdened by research (particularly, given the issues of proximity and power detailed above). This places the family doctor in the difficult position of knowing that he or she could approach patients who are likely to say yes, but having to judge whether or not those patients are already overburdened. Respect for autonomy would suggest that such a decision ought to be taken by patients themselves; but, if there is anything to the concerns raised above about the power dynamic, there is the risk that simply asking the question will incline a research-friendly patient to say yes. Balancing the risk of paternalism against the need to protect patients is not an unfamiliar problem to any doctor – but it is a problem for research in primary care in ways that it may not be for research in other contexts, simply because of the knowledge a family doctor may have.

This leads to the second use of this knowledge – gatekeeping to prevent access to certain patients, who are either perceived to be too ill, too burdened or otherwise not suitable to approach. This is more likely to be problematic when recruitment and sampling are random and aim to be representative of a population. By selectively excluding certain patients, one interferes with random sampling and potentially introduces bias. A good sampling strategy, with sufficient numbers, should serve to mitigate this risk but, that aside, this act of gatekeeping involves the family doctor using her or his knowledge of a patient to make a decision on their behalf. Again, this raises questions about finding the correct balance between autonomy and paternalism.

It is worth noting that 'paternalism' here is not being used in a pejorative sense. If it were, then that would seem completely out of kilter with current systems of research governance that routinely make decisions about who it is appropriate to approach for research participation. Paternalism may sometimes be justified. In saying that, however, in acting as a gatekeeper, primary care engages in a morally complex activity that needs to be thoughtfully considered: both by those who do it, and by those who ask it of others.

CONCLUSION

In this chapter, we have covered some select issues in primary care research ethics, but the coverage is by no means exhaustive. We have explored the extent to which primary care is obliged to participate in research and considered what factors need to be considered when making a participation decision. We have also explored some central problems in research ethics, and their particular salience in primary care, through examining the problems of proximity and power and proximity and perspicacity. The nature of the issues discussed is such that the resolution to a particular problem will depend entirely on the specific circumstances of the case. Given that, this chapter has attempted to outline some central issues, and ways of thinking about them, that might support the reader in being attentive to ethics in primary care research.

REFERENCES

1. Jamrozik K. (2004). Research ethics paperwork: What is the plot we seem to have lost? *BMJ* 329:286.
2. Annas G, Grodin M. (1992). *The Nazi Doctors and the Nuremberg Code: Human Rights in Human Experimentation.* New York: Oxford University Press.
3. Jones J. (1993). *Bad Blood: The Tuskagee Syphilis Experiment.* New York: The Free Press.
4. Slowther A, Boynton P, Shaw S. (2006). Research governance: Ethical issues. *Journal of the Royal Society of Medicine* 99(2):65–72.
5. Shaw S, Boynton P, Greenhalgh T. (2005). Research Governance: Where did it come from, what does it mean? *Journal of the Royal Society of Medicine* 98:496–502.
6. Jones R. (1999). The ethics of research in general practice. In Dowrick C, Frith L. (eds.), *General Practice and Ethics: Uncertainty and Responsibility.* London: Routledge. pp. 141–155.

7. Ives J, Draper H, Damery S, Wilson S. (2009). Do family doctors have an obligation to participate in research. *Family Practice* 26:543–548.
8. Draper H, Wilson S, Flanagan S, Ives J. (2009). Offering payments, reimbursement and incentives to patients and family doctors to encourage participation in research. *Family Practice* 26(3):231–238.
9. Wilson S, Draper, H, Ives, J. (2008). Ethical issues regarding recruitment to research studies within the primary care consultation. *Family Practice* 25:456–461.
10. Ibid., 544.
11. Ibid., 545.
12. Ibid., 454.
13. Kant I. (2002). *Critique of Practical Reason.* W. Pluher (trans.). Indianapolis, IN: Hackett.
14. Kraut R. (2009). *What is Good and Why: The Ethics of Well-being.* Harvard University Press. Cambridge, MA.
15. Manson N, O'Neil, O. (2007). *Rethinking Informed Consent in Bioethics.* Cambridge: Cambridge University Press.
16. Beauchamp T, Childress J. (1994). *Principles of Biomedical Ethics.* 4th ed. New York: Oxford University Press.
17. Draper et al., 2009, *op. cit.*, 459.

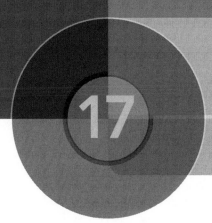

Integrating ethical theory with musculoskeletal primary care practice

17

CLARE DELANY

Physiotherapy primary care practice is very similar to a general medical practice model of care. People are either referred to see a physiotherapist from their doctor or medical specialist for a specific physical problem or they may independently seek out the services of a physiotherapist. In both of these situations, the physiotherapist works as a primary practitioner and is responsible for assessment, diagnosis and appropriate management of the patient's condition.

In this chapter, I describe the delivery of care in physiotherapy primary practice settings, focusing predominantly on musculoskeletal-based clinical work, drawing broadly from discussions in physiotherapy literature and more specifically, from an empirical study of physiotherapists communicating with their patients in primary practice treatment settings. I analyse the relationship between visible elements of physiotherapists' communication with their patients with underpinning ethical theories and values concerning clinical communication. Based on the descriptions of the visible elements of communication, I posit that physiotherapy musculoskeletal-based primary practice has a predominant focus on the delivery of efficient, targeted, structured and evidence-based treatment. I conclude the most visible ethical value driving physiotherapy treatment is beneficence. Whilst this is an important and proper focus, I contend that such a focus tends to overlook and as a consequence, to neglect other equally important ethical dimensions of this area of physiotherapy primary practice, in particular the principle of respecting and enhancing a patient's autonomous participation in the treatment encounter. In the final section, I propose theories and conversational habits which might assist in strengthening the connection between the ethical basis of communication in physiotherapy primary practice and the words used and overall discourse of musculoskeletal physiotherapy practice.

AN ETHICAL FRAMEWORK FOR ANALYSING CLINICAL PRACTICE

I have previously described an 'iceberg' framework[1] as a way to conceptualise therapist/patient communication from the comparative perspective of external or above-surface actions – what is outwardly visible in the clinical encounter – with a corresponding internal or below-surface perspective, representing possible practice paradigms and ethical theories informing the visible, above the surface elements.

In this simplified model (Figure 17.1), the top section of the iceberg represents what is visible, what physiotherapists in primary clinical practice settings actually say and do and how they communicate with their patients. Below the surface are the less visible practice paradigms and ethical values which either explicitly or implicitly guide clinical practice decisions and actions. These reflect a particular clinical and practice orientation. Physiotherapy codes of ethics[2–4] (below surface level 2) are derived from the four biomedical ethical principles advocated by Beauchamp and Childress[5] (level 3). The principles outline ethical obligations to ensure treatment is beneficial, does not cause harm; respect client autonomy and is just. The genesis of these principles and codes of conduct are foundational ethical theories (level 4), including deontology[6–8] and utilitarianism.[9] The central theoretical focus of deontology is to do one's duty. From this basis, the right thing to do derives from a universal duty to respect other human beings. Respecting a patient's autonomy by obtaining their informed consent to treatment and by providing information about risks and benefits and alternatives of proposed treatments aligns more closely with the idea of deontology. Whereas making decisions about the most appropriate and beneficial treatment (with or without a patient's contribution or autonomous choice) is commonly aligned with a utilitarian justification of an action being the right action to take because of predicted clinical benefit. In utilitarian theories, the rightness or wrongness of an action is based on the consequences of performing it.

The key assumption of the iceberg model is that there is a relationship between the decisions and actions a practitioner takes when conversing with their patient and setting the clinical communication agenda, and his/her understanding of underlying bioethical principles and theories.[10,11] In their seminal paper, Emanuel and Emanuel[12] discuss how underlying ethical values might manifest in clinicians' conceptions of their professional roles including how they go about communicating with, and sharing decisions with patients. Table 17.1 provides an adapted version of Emanuel and Emanuel's ideas and illustrates how a clinician's overt patterns of clinical communication (what he or she says and does within the clinical encounter) represent value-based assumptions about professional and patient roles. The four types of communication (Table 17.1), and their underlying ethical assumptions about patient contribution and

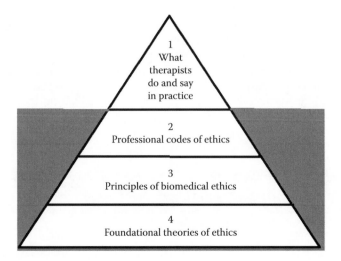

Figure 17.1 The iceberg model.

Table 17.1 Intersection between ethical values, assumptions and communication styles

Types of communication	Assumptions about patient values	Clinician's obligations and role	Patient's obligations and role
Paternalistic Clinician leads the conversation and decides what is best for the patient.	Patients have **objective values** which are shared with the clinician.	**In their role as their patients' guardian,** clinicians are obliged to act in the best interests of their patients, independent of patient's current preferences.	**Patient's role is to agree** with objective medical values.
Informative Clinician provides information to the patient about options for treatment.	Patients know **their own values** which are defined and fixed or stable.	**In their role as the competent and technical expert,** clinicians provide factual information to their patients and implement the patient's selection.	**Patient's role is to choose** between available options of treatment as presented by the clinician.
Interpretive Clinician provides information and assists the patient to make sense of the information in relation to their own values and concerns.	Patients may have **conflicting or not fully formed values** that may require elucidation.	**In their role as patient advisor or counsellor,** doctors provide both factual information and they help to interpret relevant patient values.	**Patients are expected to develop a level of self-understanding** relevant to proposed clinical care.
Deliberative Clinician provides information and identifies the values inherent in the proposed clinical options to assist the patient evaluate how they relate to their own values and goals.	Patients' values **are open to development.**	**In their role as their patients' teacher or friend,** doctors provide factual medical information and the values underlying medical choices.	**For patients, autonomy comprises moral self-development as** it is relevant to medical care.

Source: Adapted from Emanuel, E.J., and Emanuel, L.L., *JAMA*, 267(16), 2222, 1992.

choice, will be used to guide the analysis of examples of communication in musculoskeletal physiotherapy primary practice presented below.

PHYSIOTHERAPY PRIMARY CARE PRACTICE

The practice of physiotherapy encompasses assessing and managing a range of neuro-musculoskeletal conditions including acute/short-term injuries; chronic conditions such as osteo-arthritis, back pain and many other disorders of the neuro-musculoskeletal system. A unifying concept across different areas of physiotherapy practice is a concern with movement.[13] For example, the World Confederation for Physical Therapy defines physiotherapy as:

> … services to individuals and populations to develop, maintain and restore maximum movement and functional ability throughout the lifespan. This includes providing services in circumstances where movement and function are threatened by ageing, injury, pain, diseases, disorders, conditions or environmental factors. Functional movement is central to what it means to be healthy.[14]

Despite this overarching definition, there are also fundamental differences in the aims, focus and treatment regime between different speciality areas of physiotherapy. It is important to acknowledge that in this chapter, I take a narrow slice of a highly diverse health discipline, focusing closely on the area of musculoskeletal practice.

THE MUSCULOSKELETAL PRIMARY PRACTICE SETTING

A physiotherapy primary practice setting may be a privately owned business or public outpatient clinic. Treatment sessions are usually scheduled for approximately 20–30 minutes. Musculoskeletal physiotherapy practice in this setting is characterised by a focused assessment which seeks to identify and specify the nature, severity and extent of a patient's condition. Treatment is then linked to the assessment findings and progress is measured via reassessment of baseline diagnostic and symptomatic measures. 'Objective' assessment comprises questions framed by the therapist and directed to specific features of the patient's condition. 'Subjective' assessment involves questions which allow the patient to describe the nature, history, behaviour and functional impact of the problem.

This structured clinical reasoning approach involves methodically gathering information to form hypotheses, followed by logically and individually testing the hypotheses. The approach represents an established practice paradigm, namely 'the scientific/experimental/positivist' paradigm' using hypothetico-deductive clinical reasoning, and focusing on objective and predictable types of knowledge in practice' (p. 434).[15] The aim of such an approach is to obtain an accurate and justified diagnosis and to enable a logical and evidence-based progression of treatment. The approach was first developed as a hypothesis-oriented model by Rothstein and Echternach.[16] The language used in this approach reflects objectivity and precision.[17]

Table 17.2 summarises the essential steps within this model.[18] Although there have been several studies and related discussions in the physiotherapy clinical reasoning literature that

Table 17.2 Hypothesis-oriented model of clinical reasoning

1. Collect initial data by interview or subjective examination.
2. Generate a problem statement and establish functional or disability-related goals.
3. Collect further data by physical examination.
4. Generate hypotheses related to achievement of goals.
5. Plan how you will re-evaluate for ongoing examination of impairment.
6. Plan treatment strategy based on hypotheses.
7. Plan tactics (specifics of treatment) to implement strategy.
8. Implement treatment.
9. Reassess to check whether goals have been met.
10. Continue to modify treatment, or generate new hypotheses accordingly.

Table 17.3 Demographic profile of patients and therapists

Physiotherapist details	Patient details
• 11 male, 6 female • Years since graduation (4–25) • 9 with postgraduate qualifications in manipulative therapy	• 11 initial visits, 6 return visits • Acute back pain (6), chronic back pain (4), sports injury (6), shoulder injury (1)

have expanded and elaborated on this early model,[19–21] it nevertheless represents the basic structure and approach underlying physiotherapy clinical reasoning.

In the next section, I draw from data comprising transcripts of physiotherapy primary practice treatment to examine the features of communication between a therapist and a patient within a typical primary practice treatment encounter. The goal is to identify the (above surface) features and the focus of clinical communication in this area of clinical practice.

SPECIFIC EXAMPLES OF PHYSIOTHERAPY COMMUNICATION IN THE PRIMARY PRACTICE SETTING: AN EMPIRICAL STUDY

The empirical data drawn from a qualitative study of a purposive sample of 17 physiotherapists working in primary practices in Victoria, Australia. Ethics approval was obtained from The University of Melbourne Department Human Research Ethics Group in 2005. Therapists were recruited from a publicly available list of primary practices in Victoria, Australia. The practitioners agreed to have a single treatment audiotaped and then to be interviewed following this treatment (Table 17.3). The results of the interview data have been previously published.[1] In this chapter, I report unpublished findings from the audiotaped treatment sessions.

Each audiotape of a treatment session was transcribed in full and analysis of the data was based on grounded theory methods of categorising, coding and grouping the data.[22] The aim was to generate both a description and a theoretical explanation of the type of communication occurring within the therapeutic encounter. Quotations below use pseudonyms for the participating therapists and provide representative examples of the described themes.

The analysis of these data was guided by two main questions:

1. What is the nature of the clinical communication between the therapist and the patient?
2. What ethical ideals and assumptions about clinical practice underpin the types of information exchange and communication between the therapist and the patient?

KEY FINDINGS

Therapists' communication with their patients conformed to a recognisable structure and style with three distinct phases consisting of assessment, diagnosis and treatment. During the assessment phase, therapists sought information from their patients about the nature and history of their problem, including its impact on their lifestyle and functional abilities. This was followed by a phase of physical assessment. In the diagnostic phase which followed, the therapist's clinical reasoning and diagnostic thought processes were communicated to the patient. Giving the patient information about the treatment and advice about self-management strategies was the final phase of the treatment encounter.

One therapist's communication, Joseph, is featured below to illustrate the structured nature of the clinical interaction. The structure of Joseph's interaction stood out for its clarity and order.

The same structure was visible, although more flexibly packaged, in all other treatments. Joseph's use of scientific and reductionist language is an exemplar of a typical hypothesis-oriented or hypothetico-deductive approach.[21]

The patient in this treatment was a woman who presented with thoracic back pain. Table 17.4 provides a chronological list of the questions Joseph asked to his patient in the

Table 17.4 Initial assessment

1. Ok. Right. How can I help you then?
   Um, it's a similar problem to what I came with last time. I don't know if you have it there - I've just had a baby, five weeks ago.
2. Five weeks ago, yes.
   Yeah. And it was a caesarian.
3. Ok, yep.
   I've recovered really well, that's fine, but I can feel my back is quite sore and I had some work in the hospital as well. Umm, in two places this time. One, I think, around about here ...
4. Yep. Around about there.
   And it's similar to what I had last time and it feels as if it locks. The times I've come before it's actually locked and you've been unable to unlock it. This time it hasn't locked yet, but I can feel it starting to.
5. What sort of pain?
   Um, it's like a sharp pain.
6. Is it there all the time?
   No. Umm
7. So it just comes back.
   Sort of when I twist, when I'm twisting or moving.
8. Twisting and moving.
   Yeah.
9. What do you mean by moving?
   Umm, more probably when I'm lifting. Probably the baby.
10. The baby.
    Yeah, lifting the baby.
11. Ok. So does it happen every time you lift the baby?
    (pause) No, but it's getting more.
12. More?
    It is increasing, yeah.
13. So how long did it take before that pain settled?
    Umm, it was virtually a couple of days after I had the baby it started. So...just in that one spot. And the other thing is...just in here around my shoulders, my whole pregnancy I had a pain. I'll show you on here (laugh) Um, sort of right in here.
14. Around the
    Yeah, especially my left hand side.
15. Yep. Around about there.
    The whole pregnancy, my husband would constantly rub it at night.
16. Mmm.
    And I can still feel it, like I can still feel really tight.
17. On both sides?
    On both sides.

assessment phase of the treatment (the patient's responses are in italics below each of Joseph's numbered questions). There were in fact 70 questions in this phase of Joseph's assessment. I have included the first 17 only as they provide a representative sample of their style and content.

In Table 17.4, the questions are directed at defining and clarifying the site of pain (see e.g. questions 4, 9 and 11), establishing the cause and assessing the nature of the pain (Q5) and seeking the extent of the pain (Q6). The questions are a mix of both open (Q's 1, 5, 9) and closed questions, but the focus is clearly to define and classify the patient's symptomatology. It is particularly noticeable here that the patient's responses are mostly reduced to simple and non-expansive answers. Although the patient on several occasions began to tell her story or her interpretation of her problem (Q's 3, 4, 13), the questions from Joseph mostly focused on his more specific agenda. They do not follow the content introduced by the patient at the time it was introduced.

Following examination of the patient's movements, Joseph used palpation of the joints of the spine to further locate the source of the pain. This palpation of his patient's joints and spinal muscles merged into the actual treatment, involving mobilisation by physical pressure on particular spinal joints. The role of the patient during the treatment phase of the encounter shifted from answering questions to providing feedback about the physical effects of the treatment. Throughout these phases of treatment, Joseph is clearly in charge of the direction and focus of the communicative agenda.

Joseph's treatment highlighted two further phases of the clinical communication structure, common to all other participants in the research. They involved giving advice (Table 17.5) and instructing the patient on strategies for self-management (Table 17.6). In a study of discourse and decision-making in medical encounters, Elwyn et al.[23] collapsed these two phases into a single phase where 'decisions are made and future management agreed' (p. 478).

Although patients presented with a range of conditions, the communication structure and pattern was generally consistent across the data in this study. This structured approach to treatment is not a surprising finding of physiotherapy practice. It forms a core component of undergraduate and postgraduate physiotherapy programmes and it has been described in previous[24–26] and more recent studies of physiotherapy interactions.[17]

Table 17.5 Advice

165.	All right and then we will talk about some stretching exercise, both to your upper back.
	Yep.
166.	And also your chest.
	Yep.
167.	Because I find that maybe the way that you, you know, holding your baby and feeding your baby, that's one thing. Another one is that taking the pram in and out of the car, pushing and pulling the pram.
	Yep.
168.	All right .So that's another something that we have to discuss. Just stay where you are. I'll get you the hotpack. (pause) So did you feel the pain worse after the operation, I mean, propped up in the bed for a few days?
	Yes, very much.
169	Did you feel worse that time?
	Yeah, a lot.

Table 17.6 Self-management

180. Instead of just using your, you know the upper body strength. (pause) here now? *That feels good now.*
181. Ok. Now, you may get up and get dressed then we'll go for the exercises. *Ok.*
182. (long pause) Just work those six for you. Six exercises. The first one is to stretch your chest mainly, and through your upper back. So you find a corner and then you just move a foot or two from the corner and just let yourself sink into the corner. *Uh huh.*
183. And by doing this, you feel that you are stretching over your chest and also your upper back. *Ok.*
184. Ok? And then the second one is simple. You just put your hand behind and then you further stretch over your shoulder and also your chest. Now this one is quite important actually. *Mmm.*
185. Especially for you. For breast feeding because you are holding your baby like this all the time. *Yeah.*
186. And you become tight over your chest muscle. And you are hunching your back like this, right. So what I'd like you to do, if you find a door frame or something and hold your hand there, and try to stretch your chest muscle. *Yep.*
187. All right? You can try it now. You may be amazed that, how tight it is now. *Yeah. Just sort of hold it here?*

Joseph's treatment is characterised by a tone of certainty and rationality. There is a sense that the clinical puzzle, presented at the beginning of the treatment, had been satisfactorily dealt with. Importantly, the communication approach appeared to provide an inbuilt barrier between clinician and patient, with a particular role for the patient, to listen, answer questions and perform specified movements. However, the data also demonstrate some opportunities where the patient was able to break into the communicative agenda and structure set by the physiotherapist, illustrated by two examples below.

In the first example, Saul (therapist participant 9–T9) (Table 17.7) provides opportunities for the patient in the first phase (the subjective examination) to contribute her own opinion and concerns. There is a sense of space between questions and genuine interest from the therapist towards the patient where the patient is able to complete her answers to the questions.

In the second example, Jean (T4) began the subjective examination with an open question and allowed the patient (who seemed to be quite talkative by nature) freedom to answer (Table 17.8). Within the structure and phases of the communication, Jean's role was encouraging and expansive.

These two examples highlight how therapists did encourage patients to articulate their concerns; however, such opportunities did not change the overall focus and direction of the communicative agenda, which was to achieve a therapeutic outcome, or to solve a patient's problems.

ETHICS ANALYSIS

An overall finding of this study about how therapists communicate with their patients in the primary practice musculoskeletal treatment setting was that the communication was highly structured, with

Table 17.7 Breaks in communication structure

Yeah. So where exactly is your pain?
It's sort of above the (pause) above the pelvis and also down in (pause)
Into your buttock?
Yeah.
Because that's where you had it last time when you saw Narelle
Oh right, ok.
Yeah. Does it feel like it's the same sort of problem?
Yeah. Um…I thought for a little while that I was having um (pause) kidney problems but I think it's
just my back
Yeah, because it was higher for a while wasn't it?
Yes
Closer to your waist?
Yes
But that's now resolved?
Yes
Saul – T9 – 10 – 15

Table 17.8 Break in communication structure

How have you been since last week?
Well after my workout with you, that night it was terrible, I got home and I (pause) before I went to
bed I did those…the exercises and might have done it too much, I'm just not sure (pause) um, you
know (pause) there was the one where you put your foot on another, and that was a bad night, but
then the night before last I found I could lie on my side. That's the first time I've done that since
the 20th of February. So that was (pause) last night it wasn't bad either. So, I have two reasonably
good nights and I don't know if it's that particular exercise. And whenever I think of it I'm doing my
tummy pulling, but I found that very difficult to do but you said do it when you're bending over
(pause) well, you know, you just sort of (pause) I just don't seem to have the (pause) enough
(pause) I do it, you know, if I'm standing up, you know I can do it good and I can do it when I'm
sitting down coming in on the train I'm thinking of it.
Good.
You, know. I'm thinking of my posture a lot more too.
Well done. It will probably get easier to do it when you're doing activities as well and I guess it's, as
   much as anything it's almost on the return from bending over that you need to draw the tummy in
   to support the spine.
Mmmm.
So that's (pause)
When I'm doing the dishes (pause) well (pause) you know, I suppose it's the height or something,
but I feel, you know, that it's all falling forwards, you know, so that I can understand why you are
telling me to think of my posture.
Good.
Jean – T4 – 1 – 5

an emphasis on therapists directing the content and focus of the enquiry and solving patients' physical problems. The key question driving the ethical analysis of this communication was:

- What ethical ideals and assumptions about clinical practice underpin the types of information exchange and communication discourse between the therapist and the patient?

I suggest that the most visible ethical framework underpinning therapists' communication with their patients is one of beneficence. Therapists focused on accurately pinpointing the patient's presenting problem and assessing and providing a treatment within the available time frame. The focus and structure of the conversation aligned more closely with the paternalistic and informative models rather than the interpretive and deliberative models proposed by Emanuel and Emanuel (Table 17.1).[12] The phases of therapists' communication, which incorporated disclosure of information and explanation of clinical reasoning and treatment justification, were similar to the features of Howard Brody's[27] model of transparent communication where the therapist communicated their thinking and reasoning to the patient.

Although there were examples of breaks or gaps in the structure where patients were able to express their views and opinions, the dominant communication process was therapist-driven. This clinical focus and communication structure has been similarly identified in more recent studies of the physiotherapy primary practice treatment setting.[17,28,29] From an ethical perspective, the style of communication was less inclusive of ethical values such as promoting patients' autonomy through acknowledgement of their values, beliefs and contributions to the communication.[30,31]

Instead, the communication seemed to have the effect of limiting patients' autonomous contribution and shutting out conversation about their values and goals. The structure shows little alignment with models of ethical communication such as patient centredness where the patient and their individual concerns and circumstances are more centrally located within the treatment interaction[17,32], or shared decision-making where, according to Charles et al.[33], both parties (clinician and patient) take steps to participate in the process of treatment decision-making and both parties agree to the decision (p. 682). This is not to suggest that the practitioners in this study were completely unaware of these dimensions within the clinical encounter.[1] However, their taped interactions, recorded in one treatment encounter, demonstrate a very focused and clinician-driven conversation.

SUGGESTIONS FOR ENRICHING MUSCULOSKELETAL PHYSIOTHERAPY PRACTICE WITH ETHICAL THEORY

The bottom layers of the iceberg model (Figure 17.1) provide important concepts for reframing clinical communication in musculoskeletal physiotherapy practice. Using the ethical meaning of autonomy to guide communication in clinical practice means that a therapist needs to be aware of not only their patient's freedom to make a choice and contribute their views and values, but also their capacity to do so. At level 4, (Figure 17.1), Immanuel Kant's theories of autonomy highlight the importance of each person's inherent ability to reason and reflect as a basis of action.[6] John Stuart Mill defined autonomy according to its value in maximising happiness, emphasising a person's individual right to be free from interference in attaining what they regarded as well-being and happiness.[9] Applied to the specific and practical sphere of the healthcare context, Gerald Dworkin draws from these theories to suggest particular attention should be given to autonomy because of the embodied nature of people.[7] That is, 'the care of our bodies is linked with our identities as persons' and whatever 'goals or values we have are tied up with the fate of our bodies' (p. 113). By this, Dworkin is suggesting that as 'one's body is irreplaceable and inescapable' and because one's body 'is me', then it follows that 'failure to respect my wishes concerning my body is a particularly insulting denial of autonomy' (p. 113).

If Dworkin's account of autonomy was regarded as the supporting theoretical framework for informed consent specifically and communication more generally, then respecting patients' autonomy would involve the therapist explicitly seeking information from the patients about themselves and their perspectives rather than setting the communicative agenda according to a clinically defined perspective.

From this theoretical account of respect for autonomy, a patient's capacity and willingness to act autonomously depend not only on sharing information related to a specific decision but also on an awareness of more subtle barriers such as the influence of therapists' goals, treatment structure and the therapeutic relationship established within the clinical interaction itself.[34] To create an atmosphere of respect and partnership, Shaw and De Forge[15] suggest therapists' need to adopt a more 'tentative' (p. 427) approach to their knowledge, and practice claims to allow for other sources of knowledge, perspectives and views about clinical reasoning processes and clinical communication. This requires embracing the concept of professional reflexivity.

The term 'reflexivity' has traditionally been referred to research settings as a type of scrutiny and awareness of not only the research practices but also the factors that influence the researcher's construction of knowledge, such as their individual interpretations and ways of presenting findings.[35] Rice and Ezzy[36] describe reflexive research as a process of acknowledging 'that the researcher is part and parcel of the setting, context and culture they are trying to understand and analyse' (p. 41). I suggest that this same type of reflexivity is necessary for physiotherapists in considering their communication style with their patients. The ethical values and goals of practice that implicitly influence the methods of communication have a flow-on effect on a patient's actual ability to contribute autonomously in the clinical interaction. Therefore, in order to put into practice the ideals of an 'ethically enriched' communication process, physiotherapists need knowledge of the defining features and elements of theories of autonomy, beneficence and justice as well as knowledge of how their own clinical practice paradigms intersect with ethical theory. This reflexive and critical scrutiny of themselves and their ways of practising clinically and ethically are crucial.

ETHICAL VALUES AND HABITS OF CONVERSATION IN THE CLINICAL ENCOUNTER

Within the clinical encounter, and in the area of the iceberg which is visible and above the surface (Figure 17.1), imbuing clinical communication with ethical values requires practitioners to use specific words[37] and adopt particular conversational habits[34] which open up the agenda to allow the patient to contribute. Heritage et al.[37] studied the impact of using the words 'any' or 'some' within questions, inviting patients to express concerns beyond the primary reason for visiting the doctor. They found that if the question was posed as 'Is there something else you want to address in the visit today?' (the word 'some' has positive linguistic associations), patients were significantly more likely to express their unmet concerns than if the questions was posed as 'Is there anything else you want to address in the visit today?' ('any' has negative linguistic associations). Matthias et al.[34] delineated four categories of behaviours which critically influence whether patients are able to contribute their perspectives and share their real concerns in a clinical encounter. The first is to invest in the beginning of the encounter by creating a welcoming atmosphere to set a communication agenda where patient and clinician co-create priorities or areas of concern. The second habit is to elicit the patient's perspective by asking for their opinion and concerns and expectations of the treatment. The third habit is to express empathy by demonstrating an understanding and acknowledgement of the patient's experiences. The final habit is to invest in the end of the encounter by ensuring that the patient understands the diagnosis or treatment plan. This might be done by asking the patient to repeat in his or her own words, the clinician's instructions or information.

In the data presented in this chapter, there were some examples of eliciting the patient's perspective. However, there were few examples of demonstrating empathy, setting an agenda of partnership and shared decision-making. Instead, the data highlights a tendency for the musculoskeletal practitioner to tightly control the treatment and communication agenda. These findings resonate with the discussion about doctor/patient communication in Jay Katz's book *The Silent World of Doctor and Patient*.[38] Katz refers to 'doctors' millennia-long tradition of solitary decision-making' (p. 85). Resistance to change, according to Katz, is not solely based on unwavering certainty that 'clinician knows best', but on an awareness (conscious or subconscious) of the tensions inherent in sharing decisions with patients, such as the pervasive belief in professional authority and freedom from lay control. According to Katz, the values of the clinician are often homogenised to a catch-all phrase of 'medical judgment' and that this should be examined, or at the very least clinicians should be aware of the values behind the treatment he or she is proposing (p. 98). Moreover, he maintains that clinicians have previously tried to justify their preference for patients' trusting silence rather than conversation, in the belief that physicians and patients have an identical interest in medical matters, and this resonates with the assumptions of the informative and paternalistic models of communication (p. 98).

In framing his conversation model, Katz suggests a need for active reflection on values and motivations held by health professionals, and how they may influence communication (with a particular focus on obtaining informed consent). He points to four broad areas for reflection contained within the idea of a conversation model (p. 102). Firstly, that there is no single way of living with health or illness, or (translated to physiotherapy terms) disability or dysfunction. Alternative choices in medicine (and physiotherapy) must therefore be explained. Secondly, both physicians and patients bring their own vulnerabilities to the decision-making process, and as such 'both are authors and victims of their own individual conflicting motivations, interests and expectations' (p. 102). The third area is that parties should relate to each other as equals, rather than from the obvious and traditional pattern of parent-like caregiver and child-like receiver of care. Finally, there should be a willingness to explore both reasonable and non-reasonable decisions, values and judgments on the part of both the clinician and the patient.

CONCLUSION

In physiotherapy practice, there is a strong tradition of practice epistemologies based on biomechanical views of the body.[39] This has in turn shaped the communication strategies employed as part of the clinical reasoning process. In this chapter, I have sought to illuminate communication in primary practice musculoskeletal physiotherapy practice by exploring examples of clinical conversations and proposing possible underlying ethical assumptions. Musculoskeletal physiotherapy practice is a tightly focused clinical practice area, which draws strongly from deductive and diagnostic models of clinical reasoning. A prominent ethical focus is one of the physiotherapists benefitting the patient. Whilst this is an important and expected component of healthcare, I suggest there is room to include a richer substrate of ethical theory into such focused clinical interactions. Making room requires firstly, a greater understanding and awareness of the values and assumptions which underpin clinical practice, and secondly, an expanded conception (informed by theory and models of behaviour) of how respect for patient autonomy can be incorporated into everyday clinical communication.

REFERENCES

1. Delany C. In private practice, informed consent is interpreted as providing explanations rather than offering choices: A qualitative study. *Australian Journal of Physiotherapy* 2007;53:171–7.
2. *Australian Health Practitioner Regulation Agency—Home.* Available from: https://www.ahpra.gov.au/ (accessed July 24, 2017).
3. *APA | Code of Conduct.* Available from: https://www.physiotherapy.asn.au/APAWCM/The_APA/About_The_APA/APACode_of_Conduct.aspx?hkey=f2b9eddb-d561-4ad8-a2c0-6c6d0391c6c5 (accessed July 24, 2017).
4. *Code of conduct | The Chartered Society of Physiotherapy.* Available from: http://www.csp.org.uk/tagged/code-conduct (accessed July 24, 2017).
5. Beauchamp TL, Childress JF. *Principles of biomedical ethics.* New York: Oxford University Press; 2001.
6. Kant I. Groundwork of the metaphysics of morals (1785). In: Gregor M, editor. *Immanuel Kant groundwork of the metaphysics of morals.* Cambridge: Cambridge University Press; 1998.
7. Dworkin G. *The theory and practice of autonomy.* Cambridge: Cambridge University Press; 1988.
8. Young R. *Personal autonomy beyond negative and positive liberty.* London: Croom Helm; 1986.
9. Mill JS. *On liberty.* McCallum, editor. Oxford: Basil Blackwell; 1948.
10. Hope R, Savulescu J, Hendrick J. *Medical ethics and law: The core curriculum.* Elsevier Health Sciences, Edinburgh. 2008.
11. Edwards I, Delany C. Ethical reasoning. In: Higgs J, Jones M, Loftus S, Christensen N, editors. *Clinical reasoning in the health professions.* 3rd ed. Boston, MA: Elsevier; 2008, pp. 279–89.
12. Emanuel EJ, Emanuel LL. Four models of the physician-patient relationship. *JAMA* 1992;267(16):2221–6.
13. Wikström-Grotell C, Eriksson K. Movement as a basic concept in physiotherapy—A human science approach. *Physiotherapy Theory and Practice* 2012;28(6):428–38.
14. World Confederation for Physical Therapy. *Policy statement: Description of physical therapy.* London: WCPT; 2011.
15. Shaw JA, DeForge RT. Physiotherapy as bricolage: Theorizing expert practice. *Physiotherapy Theory and Practice* 2012;28(6):420–7.
16. Rothstein JM, Echternach JL. Hypothesis-oriented algorithm for clinicians a method for evaluation and treatment planning. *Physical Therapy* 1986;66(9):1388–94.
17. Hiller A, Guillemin M, Delany C. Exploring healthcare communication models in private physiotherapy practice. *Patient Education and Counseling,* **98**(10): 1222–1228. 2015.
18. Jones M, Jensen G, Rothstein JM. Clinical reasoning in physiotherapy. In: Higgs J, Jones M, editors. *Clinical reasoning in the health professions.* Oxford: Butterworth-Heinemann; 1995, pp. 72–87.
19. Edwards I, Jones M, Carr J, Braunack-Mayer A, Jensen GM. Clinical reasoning strategies in physical therapy. *Physical Therapy* 2004;84(4):312–30.
20. Jensen GM, Gwyer J, Shepard KF, Hack LM. Expert practice in physical therapy. *Physical Therapy* 2000;80(1):28–43.
21. Smart K, Doody C. The clinical reasoning of pain by experienced musculoskeletal physiotherapists. *Manual Therapy* 2007;12(1):40–9.

22. Charmaz K. *Constructing grounded theory*. Los Angeles, CA: Sage; 2014.

23. Elwyn G, Edwards A, Kinnersley P. Shared decision-making in primary care: The neglected second half of the consultation. *The British Journal of General Practice* 1999;49(443):477–82.

24. Haswell K, Gilmour J. Basic interviewing skills: How they are used by manipulative physiotherapists. *New Zealand Journal of Physiotherapy* 1997;25:11–15.

25. Thornquist E. Diagnostics in physiotherapy–processes, patterns and perspectives. Part II. *Advances in Physiotherapy* 2001;3(4):151–62.

26. Parry R. The interactional management of patients' physical incompetence: A conversation analytic study of physiotherapy interactions. *Sociology of Health & Illness* 2004;26(7):976–1007.

27. Brody H. Transparency: Informed consent in primary care. In: Arras J, Steinbock B, editors. *Ethical issues in modern medicine*. 5th ed. Mountain View: Mayfield Publishing Company; 1989, pp. 94–100.

28. Praestegaard J, Gard G. Ethical issues in physiotherapy–Reflected from the perspective of physiotherapists in private practice. *Physiotherapy Theory and Practice* 2013;29(2):96–112.

29. Solomon P, Miller PA. Qualitative study of novice physical therapists' experiences in private practice. *Physiotherapy Canada* 2005;57(3):190–8.

30. Charles C, Gafni A, Whelan T. Decision-making in the physician–patient encounter: Revisiting the shared treatment decision-making model. *Social Science & Medicine* 1999;49(5):651–61.

31. Delany C. Making a difference: Incorporating theories of autonomy into models of informed consent. *Journal of Medical Ethics* 2008;34(e3):1–5.

32. Kidd MO, Bond CH, Bell ML. Patients' perspectives of patient-centredness as important in musculoskeletal physiotherapy interactions: A qualitative study. *Physiotherapy* 2011;97(2):154–62.

33. Charles C, Gafni A, Whelan T. Shared decision-making in the medical encounter: What does it mean?(or it takes at least two to tango). *Social Science & Medicine* 1997;44(5):681–92.

34. Matthias MS, Salyers MP, Frankel RM. Re-thinking shared decision-making: Context matters. *Patient Education and Counseling* 2013;91(2):176–9.

35. Guillemin M, Gillam L. Ethics, reflexivity, and "ethically important moments" in research. *Qualitative Inquiry* 2004;10(2):261–80.

36. Rice PL, Ezzy D. *Qualitative research methods: A health focus*. Melbourne: Oxford University Press; 1999.

37. Heritage J, Robinson JD, Elliott MN, Beckett M, Wilkes M. Reducing patients' unmet concerns in primary care: The difference one word can make. *Journal of General Internal Medicine* 2007;22(10):1429–33.

38. Katz J. *The silent world of doctor and patient*. Baltimore, MD: JHU Press; 2002.

39. Nicholls D, Holmes D. Discipline, desire, and transgression in physiotherapy practice. *Physiotherapy Theory and Practice* 2012;28(6):454–65.

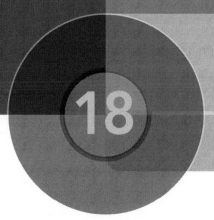

Power, prejudice and professionalism: Fat politics and medical education

18

JONATHON TOMLINSON

INTRODUCTION

The importance of knowing what patients think about professional attitudes and the experience of care has been highlighted by a *British Medical Journal* feature called, 'What your patient is thinking'.[1] In the first article in the series, the author describes how she is seen by health professionals 'as a fat person first and an individual second'. As the many rapid responses to the article demonstrate clinicians struggle to fulfil their duties to address patients' presenting concerns at the same time as attending to their risk of future disease. The attitudes and behaviour of medical students and health professionals towards patients, society and each other are core features of professionalism but also reflect both social and professional morality. Professionalism in practice is not fixed or defined by health regulators or professional colleges, but is challenged by our work and openly debated on social media by professionals with patients and the public. It is richer, more nuanced and more sensitive for it. Taking attitudes to obesity and obese patients as an illustrative case, I want to draw attention to the ways in which obesity, like many other risk factors for disease, remains a moral issue even though we attempt to treat it as a clinical issue. I discuss ways that can be used to help professionals raise awareness, insight and understanding of the moral attitudes that pervade our practice and how they relate to power and professionalism with reference to obesity and beyond.

TERMINOLOGY

The terms 'overweight', 'fat, obese', and so on mean different things to different people and in different contexts. In a clinical context, overweight, obese and severely obese each refers to a specified range of body mass index (BMI) values. The term 'morbid obesity' is equivalent to 'severe obesity' and denotes a BMI above 40. 'Grossly overweight' is a colloquialism also used unreflexively by professionals is if it were a clinical definition, specifying a BMI. Surveys of overweight patients and parents of overweight children have shown that in discussions with health professionals, they prefer terms like 'overweight' or 'weight problem' to 'obesity' or 'fat', or 'large size'.[2,3] Among 'fat activists', though the term 'fat' has been appropriated, and because this is about how power and politics interact with medicine, I have included 'fat' in the title and used it in the text aware that it may be perceived as pejorative if used by a medical professional or a thin person.[4] I also recommend reflecting on one's own perspectives and setting an example through role modelling. With this in mind, I hereby declare that I am a healthy, affluent, male, white doctor with a BMI of 25 who lives in close proximity to sporting facilities and cheap, nutritious food. I'm fortunate enough to have been a thin child who had a secure childhood in which home-grown food and sport were encouraged. I have had favourable social determinants of health.

I will use the terms referred to by the authors I am citing, but I am aware that there are no universally acceptable terms.

The literature refers to prejudice, bias, stigma and shame often interchangeably though they are not the same. For consistency, I have used prejudice except where specified.

PROFESSIONALISM AND MORAL OPPROBRIUM

Professionalism refers to the development of professional values, character and behaviour and is most effectively learnt through the interaction of students with role models as they go through their training.[5] One major limitation of this approach is its inward gaze and emphasis on learning from each other, rather than from the patients and communities that we are expected to serve.[6] Medicine is more than an applied science; it is a moral and social practice. It is informed by science no more or less than it is by values and culture of the profession and society beyond.[7]

Professional prejudice is particularly strong where patients are thought to have brought illness upon themselves or contributed to it, if they fail to do their bit by complying with medical advice and treatment, if they are difficult or impossible to treat or if their perceived weaknesses remind professionals of their own.

Prejudice against overweight patients is as prevalent among medical students, doctors and other health professionals as it is among the general public, and the more overweight patients are, the less respect their doctors show them. Even doctors who specialise in working with obese patients are as prejudiced as their peers. Although prejudice, stigma and anti-fat bias have been defined differently by various studies, they are usually characterised by a tendency to overemphasise individual behaviour while neglecting other factors.[8–13]

Self-identified 'fat' social scientist, Sophia Apostolidou, describes two categories available to fat people: 'the careless, or *immoral* lacking in self-respect 'fatties' who, despite their better knowledge, continue to criminally abuse their 'freedom'… and the *irrational* 'fatties, … guilty of 'fatlogic''.[14]

These categories of irrationality and immorality recur in the medical literature. For example, in the UK and the United States, primary care physicians reported viewing obese individuals as non-compliant (irrational) and weak-willed, and sloppy and lazy (immoral).[15] Over half of the US doctors also described them as unattractive, thereby failing in their moral duty to make themselves visually appealing. When prejudice is explicit and not just implicit, it is openly expressed and severely obese patients are more likely than any other group to bear the brunt of medical professionals' derogatory humour.[16]

CAUSES OF PREJUDICE

It is a popular assumption shared by public and professionals that being overweight or obese is the consequence of eating too much and exercising too little, the punishment shared by people guilty of the twin sins of gluttony and sloth. Modern narratives about an epidemic of obesity hold them to blame for overwhelming health services and under-mining the economy. In countries with higher rates of obesity, where there is more public discourse, prejudice is more prevalent.[17] Although in England, rates of obesity are falling in children and have been rising very slowly in the last 10 years in adults,[18] concerns have risen to the level of a moral panic, characterised by a *concern* about the threat to the econ-omy and health services, *hostility* in the form of moral outrage towards those responsible, *consensus* that something must be done, *disproportionality* in reports of harm and *volatility* in terms of panic.[19] Public health campaigns have fanned the moral panic by using the 'pedagogy of disgust'.[20] Not primarily pedagogic (educational), these campaigns attempt to provoke emotional responses which 'may include shame and humiliation, concern about appearing unattractive or sexually undesirable – and disgust'. Lupton links the emotional aspect with its moral counterpart:

> "Disgust is an unreasonable emotion because it projects our fear and anxiety about
> physical decay and death onto certain individuals and social groups, people who are
> already marginalised and stigmatised. Instead of attempting to reduce their social
> disadvantage, our disgust positions them as inferior. We turn away from them."

Medical prejudice reflects students' sense of self. Psychoanalyst David Bell notes the tendency to locate our weaknesses or vulnerabilities in others and project hostility towards these traits onto the people who possess them.[21] Medical students are selected for and tend to value highly traits that are necessary for successful entry into medical schools and their career. These include being self-directed, independent, rational and highly motivated. They internalise not only these traits but also the associated assumptions that success has far more to do with self-discipline and hard work, than social advantage, genetic-inheritance or good luck. Hostility, in the form of derogatory and cynical humour directed at over-weight patients may be a reflection of how students view themselves when they lack moti-vation or self-discipline.[16]

Another source of medical prejudice is due to health professionals' perceived helplessness in the face of overweight patients. This can come from their failure to help patients lose weight, in part because access to effective community programmes where social determinants might be addressed is limited. Weight-loss drugs which are easily accessible are expensive, marginally effective, have considerable side-effects and are often banned or restricted on safety grounds shortly after introduction.[22,23] Helplessness also stems from frustration that their therapeutic interventions, for example, surgery in morbidly obese patients, are more difficult and carry greater risks or are less effective.[24] Prejudice is exacerbated by frustration and obese patients are blamed for medicine's failings.

RATIONALITY, CHOICE AND EDUCATION

One policy response to the problem of *fatlogic* – the failure to act rationally – is to focus on individual behaviour, rather than the social conditions that shape the choices people make. A debate from the House of Commons in April 2014 illustrates the UK government's approach. In response to a question about reducing the amount of sugar in children's diets, the Under Secretary of State for Public Health stated, 'The Government believe we need to give people information. The Opposition believe in a top-down, state-driven approach'. Information alone does not address the social and economic circumstances that constrain choice.

Citizens are urged to understand obesity as a problem of individual biology and economic responsibility through the use of 'biopedagogies'.[25] Biopedagogies revolve around the moral regulation of bios or life whereby political power is exerted by moral pressure through regimes of scientific truth mediated by medical experts.[26] For example, when Daily Mail Doctor Ellie Cannon asserted that fat is 'quite simply a health issue', she implicitly denied obesity any political, social or other status. 'Fat', she wrote,

> "truth be told, is neither a feminist nor a cosmetic issue. It is, quite simply, a health issue. And we shouldn't allow ourselves to be steered into losing sight of that fact".[24]

MEDICALISING OBESITY

When Cannon defines obesity as 'simply' (and solely) a medical issue, she not only defines fat people as diseased but also defines what they are not, that is, for example, healthy, athletic, feminine, masculine, erotic, powerful or beautiful. Medicalisation raises the causative status of individual biology and behaviour relative to other social and economic factors such as sugar subsidies, fast-food advertising and car culture. Little is taught to medical students about the impact of adverse childhood experiences, in spite of their very strong association with obesity in adulthood.[27] In addition, medicalisation presents obesity as a *cause of* social and economic problems such as overwhelmed health systems and underperforming economies.[28] Medical students are taught very little about professional power or patient powerlessness and tend consequently to view empowerment as something doctors do with patients in a consultation, rather than a consequence of the social determinants of health.[29]

Medicalisation redefines risk factors as diseases, reduces the thresholds at which they are defined and widens the range of associated harms. Medicalisation is claimed to increase medical power but can lead to doctors feeling powerless in conditions like obesity when there is little they can do. Nevertheless, obesity has been medicalised to such an extent that there are few medical conditions for which it cannot be associated and therefore, blamed. Blame is medicalisation's remoralising tendency with the result that people draw on its medical impact to legitimise their prejudice by blaming obese patients for being a burden.

PATIENT RESPONSES TO STIGMA

A lot of the time professionals are unaware of their attitudes towards obese patients perhaps because 'prejudice tends to go unchecked when it operates by way of stereotypical images held in the collective social imagination'.[30] Unsurprisingly, however, patients pick up on it, with over 50% of patients reporting inappropriate comments from their doctor and over 80% of patients attending a dietetic clinic agreeing that 'weight is blamed for most medical conditions'.[31]

Clinicians exercise pastoral power, which means that more often than we realise, we exert moral approval or disdain upon our patients. Disapproval 'mobilises effects of shame and guilt'. When patients feel ashamed or stigmatised by health professionals, they trust them less and are less likely to reattend, which may even be the professional's conscious (or subconscious) aim.[32,33]

Another consequence of being made to feel ashamed is that patients who feel stigmatised because of being overweight or obese tend to comfort eating and gain weight.[34]

INTERVENTIONS TO REDUCE MEDICAL STUDENT PREJUDICE

A small number of interventions have been tried with modest benefits. Students who were shown a short film about weight bias in healthcare showed improvements in beliefs and attitudes towards obese patients.[35] A mixture of video, audio and written components resulted in first-year students being less likely to blame patients for being overweight a year after the intervention.[36] Students who read articles about stigma and communication before meeting a 'standardised obese patient' for 8 minutes showed small but significant improvements in stereotyping and empathy and large improvements in confidence in communication immediately afterwards but the stereotyping returned to baseline at 1 year.[37]

Other interventions to increase sensitivity and empathy in medical students have been tried with modest benefits.[38,39] If empathy is conceived as an emotional response in which judgement is suspended, interventions are unlikely to be successful, because critical judgement is part of nature and clinical practice. A better approach might be to raise insight and awareness about what emotions and moral judgements are already involved in clinical practice.[40] In discussing their study about patient-centred behaviour in medical students, Bombeke et al. concluded that 'raising students awareness of their personal attitudes might be a better learning goal than teaching better attitudes' because students may resist attempts to force them to be patient-centred.[41]

PROFESSIONALISM AND MEDICAL EDUCATION

The challenge is to help develop and sustain professional attitudes and behaviour which are resilient and responsive in the face of pressures of training, work and wider society. It is generally accepted that professional identity formation is a process of enculturation within which medical education plays a role along with the hidden curriculum and students' previously held vales. Understanding obesity as not only a medical but also a social, political issue can illuminate ways in which medicine is a moral practice. Thinking about medicine this way, as teachers, we should make explicit medicine's political and moral dimensions. One way we can do this is by encouraging students to explore the experiences of people for whom obesity is not simply or solely a medical issue.

In medical education, patients are allowed to speak or teach only when they are invited to by clinicians and educators. Only certain types of patients are invited, for example, those whose medical problems exemplify the dangers of being overweight. What patients are allowed to talk about is often restricted to the facts the doctor or student wants to know, in order to complete a medical history. This control of patients' narratives is described by philosopher Havi Carel as 'epistemic injustice'. According to Carel, testimonial justice requires us to let patients tell their own story and hermeneutic justice requires us to invite patients to offer their own interpretations; epistemic justice requires both. Injustice results because of differences in power between patients and professionals, a lack of awareness that injustice exists and a lack of resources, especially time.[30]

Epistemic justice enables patients to share their lived experiences, what Carel also calls phenomenology or embodied experiences, for example, what it's like to be on the receiving end of social and professional attitudes, as a fat person. More is needed, in part because patients may never feel comfortable telling us what they really think, but also if we are to appreciate patients' experiences not only as patients but also as people of culture, gender, history, and so on. We need to examine narratives from outside the consulting room. In *Illness as Narrative*, Ann Jurecic explains,

> If one of the consequences of modernity is that we no longer depend on traditional explanations for suffering, loss and morality, and if doctors' offices and hospitals cannot function as spaces where personal meaning can be developed, then the existential questions about human fragility and significance have to be asked and answered elsewhere.[42]

The internet offers spaces for other voices, for example, the 'Fat health' blog where patients share stories about being ashamed by healthcare professionals, and Lashings of Ginger Beer Time (LGBT) blog about gender, queer and transpolitics and fat acceptance.[43] The LGBT blog invites 'guest posts from people with lived experiences we haven't explored', explicitly highlighting the role of digital spaces for epistemic justice. Encouraging students to engage with social media by reading blogs like this can help them explore narratives, not only in relation to obesity but other experiences of health and illness, for example, blogs written by people with mental illnesses, cancer or diabetes.

The aim of this critical engagement is described by Dasgupta as narrative humility.

> Narrative humility acknowledges that our patients' stories are not objects that we can comprehend or master, but rather dynamic entities that we can approach and engage with, while simultaneously remaining open to their ambiguity and contradiction, and engaging in constant self-evaluation and self-critique about issues such as our own role in the story, our expectations of the story, our responsibilities to the story, and our identifications with the story – how the story attracts or repels us because it reminds us of any number of personal stories.[44]

Such an approach to medical education is designed to reveal medicine's controlling tendencies, not only with regard to obesity and fat-politics but also towards other patients and conditions. It compliments evidence for teaching professionalism, which favours a mixture of role-modelling and reflective practice. Reflection requires the dissonance that comes from realising one's attitudes and behaviour aren't what you thought they were and a commitment to consider seriously why that is. The fact that so few professionals are aware of their fat prejudice emphasises the importance of a thick conception of reflective practice in which insight is gained through the critical analysis of knowledge gained from personal reflection, patient narratives, peer discussion and academic and other literature.

A positive conception of professional power is that power and knowledge are co-created by patients and professionals through 'therapeutic alliances' through which kindness, commitment, interpretation, bearing witness and advocacy all play important roles. Power is not only a malign force, as even Foucault argued, 'It needs to be considered as a productive network that runs through the whole social body much more than a negative instance whose function is repression'.[45] Mol has argued that medical power is both structural and symbolic and socially conferred and is a necessary part of the therapeutic relationship, especially in the care of patients with chronic conditions.[46]

Role modelling is a particularly problematic aspect of professionalism training for the simple reason that most role models that students are exposed to are outside the jurisdiction of the medical school. Learners experience good as well as bad role models and complain that they are not exposed to enough good ones, for example, 34% of medical students complained that a lack of role models was a barrier to learning about empathy.[47] Attributes that students value in their role models include not only value clinical competence but also teaching skills, concern for the doctor–patient relationship and attention to the social determinants of health.[48] The problem of how to increase students' exposure to good role models arises partly because of the unchallenged assumption that role models are people students should look up to. In practice, this refers to an authoritarian hierarchy which makes it hard for students to challenge behaviour that is perceived to be unprofessional. A second problem is the concept of poor role models as bad eggs, and professionalism as an issue of individual behaviour rather than a team or institution-based set of values and behaviours. One potential solution is for role modelling to be learnt as an aspect of professionalism by all clinicians in facilitated, non-hierarchical, small discussion groups. This gives greater emphasis to the importance of teamwork, shared responsibility and learning and mutual support that makes participants active in their own professional identity formation. Within this it is implied, but can also be made explicit, that students and clinicians *all* act as role models to those around them. A model of group support that enables staff of all backgrounds and levels to come together and talk about how they are affected by caring for the same patients, called Schwartz rounds, is already taking place at over 300 English NHS institutions at the time of writing – and is being steadily spread to other institutions.[49]

CONCLUSIONS

By presenting medical student and physician attitudes towards obesity, I have argued that the medicalisation of obesity shows that medical professionals share and contribute to a remoralising of social attitudes. In their relationships, they have the power to control the stories that patients are allowed to tell, restricting them to particular medical narratives to the exclusion of other interpretations. Without reflection, this leads to the entrenchment of attitudes, preservation of hierarchy and a lack of self-awareness. By teaching and learning about power, prejudice, epistemic justice and narrative humility, we can illuminate these problems in a way that has immediate practical benefits for patients and professionals and can make care more humane and effective.

ACKNOWLEDGEMENTS

With thanks to Professor Trisha Greenhalgh at Barts and the London, Dr Aileen Patterson at Trinity College, Dublin, and Dr Elspeth Graham at Liverpool John Moores University for encouragement, support and interest.

REFERENCES

1. Lewis E. Why there's no point telling me to lose weight. *BMJ* 2015;**350**:g6845–g6845. doi: 10.1136/bmj.g6845.

2. Wadden TA, Didie E. What's in a name? Patients' preferred terms for describing obesity. *Obes Res* 2003;**11**:1140–6. doi: 10.1038/oby.2003.155.

3. Gray CM, Hunt K, Lorimer K, et al. Words matter: A qualitative investigation of which weight status terms are acceptable and motivate weight loss when used by health professionals. *BMC Public Health* 2011;**11**:513. doi: 10.1186/1471-2458-11-513.

4. Lupton D. *Can a thin person write about fat? | This Sociological Life on WordPress.com. This Sociological Life.* 2012. http://simplysociology.wordpress.com/2012/08/27/can-a-thin-person-write-about-fat/ (accessed 6 October 2014).

5. Birden H, Glass N, Wilson I, et al. Teaching professionalism in medical education: A Best Evidence Medical Education (BEME) systematic review. BEME Guide No. 25. *Med Teach* 2013;**35**:e1252–66. doi: 10.3109/0142159X.2013.789132.

6. DasGupta S, Fornari A, Geer K, et al. Medical education for social justice: Paulo Freire revisited. *J Med Humanit* 2006;**27**:245–51. doi: 10.1007/s10912-006-9021-x.

7. Montgomery K. *How doctors think : Clinical judgment and the practice of medicine: Clinical judgment and the practice of medicine.* 1st ed. Oxford University Press; 2006. http://books.google.co.uk/books/about/How_Doctors_Think_Clinical_Judgment_and.html?id=TPg_MQEcq0gC&pgis=1 (accessed 8 December 2014).

8. Miller DP, Spangler JG, Vitolins MZ, et al. Are medical students aware of their anti-obesity bias? *Acad Med* 2013;**88**:978–82. doi: 10.1097/ACM.0b013e318294f817.

9. Foster GD, Wadden TA, Makris AP, et al. Primary care physicians' attitudes about obesity and its treatment. *Obes Res* 2003;**11**:1168–77. doi: 10.1038/oby.2003.161.

10. Blumberg P, Mellis LP. Medical students' attitudes toward the obese and the morbidly obese. *Int J Eat Disord* 1985;**4**:169–75. doi: 10.1002/1098-108X(198505)4:2<169::AID-EAT2260040204> 3.0.CO;2-F.

11. Swift JA, Hanlon S, El-Redy L, et al. Weight bias among UK trainee dietitians, doctors, nurses and nutritionists. *J Hum Nutr Diet* 2013;**26**:395–402. doi: 10.1111/jhn.12019.

12. Schwartz MB, Chambliss HO, Brownell KD, et al. Weight bias among health professionals specializing in obesity. *Obes Res* 2003;**11**:1033–9. doi: 10.1038/oby.2003.142.

13. Puhl RM, Latner JD, King KM, et al. Weight bias among professionals treating eating disorders: Attitudes about treatment and perceived patient outcomes. *Int J Eat Disord* 2014;**47**:65–75. doi: 10.1002/eat.22186.

14. Apostolidou S. *The F-word: From failed Homo-economicus to fat-posthumanist.* 2014. http://www.academia.edu/10069227/The_F_Word_From_Failed_Homo_Economicus_to_Fat_Posthumanist (accessed April 1, 2017).

15. Epstein L, Ogden J. A qualitative study of GPs' views of treating obesity. *Br J Gen Pract* 2005;**55**:750–4.

16. Wear D, Aultman JM, Varley JD, et al. Making fun of patients: Medical students' perceptions and use of derogatory and cynical humor in clinical settings. *Acad Med* 2006;**81**:454–62. doi: 10.1097/01.ACM.0000222277.21200.a1.

17. Marini M, Sriram N, Schnabel K, et al. Overweight people have low levels of implicit weight bias, but overweight nations have high levels of implicit weight bias. *PLoS One* 2013;**8**:e83543. doi: 10.1371/journal.pone.0083543.

18. HSCIC. *Statistics on obesity, physical activity and diet: England 2014.* 2014. http://www.hscic.gov.uk/catalogue/PUB13648/Obes-phys-acti-diet-eng-2014-rep.pdf (accessed April 1, 2017).

19. Campos P, Saguy A, Ernsberger P, et al. The epidemiology of overweight and obesity: Public health crisis or moral panic? *Int J Epidemiol* 2006;**35**:55–60. doi: 10.1093/ije/dyi254.

20. Lupton D. The pedagogy of disgust: The ethical, moral and political implications of using disgust in public health campaigns. *Crit Public Health* 2015;**25**:1–14. doi: 10.1080/09581596.2014.885115.

21. Bell D. Primitive mind of state. *Psychoanal Psychother* 1996;**10**:45–57. doi: 10.1080/02668739600700061.

22. Glandt M, Raz I. Present and future: Pharmacologic treatment of obesity. *J Obes* 2011;**2011**:636181. doi: 10.1155/2011/636181.

23. Doyle SL, Lysaght J, Reynolds JV. Obesity and post-operative complications in patients undergoing non-bariatric surgery. *Obes Rev* 2010;**11**:875–86. doi: 10.1111/j.1467-789X.2009.00700.x.

24. Foucault M. *The birth of the clinic: An archaeology of medical perception.* Routledge; 1973. http://books.google.co.uk/books/about/The_Birth_of_the_Clinic.html?id=05hERJhxg04C&pgis=1 (accessed 2 November 2014).

25. Rail G, Lafrance M. Confessions of the flesh and biopedagogies: Discursive constructions of obesity on Nip/Tuck. *Med Humanit* 2009;**35**:76–9. doi: 10.1136/jmh.2009.001610.

26. Cannon E. As a doctor I have to tell you that two of these models are too FAT to represent 'real women'. *Daily Mail.* 2012. http://www.dailymail.co.uk/femail/article-2224164/As-doctor-I-tell-models-FAT-represent-real-women-Women-wanting-wobbly-bits-promoting-obesity-says-outspoken-critic.html#ixzz2Av0gv1vB (accessed 16 October 2014).

27. Stevens JE. *The Adverse Childhood Experiences Study—The largest, most important public health study you never heard of—began in an obesity clinic.* Aces Too High. https://acestoohigh.com/2012/10/03/the-adverse-childhood-experiences-study-the-largest-most-important-public-health-study-you-never-heard-of-began-in-an-obesity-clinic/ (accessed 27 February 2017).

28. Link BG, Phelan J. Social conditions as fundamental causes of disease. *J Health Soc Behav* 1995;**Spec No**:80–94. http://www.ncbi.nlm.nih.gov/pubmed/7560851 (accessed 15 September 2014).

29. Donetto S. Medical students' views of power in doctor-patient interactions: The value of teacher-learner relationships. *Med Educ* 2010;**44**:187–96. doi: 10.1111/j.1365-2923.2009.03579.x.

30. Carel H, Kidd IJ. Epistemic injustice in healthcare: A philosophical analysis. *Med Health Care Philos* 2014;**17**:529–40. doi: 10.1007/s11019-014-9560-2.

31. Puhl RM, Heuer CA. The stigma of obesity: A review and update. *Obesity (Silver Spring)* 2009;**17**:941–64. doi: 10.1038/oby.2008.636.

32. Neill SJ, Cowley S, Williams C. The role of felt or enacted criticism in understanding parent's help seeking in acute childhood illness at home: A grounded theory study. *Int J Nurs Stud* 2013;**50**:757–67. doi: 10.1016/j.ijnurstu.2011.11.007.

33. Gudzune KA, Bennett WL, Cooper LA, et al. Patients who feel judged about their weight have lower trust in their primary care providers. *Patient Educ Couns* 2014;**97**:128–31. doi: 10.1016/j.pec.2014.06.019.

34. Jackson SE, Beeken RJ, Wardle J. Perceived weight discrimination and changes in weight, waist circumference, and weight status. *Obesity (Silver Spring)* 2014;22:2485–8. doi: 10.1002/oby.20891.

35. Poustchi Y, Saks N, Piasecki A, et al. Brief intervention effective in reducing weight bias in medical students. *Fam Med* 2013;**45**:345–8.

36. Wiese HJ, Wilson JF, Jones RA, et al. Obesity stigma reduction in medical students. *Int J Obes Relat Metab Disord* 1992;**16**:859–68.

37. Kushner RF, Zeiss DM, Feinglass JM, et al. An obesity educational intervention for medical students addressing weight bias and communication skills using standardized patients. *BMC Med Educ* 2014;**14**:53. doi: 10.1186/1472-6920-14-53.

38. Afghani B, Besimanto S, Amin A, et al. Medical students' perspectives on clinical empathy training. *Educ Health (Abingdon)* 2011;**24**:544.

39. Chen I, Forbes C. Reflective writing and its impact on empathy in medical education: Systematic review. *J Educ Eval Health Prof* 2014;**11**:20. doi: 10.3352/jeehp.2014.11.20.

40. Charon R. Narrative medicine: A model for empathy, reflection, profession and trust. *JAMA* 2001;**286**:1897. doi: 10.1001/jama.286.15.1897.

41. Bombeke K, Symons L, Vermeire E, et al. Patient-centredness from education to practice: The 'lived' impact of communication skills training. *Med Teach* 2012;**34**:e338–48. doi: 10.3109/0142159X.2012.670320.

42. Jurecic A. *Illness as narrative*. 2012. http://litmed.med.nyu.edu/Annotation?action=view&annid=14173 (accessed 13 October 2014).

43. LGBT. *Lashings of ginger beer time blog*. 2014. http://lashingsofgb.blogspot.co.uk/ (accessed 13 October 2014).

44. DasGupta S. Narrative humility. *Lancet* 2008;**371**:980–1. doi: 10.1016/S0140-6736(08)60440-7.

45. Foucault M, Gordon C. *Power/knowledge : Selected interviews and other writings, 1972–1977*. Pantheon Books, New York. 1980.

46. Mol A. *The logic of care: Health and the problem of patient choice*. Routledge; 2008. https://books.google.com/books?id=Val7oyGtCFsC&pgis=1 (accessed 12 March 2015).

47. Hendelman W, Byszewski A. Formation of medical student professional identity: Categorizing lapses of professionalism, and the learning environment. *BMC Med Educ* 2014;**14**:139. doi: 10.1186/1472-6920-14-139.

48. Wright SM, Kern DE, Kolodner K, et al. Attributes of excellent attending-physician role models. *N Engl J Med* 1998;**339**:1986–93. doi: 10.1056/NEJM199812313392706.

49. Point of Care Foundation. *Point of Care Foundation—Schwartz rounds*. 2013. http://www.pointofcarefoundation.org.uk/Schwartz-Rounds/ (accessed 20 October 2014).

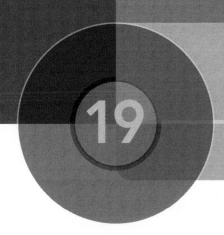

Genethics and genomics in the community

19

IMRAN RAFI AND JOHN SPICER

INTRODUCTION

In this chapter, we explore some of the aspects of what is often termed the 'new genetics' as applied to primary care (and specifically general practice) in the British National Healthcare Service (NHS). Genetics, the study of heritability, has promised much over recent years to the personalised care of patients, perhaps more than it has actually delivered. It has moved from the laboratory to the clinic and also promises to move to the community setting too, and in doing so holds challenges for all primary care clinicians. The ethical challenges of genetics (represented in the *portmanteau* term 'Genethics')[1,2] are no different in the community to anywhere else, though they may be differently described: this is the content of the chapter, along with some necessary technical issues.[3] Genomics, a more often used term in current literature and not qualitatively very different to genetics, reflects a more holistic understanding of the influence of the genome on health, science and future promise.

NEW TECHNOLOGIES 1

The 20,000 genes we carry in each cell are collectively the genome, comprising the exome (which does the protein coding) and the rest. Today, we can sequence the whole genome [whole genome sequencing (WGS)] including RNA or, being less costly, the exome [whole exome sequencing (WES)]. The methodologies and techniques behind sequencing technology can be used to identify high-risk genes such as BRCA1, associated with breast cancer, or rare gene variants such as those for developmental disorders. The findings from WGS or WES may affect reproductive choices or indeed treatment choices for various diseases in the future. It is likely that in years to come, the impact of these aspects of genomics will find a way into primary health care as our patients who undergo such tests seek help and advice, so that some understanding of what is now a large literature on genethics should be useful to a primary care clinician. Sequencing speed and accuracy is increasing and this makes determining the likelihood of pathogenicity much easier. Some costs are falling, making direct-to-consumer testing a reality, and others are extremely high, meaning that the techniques are available in the experimental and private healthcare settings only. Nonetheless, clinical utility may be difficult to determine. Variants of uncertain significance inevitably arise, the genomic equivalent of the clinically unclassifiable abnormality in a complex patient, which exemplifies a disjunction between individual genotype (the genetic code) and phenotype (the physical expression of the code).[4]

The argument can be made that genomic information is different from other kinds of biological data. It constitutes personal identity and has the potential to be predictive, diagnostic and even stigmatising.[5] Also of concern is the fact that genetic information identified by testing should not be used as a mechanism of unjust discrimination. In the United States, the *Genetic Information Non-discrimination Act* has established protection for citizens against employment and health insurance discrimination. Interestingly, it does not protect against life insurance premium loading on genetic grounds.[6] There is no concept of genetic discrimination in UK law.

In introducing DNA or RNA sequencing into mainstream healthcare practice, cost-effectiveness will be an important factor in the offering of genome sequencing through accredited laboratories, and economic analysis of clinical pathways will be necessary. In the UK, the UK Genetics Testing Network defines best practice in these areas where testing for prediction, pre-natal testing and diagnosis is needed.[7]

The mainstreaming of genomics into the UK NHS is a challenge for policymakers and educationalists which includes primary care. Accordingly, the ethical impact of these techniques in the primary healthcare setting is included in educational materials for UK general practice trainees.[8] Understanding new clinical pathways of care and the role of the non-genetics specialist can be challenging for all clinicians but having information available to primary care, enabling meaningful and informative discussions with patients exposed to genomic technology will be particularly important. Collins has usefully summarised the areas where clinicians should be mindful of the ethics of genomics, which are as follows:

The ethico-legal and social implications of the Human Genome Project[9]
- Understanding and exploring the concept of genetic variation.
- Integration of genetic technologies and information into healthcare and public health activities.
- Understanding the importance of gene–environment interactions.
- Understanding the philosophical, theological and ethical perspectives using genomic information.
- Consideration of the socio-economic factors and how concepts of race and ethnicity influence the use, understanding and interpretation of genetic information.

Applied ethical principles guide clinical management and counselling regarding reproductive choices and the use of targeted drug therapies. As genomics becomes mainstreamed into clinical practice, clinicians will need to continue to consider some of the theoretical perspectives available. For example, from the consequentialist position, a raw summation of the harms and benefits attached to a genomic intervention offers one method of ethical analysis. Inevitably, such moral calculus is necessarily constrained by deontologically derived positions such as the clinical duty of care, or the respect for autonomy. The modern principlist approach to ethical reasoning, described more fully elsewhere in this book, and characterised by respect for autonomy, beneficence , non-maleficence and justice, is perhaps more familiar when faced with decisions based on genomics information. Such principles can be addressed to some of these genomic issues: the equity of access to WGS/WES genomic technology and testing, offering and respecting patient autonomy in their decisions in managing their own genomic information will be important. The challenges for physicians will be to ensure that data are stored securely on information systems, and that discussions with patients reflect the concerns they may have around family access to genomic data or secondary access by insurance companies.

VARIATION AND UNCERTAINTY

Most relevant conditions that are presented to primary care are complex multifactorial conditions such as heart disease, cancer and mental health disorders (e.g. schizophrenia) all of which reflect gene–environment interactions, environmental or linkage to social deprivation. Inevitably, the care of patients with these conditions is an uncertain process; elsewhere in this book, we have described uncertainty as being a key feature of primary care. Uncertainty in diagnosis, for example, could be reduced in the future, as those multifactorial disorders are more accurately defined in nosological terms.

Penetrance describes the probability of an abnormal gene causing a linked phenotype and thus, highly penetrant genes exist. Examples here would include Huntington's disease. In Huntington's disease, those carrying an altered *Huntingtin* gene have a 100% chance of developing dementia in later age (in other words, it is highly penetrant and deterministic) and have a 50% chance of transmitting the altered gene to their children. So, immediately in dealing with this sort of less uncertain condition there are issues of confidentiality, of the possibility of screening pregnancies for affected foetuses and the use of preimplantation genetic diagnosis for the 'best' interests of the next generation even though this is a condition of late-onset, and so on.

Genetics by its very nature describes the variation between individuals, manifested as the phenotype. Such variation is clearly less both genetically and phenotypically in families, so it is apposite to note that this has enormous ethical importance. Quite apart from any evolutionary need, we may have to ensure the continuation of our genomes down the generations, and our genomic closeness to our relatives may imply a degree of responsibility to them also. So, those clinicians who care for families over their life course in primary care have a unique association with a clinical manifestation of their genomic 'disorders'. Thus, the decision on whether to screen the children of a Huntington's patient as above is one taken ultimately by the index case, but it can be informed by discussion with both the genetic specialist and those who know the patient and family over time. The long-term care of such a patient is inevitably coordinated by the generalist with whom he is registered, and this may have impact on such decision-making. Perhaps both should be ethical specialists?

NEW TECHNOLOGIES 2

Genomic-wide association studies (GWAS) have been used to assess rare variants in common disease using a case-control, statistical methodology.[10] GWAS has demonstrated many traits for common diseases such as inflammatory bowel disease but not much heritability was explained probably because of undiscovered rare variants.[11,12] Moreover, the public may have an overexpectation of the value of genomic data, an overexpectation which could need tempering.[13] To date, commercial companies have offered genetic diseases and pharmacogenetics data based on the result of GWAS to people who want to exercise their right (and pay) to access their own genomic information. Data have been produced on the basis of the analysis and variation at the level of single-nucleotide polymorphisms (markers of genetic similarity that are usually abbreviated to the demotic 'SNiP'). The issues around the clinical utility and validity of this sort of data and a lack of non-directive pretesting genetic counselling that occurs in the NHS may lead to subsequent re-engagement, surveillance and management through the NHS. Data validation maybe required and the potential harms of being provided with genomic information, where the clinical utility may vary or be determined to be low, need to be considered. For example, a consumer tested and being told that there is no genetic risk of obesity may lead to lifestyle choices that actually increase the risk of obesity through false reassurance, particularly where a strong family history of obesity may be present. Other than that, it is not yet clear whether there is any utility in persons knowing, for example, how much of their genome might be of Neanderthal origin.[14] Genomic knowledge has even been classed as entertainment, a challenging notion for the utilitarian.[15] As such, this sort of knowledge is analogous to the biochemical or haematological analyses provided for fee-paying patients by some private sector laboratories, and liable to be of limited effect in future healthcare.

More fundamentally, the 100,000 Genomes Project, led by Genomics England Ltd. (GEL), is an ambitious programme of translational research using next-generation sequencing technology to sequence DNA of patients affected with cancers, infectious diseases and rare diseases.

GEL have ensured a robust consent process for the 100K Project that enables healthcare professionals to manage the complexity of the data provided through sequencing, including the management of incidental findings not routinely being fed back to patients(*infra*).

Incidental findings are 'additional findings concerning a patient or research participant that may, or may not, have potential health implications and clinical significance, that are discovered during the course of a clinical or research investigation, but are beyond the aims of the original test or investigation'.[16]

The importance of an informed and voluntary consent model is of paramount importance and provides the necessary patient autonomy to participate or not. Genomic information will be seen by many as personal and sensitive, and the confidentiality of the information being generated and held will be highly important. Researchers in this setting will have a duty of care to ensure that participants have the right to withdraw. Participants would want to ensure that information governance is respected. One particular challenge for GEL would be to ensure that there is equity of access to testing. Clinicians and researchers in the project must recognise that the use of WGS may reap a benefit, and even beneficence, in terms of new diagnosis or treatment options but that the harm (maleficence) to patients or their families may be considerable through the gain of genomics knowledge that may be psychologically harmful.

Whole exome sequencing does allow targeted sequencing and minimises the number of incidental findings through the use of gene panels. These are defined areas of gene sequencing known to be associated with a particular disorder, for example, deafness or cardiomyopathy. In the case of the 100,000 Genomes Project, a set of guidelines regarding consent and insurance are operated – none of this is contentious – but there are yet no clear procedures for the handling of 'surprise' results. One might reasonably argue that the transition of such clinically relevant information via a clinician with prior knowledge of the client might be the best practice.[17] Yet, there is a duty of care to the patient and an ethical framework should be in place for any policy decision made in this setting. The management of incidental findings will need a decision on whether the laboratory reports the finding to a requesting clinician or whether the patient receives this. Arguably, it may require a prior discussion on what this might mean, including gaining knowledge that could also have an effect on other family members subject to a risk, say, of diabetes or heart disease. What is opened up here is an account of the 'ownership' of genomic information; as stated above, this kind of personal information is anything but personal, having an importance to any related individual.[18,19] For the primary care clinician, that may involve a duty of care to both the index case and family members, carrying as she does a responsibility to all.[20]

TOWARDS PERSONALISED MEDICINE

The future holds potential for an increase in phenotyping diseases and subclassifying complex diseases, exemplified by hypertension and renal disease. Analysing the value and statistical power of multiple genes all together which have been associated with a particular phenotype (e.g. heart disease) could occur more frequently.

An example of such personalised medicine is of cancer treatment based on cancer genomic profiling, tumour mutational profiling and molecular signatures of somatic mutations. All of these use information based around gene mutations on treatment options and offer the use of targeted therapies. This, however, may be restricted may be on resource grounds; the technology underlying tumour profiling of this sort is currently expensive, and probably not accessible in a resource-constrained system such as the UK NHS. Here also opens the potential for individuals not being offered therapies that have been shown to have efficacy as 'they are deemed to be genetically different'. One who is denied treatment on the grounds of genomic indication of inefficacy could be held to have suffered a double jeopardy.

Reproductive options using genomic information are expected to become increasingly available within the NHS.[21] A good example of this is the use of circulating cell-free foetal DNA analysis,[22] which will allow diagnosis of rhesus status and provide a risk of haemolytic disease of the newborn and Down's syndrome. Here, the technology allows the study of fragments of circulating DNA in the maternal circulation produced by the foetus, which is specific for that particular pregnancy. The test, a simple blood test, is non-invasive compared to the use of amniocentesis, and without the risk of miscarriage. It can provide a risk estimate of the risk of a Downs carrying pregnancy and offer a choice early in terms of continuing with the pregnancy or proceeding with termination of the pregnancy. Avoiding a live birth affected by a genetic condition such as Downs's syndrome offers reproductive autonomy but does open up many potential discussions. It can also reliably detect the genetic sex of the foetus. At the time of writing this, non-invasive prenatal testing is the subject of consideration by the Nuffield Council on Bioethics, led by a bioethicist who himself has a diagnosis of a genetic disorder.[23,24]

This includes equality of access to testing (including preimplantation testing for many genetic conditions, e.g. muscular dystrophy), prenatal testing and considering the rights of the embryo, overriding the rights of the woman, social engineering and eugenics, and procreative beneficence (the putative moral duty to have the best children possible)[25] It is relatively easy to cast the access issue in the more general ethical terms that all resource allocation decisions are made,[26] and the reader is directed to the last section of this book to consider this further. However, the advancement of personalised medicine in this genomic context may be fraught with what two authors have termed a 'capability' – based upon the degree to persons may vary in realising better health options from genetic testing.[27]

How, it may be asked, can primary care add to the ethical thinking around these complex issues? At the point of first access with the clinician, the patient subject to a decision as described in this context is in a very difficult position. Certainly in developed countries, the move to non-invasive methods of assessing the risk of serious foetal malformation is at first sight a vast improvement, as now the risk of carrying a Downs pregnancy can be assessed without risk to the pregnancy continuing. The technology underlying such a process is the field of the specialist, but its interpretation and subsequent decision-making perhaps better handled in the context of a long-term relationship between patient and clinician. Procreative benefi-cence would suggest, or even dictate, that a pregnancy that leads to an outcome worse than a better alternative is morally objectionable, and therefore, that all pregnancies of potentially malformed foetuses should be terminated. However, such a rule does not square necessarily with patients' own moral positions, which may encompass a different value to foetuses, respect for sanctity of life, disability rights or a host of other perspectives. Teasing these values out, as part of a patient decision-making process, is the stuff of primary care as well as the skill of a genetic counsellor.

WGS has been of value when looking at multiple affected family members affected by devel-opmental disorders underpinned by a genetic basis as in DECIPHER (DatabasE of genomiC variation and Phenotype in Humans using Ensemble Resources[28]). A genetic diagnosis could include a syndrome of potential complications including learning disability; however, this does not mean that there should be a loss of personal autonomy for those affected, which may include declining treatment options or taking difficult reproductive decisions. An example of this is familial hypercholesterolemia (FH): a diagnosis affecting multiple family members, and tests might include identifying family members at risk through cascade testing (which includes a DNA test).[29] In the case of FH (an autosomal-dominant condition), over 1000 gene variants have been identified and the reliance on good gene variant databases is of importance, both in terms of accurate data and also identifying pathogenic and benign variants. FH is also a disorder which has moved, in terms of its management, from the specialist to the general-ist in recent years. It is very treatable, with good evidence for benefit where the genomically identified severity can be defined. Thus, it is an example of where the laboratory, the specialist geneticist and the generalist physician, should be closely linked.

PREVENTION AND SCREENING

Predictive genomics that supports prevention can be applied either at a personal (e.g. BRCA, breast cancer gene panels, heart disease or cancer risk stratification) or population level [e.g. haemoglobinopathies, diabetes such as high-prevalence populations of maturity onset of diabetes of the young (MODY)] or stratified screening for cancer in the future.[30]

Using pharmacogenetics for predicting response to treatments, for example, studying drug targets and lessening the risk of drug adverse effects such as statin myopathy, has obvious potential value but brings an extra layer of complexity when prescribing. For example, it is known that drug metabolism shows wide genetic variation, but to complicate matters, non-coding areas may affect drug response so that WES would not identify them. The ethics of screening using genomic information is in one sense no different to other screening pro-grammes. There are guidelines on the viability of screening programmes in the UK from the UK National Screening Programme[31] – these are essentially a development of the traditional 'Wilson criteria' but they do not offer an ethical justification beyond the evidential.

However, population screening in the genomic field is not without its ethical complications, many of which will be immediately intelligible to the practitioner in primary care, necessarily in a more proximate relationship with his or her patient (and the family) than the geneticist. Great strides have been made on occasion in the elimination of genetic disease at a population level: for example, the Cyprus experience where thalassaemia has been virtually removed by means of education, screening and 'eugenic' means (such as stating which couples ought not to marry and have children).[32] Interestingly, each of these factors has been explicitly assisted by the Greek Orthodox and Muslim authorities there. Some progress also has been achieved in communities where consanguineous marriages are associated with a higher incidence of foetal malformation, mainly by the active intervention of primary care teams.[33] Such aims evidently do not value the genomically disadvantaged by avoiding their birth. Nonetheless, the state of affairs in the Cyprus example balances a healthier population over the constraints in reproductive choice.

CONCLUSION

Genomic medicine illustrates ethical issues both common to several branches of clinical care, but also dynamically distinctive ones. These distinctive issues boil down to notions of identity and agency which are to varying extents shared between genetic family members, genetically similar communities, races and ultimately human beings. An awareness of the craft of the generalist clinician in dealing with genetic disorders is arguably matched by an awareness of the craft of the ethicist: a moral craft, as it has been termed.[34] Traditionally, this moral craft has been within the domain of the genetic specialist, but will inevitably become the domain of the generalist as time goes on and research develops: the generalist being in a more long-standing and proximate relationship with his or her patient and their family.

REFERENCES

1. Lewens T. The provenance of the term is not known, but described in *What is genethics? J Med Ethics* 2004;30:326–328. doi:10.1136/jme.2002.002642.
2. Lucassen A and Parker M. The Genethics Club has probably brought the term to common parlance more than any other agency: The UK Genethics Club: Clinical ethics support for genetic services. *Clin Ethics* 2006;1(4):219–223.
3. Rafi I and Hayward J. *General practice and genomics.* https://www.genomicseducation.hee.nhs.uk/images/pdf/PHGF/phgf-general-practice-and-genomics-19Feb.pdf [accessed 16 May 2016].
4. Public Health Genetics Foundation. *Managing incidental and pertinent findings from WGS in the 100k Genome Project.* 2015. http://www.phgfoundation.org/file/13772/ [accessed 6 March 2016].
5. Fulda KG and Lykens L. Ethical issues in predictive genetic testing: A public health perspective. *J Med Ethics* 2006;32(3):143–147.
6. *A summary account from legal experts.* https://ukhumanrightsblog.com/2012/05/09/should-we-outlaw-genetic-discrimination/ [accessed 4 May 2016].
7. UK Genetic Testing Network. http://ukgtn.nhs.uk/ [accessed 21 August 2016].
8. Lukassen A. Ethical issues in genetic medicine. *InnovAiT* 2008;1(8):589–595.
9. Collins FS, et al. New goals for the U.S. Human Genome Project: 1998–2003. *Science (New York, N.Y.)* 2008;282(5389):682–689.
10. The Wellcome Trust Case Control Consortium. Genome-wide association study of 14,000 cases of seven common diseases and 3,000 shared controls. *Nature* 2007;447(7145):661–678.
11. Manolio TA, et al. Finding the missing heritability of complex diseases. *Nature* 2009;461(7265):747–753.

12. Ripke S, et al. Biological insights from 108 schizophrenia-associated genetic loci. *Nature* 2014;511:421–427.
13. Etchegary H, et al. Consulting the community: Public expectations and attitudes about genetics research. *Eur J Hum Genet* 2013;21:1338–1343. doi:10.1038/ejhg.2013.64.
14. van El CG, et al. Whole-genome sequencing in health care: Recommendations of the European Society of Human Genetics. *Eur J Hum Genet* 2013;21:580–584. doi:10.1038/ejhg.2013.46.
15. Chung MWH and Ng JCF. Personal utility is inherent to direct-to-consumer genomic testing. *J Med Ethics* 2016;42:649–652. doi:10.1136/medethics-2015-103057.
16. Ibid.
17. Genomics England. http://www.genomicsengland.co.uk/wp-content/uploads/2015/03/GenomicEnglandProtocol_030315_v8.pdf
18. Lukassen A and Clarke A. Should families own genetic information? *BMJ* 2007;335:22. doi:10.1136/bmj.39252.386030.AD.
19. McGuire, AL, et al. Ethics and genomic incidental findings. *Science* 2013;340(6136):1047–1048.
20. Dheensa, S, et al. Health-care professionals' responsibility to patients' relatives in genetic medicine: A systematic review and synthesis of empirical research. *Genet Med* 2016;18:290–301. doi:10.1038/gim.2015.72.
21. Health Education England- Genomics Education Programme. https://www.genomicseducation.hee.nhs.uk/news/item/105-the-role-of-genomics-in-assisted-reproduction [accessed 1 November 2016].
22. Norton, ME, et al. Cell-free DNA analysis for non-invasive examination of trisomy. *N Engl J Med* 2015;372(17):1589–1597.
23. Nuffield Council on Bioethics. http://nuffieldbioethics.org/news/2016/new-project-on-non-invasive-prenatal-testing/ [accessed 21 August 2016].
24. NHS Rapid Project. http://www.rapid.nhs.uk/guides-to-nipd-nipt/nipt-for-down-syndrome/ [accessed 21 August 2016].
25. Savulescu J. Procreative beneficence: Why we should select the best children. *Bioethics* 2001;15(5–6):413–426.
26. Rogowski WH, Grosse SD, Schmidtke J and Marckmann G. Criteria for fairly allocating scarce health-care resources to genetic tests: Which matter most? *Eur J Hum Genet* 2014;22:25–31.
27. Brall C and Schröder-Bäck P. Personalised medicine and scarce resources: A discussion of ethical chances and challenges from the perspective of the capability approach. *Public Health Genom* 2016;19:178–186.
28. *DatabasE of genomiC varIation and Phenotype in Humans using Ensembl Resources.* https://decipher.sanger.ac.uk/ [accessed 1 November 2016].
29. Hardcastle SJ, et al. Patients' perceptions and experiences of familial hypercholesterolemia, cascade genetic screening and treatment. *Int J Behav Med* 2015;22:92. doi:10.1007/s12529-014-9402-x.
30. *Collaborative oncology gene-environment study.* http://www.cogseu.org/ [accessed 21 August 2016].
31. *Evidence review criteria: National screening programmes. UK National Screening Committee (UK NSC) criteria for appraising the viability, effectiveness and appropriateness of a screening programme.* https://www.gov.uk/government/publications/evidence-review-criteria-national-screening-programmes [accessed 1September 2016].

32. Hoedmaekers R and ten Have H. Geneticization: The Cyprus Paradigm. *J Med Philos* 1998;23(3):274–287.

33. Darr A, et al. Examining the family-centred approach to genetic testing and counselling among UK Pakistanis: A community perspective. *J Community Genet* 2013;4(1):49–57.

34. Parker M. Scaling ethics up and down; moral craft in clinical genetics and in global health research. *J Med Ethics* 2015;41:134–137.

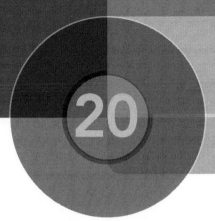

Confidentiality and forensic disclosure in the primary healthcare setting

20

HELEN SALISBURY, SHARON DIXON, AND SELENA KNIGHT

INTRODUCTION

The relationship between the patient and the clinician is built on trust, and without it the effectiveness of any clinician is severely limited.[1] That trust is based on a promise (both implicit and legally protected) that what is said in the consultation is confidential and will not be shared without permission. How else can a clinician ask about sexual history, drug use or suicidal intent and expect honest answers? The legal basis for this duty of confidentiality is not straightforward and there is no one set of laws in the UK in which it is enshrined.[1] In practice, doctors and nurses depend on their professional bodies for guidance [in the UK, these include the General Medical Council (GMC), the Nursing and Midwifery Council and the British Medical Association].

There are some exceptions to the primacy of confidentiality. In this chapter, we will explore when it may be morally and ethically right to breach this trust and where a legal requirement to keep or breach confidentially is ethically problematic. We will consider the question of consent to share information and the potential implications where a patient refuses to consent to disclosure, both where non-disclosure may risk harming the individual, and where it may pose a risk to the public. Computerisation of health data, which means that it may be accessed from multiple sites and by multiple individuals (potentially including the patient), has an impact on how clinicians act to protect patients' confidentiality. We will also look at the 2015 UK legislation around female genital mutilation (FGM) and discuss whether ethical and legal duties may conflict in this matter.

DISCLOSING CONFIDENTIAL INFORMATION IN THE PUBLIC INTEREST

The GMC in the UK advises doctors in its guidance on confidentiality that

> Confidential medical care is recognized in law as being in the public interest. However, there can also be a public interest in disclosing information: to protect individuals or society from risks of serious harm, such as serious communicable diseases or serious crime.[2]

Such advice stems from consequentialist moral theory, which proposes that the ethically correct course of action may be the one that provides the greatest overall benefit to the greatest number of people. Therefore, the moral justification for disclosing information in such a case would be that overall, the benefits to the public of information disclosure are great enough that they outweigh any potential harms that may be experienced by the individual from disclosure against their wishes.

However, the decision of whether to disclose information based on a consequentialist justification can be challenging because of the difficulties associated with accurately evaluating and weighing up the benefits and harms associated with each course of action. In particular, the guidance brings with it the challenges of considering what is meant by serious harm or a serious crime as there is no formal definition of what the word 'serious' means in either context. Clinicians need to use professional knowledge and judgment to try to form an assessment of the likelihood of the risk of significant harm, to the patient or others. This would usually not extend to crimes involving financial losses such as theft, fraud or property damage. The above guidance also suggests that doctors have a duty to inform the person whose confidential information is being disclosed, which may mean that confrontation or loss of trust is inevitable.[3]

When considering whether to breach confidentiality, some cases are reasonably clear-cut. For example, if a patient comes into a clinic brandishing a knife and states his or her intention to kill their ex-partner, it seems more than reasonable that in order to prevent a probable violent crime from being committed against another person, the doctor should report this to the authorities which could protect the patient and perhaps the intended victim as well. Famous American and British legal cases of this type have condemned clinicians who have acted in favour of confidentiality, and condoned those who have acted in favour of protecting someone from serious harm. One such case was the case of *Tarasoff* in 1976. A psychiatric patient informed his psychotherapist that he intended to kill a woman whom he specifically identified. The psychotherapist did not inform the targeted woman, and she was subsequently murdered by the patient. In the judgment, Justice Tobriner stated,

> the public policy favoring protection of the confidential character of patient–psychotherapist communications must yield to the extent to which disclosure is essential to avert danger to others. The protective privilege ends where the public peril begins.[4]

The case also prompted a 'duty to warn', whereby if 'a patient poses a serious danger of violence to others, [there is] a duty to exercise reasonable care to protect the foreseeable victim of that danger'.[5] This case may be contrasted with the British case of Edgell.[6] In this case, a patient asked his legal advisors to provide a confidential statement that the patient was no longer a risk to the public, to enable transfer to another setting. However, the psychiatrist felt this was not the case and that the patient posed an ongoing risk to the public, subsequently breaching the patient's confidentiality by informing the hospital and the Home Office of these concerns.

The court of appeal agreed that the psychiatrist had acted appropriately in breaching confidentiality as the patient posed a serious risk to the public.[7] These cases demonstrate the challenges that clinicians may encounter due to the need for them to rely on their professional judgment to appropriately balance the likely harms and benefits of disclosure against a patient's wishes.

MANY CASES IN PRIMARY CARE ARE LESS CLEAR-CUT

A patient who attends primary care and discloses cocaine abuse is clearly involved in illegal activity, buying (and possibly selling) illegal drugs as well as possible theft to fund their habit. General practitioners (GPs) in the UK are not usually required to report this to the police, although many people would consider drug use, buying drugs and theft to be 'serious crimes'. Forensic disclosure is not required in this case because cocaine abuse in itself does not pose significant immediate risk of harm to others. Consider though, whether the situation would be different if the GP knew that the patient lived with their partner and three children under the age of six. The GP might want to consider, for example, whether illegal activity such as drug selling was occurring at the home, whether the drug usage affected carrying out the responsibilities of parenting, or potentially impacted on the safety of the children. In such a scenario, breaching confidentiality may be justified because the consequences of the patient's drug habit (although not the drug use as an act in itself) is placing children at a risk of serious harm. Any healthcare professional (HCP) may be justified in breaching confidentiality and informing social services in order to ensure such children were not being placed at risk of serious harm, with a consequentialist justification that the harms associated with breaching confidentiality towards the individual patient are outweighed by the benefits of protecting the children of the family.

If the person habitually using cocaine was also a HCP, then again the GP would need to consider the impact of their usage on the safety of others, in particular their patients. Where the HCP's drug use was adversely impacting on their ability to work and therefore placing patients at risk, the GP would be professionally and morally obliged to breach confidentiality and inform the relevant services and licensing bodies (e.g. the Nursing and Midwifery Council or GMC), and take appropriate measures to safeguard patients. However, if the HCP's drug use was not affecting patient care, one would need to question whether breaching confidentiality would be justifiable, as it would be less clear whether disclosure would be in the public interest. This would be a difficult decision for the GP to make, as there may be legitimate concerns that the HCP's drug habit could worsen, potentially placing patients at risk in the future, or their drug use could prompt wider concerns surrounding the HCP's professional integrity. Care must be taken to ensure that decisions made are based on considered professional judgment, as merely a risk of potential harm to patients may not be sufficient to justify the harms associated with breaching confidentiality, particularly where there will be need to an ongoing therapeutic relationship to encourage the HCP to engage with services. Rather than breaching confidentiality in such a case, it may be necessary for the GP to seek advice from their professional body, or discuss their concerns directly with the HCP involved. Although this drug use would not be reported to the police when discovered in the context of consultation, if the patient attends a substance misuse clinic for treatment in the UK, their details will be submitted to regional or national drug misuse databases but only with their consent.[8]

Consider next the case of a woman who tells the GP that she is suffering a long history of domestic violence in the context of a controlling relationship. She may have only felt able to talk about what is happening to her because of her belief in the confidentiality of the doctor–patient relationship. She may seek assurance of confidentiality and be fearful of the consequences she may have to endure if it is discovered that she has told anyone. In this situation, there is the potential risk of harm to the woman from ongoing domestic violence, and this may be significant. Supporting a woman in this situation would normally involve assessing what she perceives to be the risk of further significant harm or injury, and informing relevant services who may be able to help. However, if the woman does not wish for, or feel ready for any further action, then domestic violence would not normally be reported to the police without her consent, even though it could be argued that a physical assault on a person is a serious crime.[9] The reason for this is that her need to trust in the safety and privacy of the doctor–patient relationship and to feel able to remain engaged with the process of seeking support and advice are extremely important, and more harm could come to her if this trust is lost through breaching confidentiality. However, there may be scenarios where the doctor feels that the risk of losing patient trust by disclosing information against her wishes are outweighed by the risk of harm from failure to intervene, for example, where there may be vulnerable individuals or children in the household. In such a situation, there would be both a moral and legal justification for such disclosure to protect others.[10]

A further challenge in such a case might be that the actions of the doctor may inadvertently result in a breach in confidentiality and thus place the patient at risk of harm. This could occur if the patient attended an appointment with their partner, or if the patient's family has home-access to their electronic healthcare records. In this scenario, the doctor would have to strongly consider their conduct during the consultation and their computer-written notes in order to avoid placing the patient at greater risk of harm. Advice may need to be sought in such a circumstance from professional indemnity bodies, or from experienced colleagues.

PATIENT CONFIDENTIALITY VERSUS PUBLIC SAFETY

These situations remind us that HCPs have a duty of care not only towards the individual patient or client, but also to other members of the public and to society. These duties are not usually in conflict with each other. However, when there is tension between the needs or wishes of the individual patient and others who could potentially be at risk because of their health or behaviour, some ethical and legal determination ought to be made as to which party should take precedence.

A common scenario in which this arises is when an individual discloses a health condition which means they would be disqualified from driving due to risk their condition poses to others. The individual in question may have important reasons for wishing to continue driving, including being able to do their job (and so be paid), to maintain independence (e.g., do their shopping) or to care for others. They may feel that not being allowed to drive will have an adverse impact on their own health and well-being. The medical guidance for conditions that preclude driving, or require ongoing assessments and monitoring, is laid out in the UK by the Driver and Vehicle Licensing Agency (DVLA), and aims to reduce the risk of accidents or injuries to other members of the public. In these situations, the statutory duty of HCPs towards the public outweighs their duty to the individual and they are required to share the relevant parts of the patient's medical information with the licensing authorities. Knowing that doctors need to report information, for example, about episodes of loss of consciousness, can lead to individuals not telling their doctors about relevant symptoms, potentially with tragic consequences. A recent example of this was in Glasgow in 2014, where a driver lost consciousness at the wheel of a garbage truck and killed six pedestrians. At subsequent judicial enquiry, it emerged that he had lied about his medical history to doctors and licensing authorities.[11] This case reinforces the benefits, or 'rightness', of acting to protect the public when clinicians become aware of factors which could compromise safe driving in accordance with statutory guidance. It also illustrates the fact that, where patients believe that confidentiality may be breached and that sharing of information with a third party (in this case the DVLA) would lead to personal adverse consequences, they may choose not to disclose important information to their doctor, resulting in a loss of opportunities for risk reduction.

ENQUIRIES FROM POLICE AND THE COURTS

On occasions, police officers ask for information held by doctors to help them with their enquiries. Regarding disclosures in the public interest, the GMC guidance advises doctors they must:

> … weigh the harms that are likely to arise from non-disclosure of information against the possible harm both to the patient, and to the overall trust between doctors and patients, arising from the release of that information.[12]

When police do ask for information in the absence of a court order it is up to individual doctors, often with advice from their colleagues and indemnity associations, to decide whether the public is best served by its release, as information should only be disclosed if this would be considered to be in the public interest.[13] If the crime is not serious, or the information is only tangential or involves information about other parties, the doctor may decide not to disclose (and may argue with the judge even if there is a court order). The situation can be further complicated if the confidentiality of the police investigation means that the doctor is not able to know all the details of the crime being investigated; in this situation, it may be difficult for the HCP to determine what information is relevant, as the amount of information disclosed should always be the minimum necessary to achieve the aim of disclosure.

One interesting area in which this has recently arisen is in the case of gun ownership. Members of the public applying for firearm and shotgun certificates in the UK must be deemed medical fit to hold a licence, and by applying for one, patients are deemed to have consented for police to contact their GP, and their GP to disclose necessary information in order to allow such an assessment to be made.[14] GPs are required to notify the police if they have concerns regarding the patient having access to a firearm, and also inform the police if the patient suffers from certain conditions, the majority of which listed are mental illnesses.[15] At the discretion of the police, GPs may be required to provide a more detailed medical report. While it is clear that GPs may have a duty to breach confidentiality if they are concerned the patient is likely to present a danger to themselves or to others by having access to shotguns, the new rules surrounding gun ownership may be ethically problematic. They raise significant moral questions about whether it is right for HCPs to disclose sensitive patient information where there has been no crime committed, and where there may be no immediate risk to the patient or the public, simply because this is a legal requirement of the gun licence application process. For example, disclosure would be required if a patient has a diagnosis of schizophrenia, but there would be no distinction between a patient who suffered with psychotic hallucinations commanding him or her to kill someone with a gun, and a patient with schizophrenia who is mentally stable. The requirement for HCPs to simply flag up all patients with a mental illness to the police is also problematic because it may exacerbate the stigma associated with such conditions, and may deter patients from disclosing their mental illness or seeking help. The requirement for GPs to notify police of concerns places great responsibility on the shoulders of the GP in terms of assessing risk, as with other cases where the degree of harm or the seriousness of the crime has to be determined by the HCP.

THE LAW AND FGM

The World Health Organization defines FGM as procedures which intentionally alter or injure the female genitalia for non-medical reasons. They describe it as a violation of the human rights of women and girls.[16] There are many adverse health consequences, both physical and psychological, for this practice and no advantages in health or hygiene. It is a cultural practice, not particular to any religion, and it is widely practiced in 28 African countries but also in the Middle East, Indonesia and Malaysia. The prevalence and type of procedure vary; in Egypt, 91% of women have been cut.[17]

In the UK, FGM has been illegal since 1985 but to date there have been no successful prosecutions.[18] There are many people living in the UK who have been cut and there are fears for the girls born into families where there is a cultural tradition of FGM. The concern is that they may be illegally operated on in the UK or, more likely, be taken abroad for the procedure.

In 2015, the *Serious Crime Act* introduced mandatory reporting of FGM in the UK: this requires that if a health or social care professional or a teacher becomes aware that a woman or girl under the age of 18 has been subject to FGM, that professional should inform the police. This is only required if the person has disclosed the FGM herself or if it has been found on examination. This is irrespective of how long prior to the disclosure the FGM took place and in which country it occurred.

If a person has been subjected to this procedure, it seems reasonable to consider that this constitutes a serious crime which, once reported, will be investigated and the people responsible will be prosecuted. Where FGM has taken place for a child under the age of 18, immediate contact with the police is required by law under the *Serious Crime Act* as there will be particular concern regarding vulnerability and safeguarding. The prosecution of parents or others responsible for FGM is intended to be protective to other girls in the family and a deterrent to other members of their community.[19] FGM clearly causes significant harm to women, and protecting other girls and women from experiencing it is crucial. There is, therefore, also a safeguarding obligation, which would justify a breach of confidentiality to safeguarding agencies, in keeping with any other situation in which a professional has concerns about a potential significant risk to a child or a young person. What is different with mandatory reporting in FGM is that professionals are legally obliged to report this first to the police before alerting safeguarding teams, though it is likely that these agencies would then work together in their response to the report.

It is worth considering the impact of breach of confidentiality on this very vulnerable patient group: some women who have suffered FGM are deeply traumatised by the experience. The PEER study reported in 2010, prior to the introduction of mandatory reporting that 'from the discussions with the women, it was clear that confidence and trust in the health services was minimal'.[20] Overcoming language and cultural barriers to build a trusting relationship with a doctor may take time and many consultations before a patient is able to talk about her experiences.

In this context, breaching confidentiality leading to police involvement and the impact of her disclosure on her family may have a very damaging effect on her trust in the medical profession. The intended deterrent effect on her community, which may make FGM less likely in future, may have the unintended consequences of preventing women and girls who have experienced FGM seeking the medical care they need in the aftermath of FGM and in pregnancy.

If the woman in question is 17 years old and was subjected to this abuse as an infant while a citizen of another country, the law requiring immediate forensic disclosure is the same but the balance of benefits and harms is altered further. If there is no risk to other girls in the family, it can be argued that the damage to the individual's trust relationship with doctors and the reduction in the wider community's confidence in the medical profession outweigh the benefits of disclosure as successful prosecution is extremely unlikely. Many argue that this legislative and punitive approach to the problem of FGM is likely to drive the practice underground and delay its eradication, advocating instead a focus on engagement with community and religious leaders and education about the health risks of FGM.[21–23] There are also questions about the ethics of treating FGM as legally different from other forms of abuse against women and children.

The GMC guidance is clear that we should disclose information when the law requires us to do so; however, we are also charged to weigh the risks and benefits of disclosure to the individual and to consider the damage that disclosure may cause to the overall trust between patients and doctors.

In most situations, doctors are given discretion to weigh up the likely benefits and harms of forensic disclosure, as in the case of domestic abuse described above. In the case of FGM, the *UK Serious Crime Act* has taken away this discretion, and doctors are obliged by law to disclose information to the police without patient consent even if they believe the harms, in the form of damage to trust, outweigh any possible benefits. It appears doctors have conflicting ethical and legal duties.

CONCLUSIONS

Healthcare professionals start from the position that what patients tell them is shared in confidence and regard this as an essential element of the trust relationship that they have with them. Nevertheless, there are clearly times when they should and must break this confidentiality, usually to protect a person from risk of serious harm. In most situations, this is a matter of professional judgment, with guidelines and advice from professional bodies to aid these decisions. However, in specific areas, the law is more clearly delineated, for example, in the case of firearms licensing and FGM in the UK, the results of which may sometimes conflict with HCPs judgments of the balance of harms. The potential hazard is that losing trust leads to non-disclosure of relevant clinical information and opportunities to protect the patient or others are lost, as demonstrated by the bin lorry case.

These situations are challenging and often there is no clearly 'right' answer; it is important that HCPs reflect on each case carefully and colleagues support each other in making the difficult decisions needed.

REFERENCES

1. O'Brien J and Chantler C. 2003. Confidentiality and the duties of care. *Journal of Medical Ethics* 29: 36–40. DOI: 10.1136/jme.29.1.36.
2. General Medical Council. 2009. *Confidentiality.* Paragraph 36 (disclosures in the public interest). GMC, London.
3. Ibid., Paragraph 39 (disclosures in the public interest).
4. *Tarasoff v Regents of the University of California* [1976] 17 Cal. 3d 425, 442.
5. Ewing CP. 2005. Tarasoff reconsidered. *Judicial Notebook* 36(7): 112.
6. *W v Egdell* [1989] EWCA Civ 13, *W v Edgell* [1990] 1 ALL ER 835.
7. *W v Edgell* [1990] 1 ALL ER 835.

8. Public Health England. 2013. [online]. *National Drug Treatment Monitoring System*. Available at: http://www.nta.nhs.uk/uploads/ndtmsconfidentialitytoolkitv6.3.pdf [accessed 29 July 2016].

9. General Medical Council, 2009, *op. cit.*, Paragraph 51 (disclosures to protect the patient).

10. Shakespeare J and Davidson L. Date unknown. *Domestic Violence in Families with Children* [online]. Royal College of General Practitioners. Available at: http://www.rcgp.org.uk/policy/rcgp-policy-areas/~/media/Files/Policy/A-Z-policy/Domestic%20Violence%20in%20families%20with%20children.ashx [accessed 14 July 2016].

11. BBC. 2015. *Glasgow Bin Lorry Crash: Family to Prosecute Harry Clarke* [online]. *BBC*, 7 December. Available at: http://www.bbc.co.uk/news/uk-scotland-glasgow-west-35025408 [accessed 13 July 2016].

12. General Medical Council, 2009, *op. cit.*, Paragraph 37 (disclosures in the public interest).

13. General Medical Council, 2009, *op. cit.*, Paragraph 22 (disclosures to the courts or in connection with litigation).

14. Home Office. 2016. *Guide on Firearms Licensing Laws*. Section 10.22. Home Office, London.

15. Ibid., Appendix C.

16. World Health Organization. 2016. *Female Genital Mutilation*. World Health Organization, Geneva.

17. UNICEF. 2013. *Female Genital Mutilation/Cutting: A Statistical Overview and Exploration of the Dynamics of Change* [online]. UNICEF. Available at: http://www.data.unicef.org/corecode/uploads/document6/uploaded_pdfs/corecode/FGMC_Lo_res_Final_26.pdf [accessed 14 July 2016].

18. Ministry of Justice/Home Office. 2015. *Serious Crime Act 2015. Factsheet—Female Genital Mutilation.* Ministry of Justice/Home Office, London.

19. Home Office. 2015. *Mandatory Reporting of Female Genital Mutilation—Procedural Information*. Home Office, London.

20. Hussein E and Foundation for Women's Health Research and Development (FORWARD). 2010. *Women's Experiences Perception and Attitudes of Female Genital Mutilation* [online]. The Bristol PEER study. Available at: http://www.forwarduk.org.uk/wp-content/uploads/2014/12/Womens-Experiences-Perceptions-and-Attitudes-of-Female-Genital-Mutilation-The-Bristol-PEER-Study.pdf [accessed 14 July 2016].

21. Bewley S, Kelly B, Darke K, Erskine K, Gerada C, Lohr P, and de Zulueta P. 2015. Mandatory submission of patient identifiable information to third parties: FGM now, what next? *British Medical Journal* 351: h5146.

22. Naftalin J and Bewley S. 2015. Mandatory reporting of FGM. *British Journal of General Practice* 65(638): 450–451. DOI: 10.3399/bjgp15X686437.

23. Mathers N and Rymer J. 2015. Mandatory reporting of female genital mutilation by healthcare professionals. *British Journal of General Practice* 65(635): 282–283. DOI: 10.3399/bjgp15X685141.

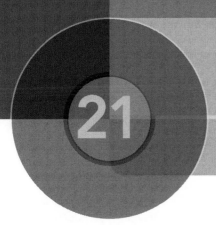

Mental health and ethics in primary care

SELENA KNIGHT, ANDREW PAPANIKITAS, AND JOHN SPICER

INTRODUCTION

Healthcare professionals (HCPs) working in primary care settings commonly encounter patients with mental illnesses. In many cases, the illness may have little impact on the consultation, decision-making and responsibilities of the HCP. However, patients with mental illness may present to primary care settings in a number of ways, and each individual situation may raise its own ethical challenges.

In this chapter, we explore some of the ethical issues which HCPs may encounter when caring for patients with mental illness in a primary care setting. We discuss the diagnosis of mental illness in primary care, considering the wider benefits and harms of making such a diagnosis. We reflect on confidentiality as a much rehearsed ethical topic in the context of mental health, because of the social stigma associated with psychiatric illness and because patient-centred confidentiality is a predominant concern in Western medicine. We examine the ways in which the HCP–patient relationship can be ethically distorted by mental illness and the consequent justice issues that arise when illness makes interaction with healthcare services chaotic. We conclude by reflecting on the multiple roles that an HCP may have when caring for patient with mental health needs and the fine line between paternalism and abandonment, between HCP as carer and as societal guardian.

ON THE ETHICS OF DIAGNOSIS

A problem which we acknowledge but do not dwell upon is that mental illness is epistemologically problematic. For some, mental illness is an illness to be treated like any other. For others, it may be considered to be less an illness and more a construct of our attitude towards what is expected of us as citizens.[1] Currently, the formal diagnosis of a specific mental illness requires using either the World Health Organization's *International Classification of Diseases* (ICD)[2] or the American Psychiatric Association's *Diagnostic and Statistical Manual of Mental Disorders* (DSM).[3]

These manuals provide diagnostic criteria, primarily focusing on symptoms, duration and impact on the patient's life, to enable a formal diagnosis. The development of these manuals has standardised the diagnostic process, ensuring coherent choices of treatment, and enabling research. Despite advances in neuropsychiatry, however, mental illnesses often do not yet have the same evidential basis as 'organic' health problem in terms of an observable pathophysiological process in the body.

In primary care, diagnosing a mental illness is not necessarily straightforward.[4] Patients may present with non-specific physical symptoms such as fatigue, reduced appetite or general apathy, causing diagnostic uncertainty as to whether such symptoms represent a physical illness or mental illnesses such as depression. Alternatively, patients may present with another health problem, but their conduct or behaviour may prompt the HCP to consider the possibility of an undiagnosed mental illness. Patients may present with mood disturbance, and it may be difficult for the HCP to determine whether this is simply a 'normal' and appropriate emotive response, for example, following a significant life event such as a bereavement or redundancy, or whether it is pathological and indicative of an underlying mental illness necessitating an intervention.

In some situations, the question faced by HCPs might not be 'can I make a diagnosis', as the DSM and ICD facilitate this in their provision of clear, time- and symptom-specific diagnostic criteria. Rather, the question faced may be 'should I make a diagnosis?', particularly where such a diagnosis has the potential to result in harm and may convey little benefit to the patient. In such cases, HCPs are required to make assessments and decisions outside their perceived normal clinical remit of simply making the diagnosis, by being required to additionally evaluate potential harms and benefits which may ensue for the individual patient, and for a wider society.

In some cases, a formal diagnosis of a mental illness may be clearly beneficent. It may provide eligibility for beneficial medical or psychological treatment, or financial or employment support. The formal recognition of symptoms may encourage patients to acknowledge and recognise the impact of their difficulties, and subsequently enable them to accept treatment. Making a diagnosis may be seen as good from a consequentialist perspective, as formally diagnosing and treating the mental illness may eventually enable the patient to return to normal life and become a functioning citizen able to participate in and contribute to society. Potential distress is reduced not only to the patient but also to those who interact with them and inappropriate use of resources such as emergency services might be reduced.

However, making a diagnosis of mental illness can also result in foreseeable harm. One consequence of receiving such a diagnosis is that it legitimises the sick role for the patient. Whilst this does offer the benefits outlined above, patients may use their newfound diagnosis to define themselves as someone who is 'ill', and subsequently devolve themselves of responsibilities such as caring responsibilities, engagement with education or employment and financial responsibilities.[5] It may even excuse behaviour which societal consensus might regard as reckless, immoral or illegal. In many countries and historically in the UK, a diagnosis of 'insanity' has saved many people from judicial execution on the justifiable basis that if someone is not responsible for their actions, they should not be held accountable for them. Whilst the general idea of the 'sick role' may benefit the patient as an individual (and we are not saying that this is wrong *per se*), questions may arise as to how this fits into the justice systems that are created for the benefit of society as a whole.

Secondly, the medicalisation of aspects of mental health through a formal diagnosis may result in some patients receiving benefits which might be viewed as unjust in wider society terms. A university student experiencing hyperactiveness and poor concentration may receive a diagnosis of Attention Hyperactivity Deficit Disorder (ADHD) and subsequently be treated with methylphenidate, a drug commonly associated with improved concentration and performance. If, for argument's sake, we assume that the medication works flawlessly and without side effects, an unintended but foreseeable outcome of this treatment may be improved performance and grades. Whilst some questions about enhancement of performance in competitive settings are best answered through societal debate and consensus, an HCP may question whether treatment of a condition or enhanced performance motivates the diagnosis. Whilst healthcare traditionally has concerned itself with correcting deficits, treatment that represents a net enhancement raises the question of whether others should be denied a similar opportunity who do not have the condition as severely, or even at all. The question then is whether HCPs should administer such medication.

Thirdly, the provision of a diagnosis of mental illness may have a significant adverse impact on a patient's sense of personhood and autonomy, both immediately, and in the future. The personal nature of the symptoms experienced by those with mental illnesses may cause a patient to call into question aspects of their identity, impacting on their perception of self and personhood. Once a diagnosis of a mental illness has been formally made, future decision-making by the patient may be at risk of being called into question. For example, if a patient has low mood and receives a formal diagnosis of depression, a later decision to refuse chemotherapy might be scrutinised in more depth than would otherwise be the case. The HCP may have concerns that the decision has been influenced by the patient's depression or possible underlying suicidal ideation, rather than simply the patient deciding they would rather avoid the significant side effects associated with chemotherapy. As another example, a patient formally diagnosed with dementia may have future decisions called into question because of presumed cognitive impairment. Importantly, such decisions may not only be those regarding their health but may also extend to include decisions surrounding finances, accommodation and nursing care. Unlike physical illnesses for which a cure may be objectively defined through normalised blood results or radiological resolution, the personal and subjective nature of the symptoms of mental illness make it far more difficult to determine the point at which a patient has been 'cured'. As a result, it may not be easy for patients to shed a diagnosis of mental illness, and thus, HCPs have a responsibility to carefully consider the future impact their diagnostic decision-making may have.

By being in a professional position to give patients a formal diagnosis of a mental illness and legitimise the sick role, primary care HCPs act as 'social arbiters' to the responsibilities and benefits of such patients.[6] The wider impact on the patient in terms of their ensuing illness behaviour may be socially defined, and may vary according to the cultural and social expectations of the society in which they reside.[7] HCPs have the power to not only label the patients' thoughts, feelings and emotions as being a consequence of a mental illness but also to disregard and disempower such patients by defining their symptoms as being within the normal range of emotions and not pathological in nature. The ethical challenge for such HCPs is to determine whether making a diagnosis of a mental illness is truly in the patient's best interests by weighing up the potential benefits and harms such a diagnosis will bring, not only to the patient but also to the society as a whole.

CONFIDENTIALITY AND MENTAL HEALTH

The importance of respecting patient confidentiality is clearly demonstrated in professional guidelines and case law, and is also viewed as a morally desirable behaviour for HCPs. However, the duty to maintain confidentiality is not absolute, and situations may arise where an HCP feels it may be necessary to breach confidentiality, most commonly where the benefits of main-taining confidentiality are outweighed by a significant risk of harm to the patient or to others associated with not sharing such information.

Such situations are not isolated to only those with physical illnesses but may also be found with patients with mental illnesses. One example may be where an HCP learns of a patient's occupation, and becomes concerned that a deterioration in their mental state could place the public at risk.[8] Obvious occupations not only include doctors, HCPs and pilots,[9] but may also include those such as bus drivers, police or teachers. If an HCP has serious concern that the patient's mental illness is adversely impacting on their ability to perform their job to such a degree that the public are being put at risk, most would agree that they have a professional and moral responsibility to encourage the patient to disclose their condition to their employer to enable them to take appropriate actions to minimise or mitigate the risk, such as offering the patient time off from work, or amending their duties.

In many cases, the patient will oblige, but there may be situations where a patient's men-tal status means they lack insight into their condition and thus refuses to consent to dis-closure of such information. Here, the HCP may have a moral and professional duty to breach patient confidentiality and disclose such information to the appropriate party. This is recognised in professional guidelines such as those of the General Medical Council (UK), which states that

> personal information may ... be disclosed in the public interest, without patients' consent, and in exceptional cases where patients have withheld consent, if the benefits to an individual or to society of the disclosure outweigh both the public and the patient's interest in keeping the information confidential.[10]

As with breaching confidentiality in patients with physical illnesses, the justification for such action is rooted in utilitarian theory, and requires an assessment of the overall balance of benefits and harms. However, in patients with mental illness, there may be additional factors requiring consideration in deciding whether breaching confidentiality is ethically justified. Patients with mental illness may have a particularly close relationship with their primary care HCP because of the personal, sensitive and chronic nature of their disease. Significant time and effort may have been invested by the HCP to establish a positive and trustworthy relationship with them, and breaching confidentiality may damage or even lead to the total breakdown of this important therapeutic relationship. This may have catastrophic adverse outcomes for the patient in terms of their ongoing engagement with services and treatment and prognosis. Therefore, there may be scenarios in which an HCP decides not to breach confidentiality if he or she deems that such a breach will result in unjustifiable harm to the HCP–patient relationship In such situations, the HCP may take responsibility for significant risk and may wish to share this burden with other people involved in the care of such patients.

The position of HCPs specifically in primary care can also raise unique challenges in rela-tion to confidentiality. One such challenge is the potential interaction between the HCP and the patient's relatives. In a primary care setting, it would not be unusual for the patient's rela-tives to be registered under the care of the same HCP as the patient, and ethical dilemmas may arise as a result of this. Relatives may ask the HCP for information about the patient's mental illness, and it is accepted that it would generally not be appropriate to breach confidentiality in such circumstances. However, a relative attending an appointment may provide the HCP with a unique opportunity to obtain a collateral history regarding the patient with mental ill-ness. Such a collateral history may be valuable in helping the HCP formulate a better picture of the patient's mental state, and enabling him or her to make more informed decisions regarding their care. However, the prying of such information is ethically problematic, as it violates the privacy of the individual patient, and may inadvertently lead to a breach in the patient's confidentiality. This will be particularly the case if patient is unaware of the conversation between the HCP and the relative, although this might be the only way in which the HCP is able to acquire such information, particularly if the patient themselves does not engage well with the primary care HCP.

An alternative source for a collateral history for a patient with a mental illness may be through social media. Many people have public profiles on social media forums which may be accessible to HCPs. Is it ethically justifiable for an HCP to use such forums to access patient information? Changes in behaviour, for example, posting pictures on a social media profile of recklessness or drunkenness, might alert the HCP to a significant deterioration in a patient's mental status. Accessing the patient's social media profile may provide the HCP with crucial information not obtainable through any other means, and may prompt the HCP to review the patient, and make changes to their treatment which could provide great benefit. However, accessing and using sources of information such as social media profiles raise significant ethical issues.[11] Similarly to using relatives as collateral history-givers, the invasion of the patient's privacy through the intrusion into their personal sphere, outside the accepted confidential space of the consultation room, violates the patient's privacy and instinctively causes a sense of moral unease. Accessing such information also risks blurring professional and personal boundaries between the HCP and patient.[12] Although patients may post information on social media forums knowing that this is a public space, it is unlikely that they do so with the forethought that such information may be accessed by their HCP and used in decision-making. Should the patient become aware that this information is being accessed and used in such a way they may feel a sense of violation, and this may have significant adverse effects on their relationship with the HCP.[13] That said, even if the patient remains unaware that the HCP has accessed such information, there is still an instinctive feeling of dishonesty associated with such behaviour and clinicians would need to very carefully consider whether this is morally justified by the benefits they may gain through becoming privy to such information.

RESTRAINT AND COERCION

Significant ethical challenges can arise in the management of patients with mental illness, particularly where there may be disagreement between the HCP and the patient around their care and they refuse treatment.

Some patients with mental illnesses may be so acutely unwell that refusing treatment may place their life, or the lives of others, at significant risk of harm. Here, the threat of formal detention ('sectioning') may prompt them to accept treatment, which in England and Wales is legislated by the *Mental Health Act 1983* (amended in 2007). The Act permits involuntary detention for assessment, provided the person is 'suffering from a mental disorder of a nature or degree which warrants their detention in hospital'[14] and that detention is 'in the interests of their own health or safety or with a view to the protection of others'.[15]

This stylised legal language foregrounds both the need for a diagnosis, of sorts, and the utilitarian judgement that such in infringement of liberty rights is justified by detention. Full details of legal constraints and processes will vary around the jurisdictions of the world, but not by much. In the Act above, most commonly a doctor with prior knowledge of the patient, such as their primary healthcare clinician, plays a part in the assessment for detention. They may be well placed to provide evidence which justifies coercive care, and supports the decision that detention against the patient's will is in their best interest and necessary under the relevant legal definitions. Acting as the 'usual doctor', the primary care professional's knowledge of the patient's wider circumstances places them in a better position to take into account broader factors which might be relevant in the assessment process, such as prior wishes, the patient's previous experiences of services, family support, and so on. In comparison, the 'expert doctor' who may also be involved in the legal process of 'sectioning' is likely to be a psychiatrist, who aside from formally assessing the patient for detention may have little prior knowledge of them as an individual. The role of the two different professionals in this process highlights the ethical challenges that might be encountered in determining best interests. On one hand, the 'usual doctor' is likely to consider far broader, non-medical factors. They are also likely to maintain an ongoing relationship with the patient beyond their detention. This may mean they have to take a more consequentialist approach in their decision-making in order to ensuring an ongoing trusting relationship with the patient can be continued (even if the clinician is deemed to be supporting involuntary detention). On the contrary, the 'expert doctor', with a background in psychiatry, may be primarily focused on the patient's well-being in terms of their psychiatric status, and so may have a narrower focus in their assessment, and they may be less inclined to consider the impact of detention on long-term relationships with healthcare services.

However, returning to the primary care setting, it is relatively uncommon for individual primary care clinicians to be faced with a patient who is so mentally unwell that he or she require acute admission under such a formal and restrictive measure. A more common scenario in primary care is that of a patient with a mental illness who refuses investigation, referral or treatment, but is not placing themselves or others at risk of harm serious enough to justify such an intervention. Despite the patient's refusal, the clinician may still feel that the care being refused is in their best interests, and so may feel they have a moral and professional duty to encourage the patient to accept such treatment.

One possible approach they may consider is to attempt to coerce the patient into accepting treatment. Coercion may take many forms ranging from the subtle nudge, such as over-exaggerating the expected benefits of treatment, to a more aggressive approach, such as alluding to a threat of formal detention should the patient not comply, perhaps even where such formal detention would not be legally justified. The approach the HCP decides to take may depend on the patient's clinical state, the nature and extent of intended benefits of the investigation or treatment being proposed and perhaps the likelihood of success of such a coercive measure.

The example of substance misuse is apposite here. In primary care, people who misuse drugs are common enough, and may draw their supply from illicit sources or even [mis]prescribed routes.

Whilst a literature has been developed on the justifications for coerced treatment in specialist services, there is very little on the ethics of persuasion, encouragement or indeed coercion into treatment or treatment moderation where patient care is part of the holism of generalist care.[16] It has even been said that the familiarity, bred of a long-term relationship with the primary care professional, may also breed consent.[17,18] This of course may assist the primary care clinician in persuading, encouraging or nudging a substance-misusing patient into a better outcome.[19]

The approaches described above are paternalistic in nature, defined by Dworkin as 'the interference with a person's liberty of action, justified by reasons referring exclusively to the welfare, good, happiness, needs, interest or values of the person being coerced'.[20] It should be noted that those clinicians who are party to such actions, be they detaining patients or attempting to coerce them, are indulging in paternalist activity – something increasingly rare in Western society. Such paternalism is considered 'soft' where the patient is of capacity, and 'hard' where he is not,[21] and such distinction is important in terms of encouraging clinicians to check and balance the proportionality of the restrictiveness of the paternalistic action against the patient's right to respect for their autonomous decision-making.

RESPECT, RESPONSIBILITY AND ABANDONMENT

There will be some situations where the patient's refusal is not sufficiently serious to warrant formal detention, but despite great effort in persuasion, the patient continues to refuse to accept treatment which the HCP strongly feels is in their best interests. Provided that the patient has capacity (and it must be stressed that patients with mental illness should still be presumed to have such capacity unless they demonstrate otherwise), such a refusal must be respected and there will be little else the HCP will be able to do other than supporting the patient in their decision-making and taking appropriate steps to minimise any ensuing harm. The HCP will need to come to terms with the moral unease that he or she is likely to experience from the patient's decision. However, by respecting the refusal, the clinician is acknowledging that patient's autonomy is of overriding importance, and that a paternalistic approach may not be justifiable in all situations. Respecting the patient's wishes may enable the clinician to maintain a trustworthy relationship with the patient, which from a utilitarian perspective may result in a more positive longer-term outcome.

One challenge faced by the HCP in such a situation will be determining how far their duty of care now extends, given the patient's refusal. The scope of the duty of care and the responsibilities of such a clinician may be difficult to define in such a situation, as there may be subtleties of the interaction between a patient and clinician that do not fit the bald 'refusal'.

For example, if a patient refuses to come to the clinic appointment at the primary care centre because of social anxiety, should the general practitioner (GP) phone them? How many times? What if they do not answer? Should they write? Should they visit them at home? If they are not at home, should they phone the patient's next of kin? But what if the next of kin is unaware of the diagnosis? Is it justifiable to go to such great lengths for a patient whose behaviour indicates they do not want treatment where primary healthcare services are so stretched?

These questions are frequently faced by primary care HCPs who ultimately retain responsibility for the patient whilst in the community, yet do not have formal powers as they would if the patient was detained under section. Such a responsibility is founded on notions of duty of care – a sound deontological principle – which even though it may be defined contractually for some doctors has to be interpreted in its practical application. Formal coercive treatment is not available to primary care clinicians under statute, and arguably is not the business of a generalist anyway. Nonetheless, in answering the rather mundane questions above, which are the stuff of everyday primary care, clinicians are faced with the challenging task of assessing patients as whole people whilst delicately balancing refusals, autonomous decisions, best interests and their own professional and moral responsibilities. Such decisions also need to be taken in the context of a wider healthcare system with limited resources, in terms of time, finances and personnel, and so how much effort is professionally or ethically required to be invested in such patients is difficult to determine.

CONCLUSION

… [primary care]..occupies an important space at the interface of users, families, communities and professional worlds, and is able to address mental physical and social aspects of care. … a low stigma setting, able to offer rapid access … a longitudinal approach where patients are never discharged … perhaps above all interpersonal continuity of care.[22]

This quote from Helen Lester, a GP and an academic who died far too young, captures the key threads of primary care as practiced in the UK and elsewhere. She ties it to the themes of mental health that we have described in this chapter.

The diagnosis of mental illness challenges our understanding of how health and illness are defined, and may alter the way we approach patients to make decisions surrounding treatment and care. The impact of a diagnosis and subsequent treatment is far broader than purely the medical, and has consequences in terms of how we treat people as members of society and how we view the principle of justice in terms of the responsibility and accountability of patients with mental illness. Added challenges encountered by primary care professionals relate to their long-term relationship with their patients and their knowledge of non-medical aspects of patients' lives, which may complicate their decision-making. Clinicians are faced with the challenge of defining best interests for patients where there are multiple confounding factors, coupled with the need to consider not only the patient's wishes but also their vulnerability and how this may adversely impact them.

Primary care health professionals cannot avoid the ethical dilemmas so described but their analysis may help their clinical practice as advocates, societal guardians, resource arbiters and even occasionally, paternalists.

REFERENCES

1. Rogers A and Pilgrim D. (2014). *A Sociology of Mental Health and Illness.* 5th edition. Oxford: Oxford University Press.
2. World Health Organization. *The ICD-10 Classification of Mental and Behavioural disorders: Clinical Descriptions and Diagnostic Guidelines.* Available from: http://www.who.int/classifications/icd/en/bluebook.pdf?ua=1 [accessed 13 September 2016].
3. American Psychiatric Association. *Diagnostic and Statistical Manual of Mental Disorders.* 5th edition. Available from: https://www.psychiatry.org/psychiatrists/practice/dsm [accessed 15 September 2016].
4. Klinkman M, Dowrick C and Fortes S. (2012). Mental health classification in primary care. In: Ivbijaro G (eds.), *Companion to Primary Care Mental Health.* Section C, Chapter 2. London: Wonca and Radcliffe Publishing.
5. Misselbrook D. (2014). *Thinking about Patients.* CRC Press, Boca Raton, Florida. p. 122.
6. Ibid., 122.
7. Ibid., 131.
8. Glozier N. (2002). Mental ill health and fitness for work. *Occupational and Environmental Medicine,* 59(10), 714–720.
9. Torjesen I. (2015). The pilot, depression, and the salacious headlines that feed stigma. *British Medical Journal,* 350, h1874.

10. General Medical Council. (2009). *Confidentiality Point 37.* London: GMC.

11. Ashby GA, O'Brien A, Bowman D, Hooper C, Stevens T, Lousada E. (2015). Should psychiatrists "Google" their patients? *BJPsych Bulletin*, 39(6), 278–283. DOI: 10.1192/pb.bp.114.047555.

12. Lee Ventola C. (2014). Social media and health care professionals: Benefits, risks, and best practices. *Pharmacy and Therapeutics*, 39(7), 491–499, 520.

13. Denecke K, Bamidis P, Bond C, Gabarron E, Househ M, Lau AY, Mayer MA, Merolli M, and Hansen M. (2015). Ethical issues of social media usage in healthcare. *Yearbook of Medical Informatics*, 10(1), 137–147.

14. Mental Health Act 1893 (amended 2007).

15. Ibid.

16. Wolfe S, Kay-Lambkin F, Bowman J, Childs S. (2013). To enforce or engage: The relationship between coercion, treatment motivation and therapeutic alliance within community-based drug and alcohol clients. *Addictive Behaviours*, 38(5), 2187–2195.

17. Bowman D. (2011). *Does Familiarity Breed Consent.* Available at: http://www.mddus.com/resources/resource-type/publications/summons/2011/summer-2011-ethics-does-familiarity-breed-consent/ (accessed July 13, 2017).

18. Bowman D, Spicer J, and Iqbal R. (2012). *Informed Consent: A Primary for Clinical Practice.* Cambridge: Cambridge University Press.

19. Kabasenche WS. (2016). Forming the self: Nudging and the ethics of shaping autonomy. *American Journal of Bioethics,* 16(7), 24–25.

20. McKinstry B. (1992). Paternalism and the doctor-patient relationship in general practice. *British Journal of General Practice,* 42(361), 340–342.

21. Conly S. (2013). Coercive paternalism in health care: Against freedom of choice. *Public Health Ethics,* 6(3), 241–245.

22. Lester H, Glasby J, and Tylee A. (2004). A integrated primary mental health care: Threat or opportunity in the new NHS? *British Journal of General Practice,* 54(501), 285–291.

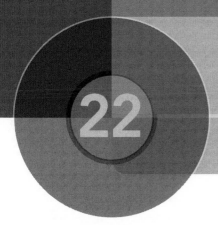

Veterans and the ethics of reciprocity in UK primary healthcare

HILARY ENGWARD

22

INTRODUCTION

In the UK, The Armed Forces Covenant states that veterans should receive priority treatment where it relates to a condition, subject to clinical need, which results from their service in the Armed Forces.[1] Those injured in service, whether physically or mentally, should be cared for in a way which reflects the nation's moral obligation to them, whilst respecting those individuals' wishes. The nature of war and the large number of soldiers surviving with injury (by contrast with previous armed conflicts in history) raise questions about the provision of medical care for injured service personnel and the nature of the government's duty of care for veterans with long-term, chronic health conditions. By extension, some of that duty is devolved to frontline healthcare services – primary healthcare in the UK. The purpose of this chapter is to explore the nature of this entitlement and moral obligation, and to consider what this might mean in relation to caring for veterans in the primary healthcare. Since primary care is often then the first point of contact between a veteran and the health services, decisions about if and how a veteran ought to be prioritised need to be articulated, including whether veterans may be distinctly vulnerable or needy.

Who are veterans? In the UK, the legal term 'veteran' encompasses anyone who has served for at least 1 day in the Armed Forces (Regular or Reserve) in uniform. In the UK, the Armed Forces community of serving personnel, reservists, their families and veterans is approximately 10 million people, of which roughly 2.8 million are Armed Forces veterans.[2] The largest age band of UK veterans is 65+ years, approximately 28% of the overall 65+ years UK population.[3] From recent wars (Iraq and Afghanistan), greater numbers of casualties survived battlefield injuries, with younger injured veterans more likely to live longer than previously due to enhanced body armour and medical evacuation,[4] and many have severe injuries to areas not directly protected by body armour, such as the head and neck. The nature of the military experience has also changed over time, with the term 'new wars' being used to characterise the nature of possible harm that deployment might incur, such as bearing witness to atrocities such as child soldiers, civilian population expulsion, exemplary violence, torture and sexual assault.[5]

In the UK, all veterans are entitled to priority access to National Health Service (NHS) hospital care for any condition, as long as it is related to their service and subject to the clinical need of others. This entitlement is set out in The Armed Forces Covenant, which outlines the relationship between the nation, the government and the Armed Forces. The covenant between the Armed Forces and society values and respects service personnel and veterans for the work they do on behalf of the nation. The enshrinement of the Armed Forces Covenant in law now places a formal obligation on the state to provide services for veterans. The nature of entitlement and the reciprocal obligation by society is however uncertain, has been subject to change during political change,[6] and has come to mean different things to different groups (such as military charities). McCartney states that there will always be a gap between what service personnel want and what the public might be willing to give.[7] Against the contemporary backdrop of deep cuts in the UK health and social service provision, the question remains as to how much the UK is willing to care for its veterans in line with other competing health and social care needs.

THE CASE FOR PRIORITY ACCESS TO HEALTH SERVICE

In the UK, the NHS provides the right to healthcare that all citizens can enjoy. Special interest groups do not gain special entitlements, and instead gain healthcare commensurate with that which is best available. However, for conditions related to military service, the Department of Health directs that veterans at their first outpatient appointment ought to be 'scheduled for treatment quicker than other patients of similar clinical priority'. Against the backdrop of competing health resources, the moral justification for some groups in society, for example, veterans, to have accelerated care over others, can be difficult to articulate, and, what makes a veteran more worthy to accelerated access to health services is unclear.

One such criterion to think about this is access based on individual medical need. At face value, this seems reasonable as it suggests that access to services can be based on objective scientific and clinical knowledge. However, medical need in itself is not neutral and confers notions of preference or value. For example, prolongation of life, elimination of disease and improved quality of life are all medical needs, but how these are to be ranked in relation to each other is unclear. If, however, the level of need which a veteran has is the same as that of another member of the general public, but the veteran is given priority, then 'need' cannot be the rationale for the veteran's priority. All other things being equal, the priority must stem from the veteran status as a veteran. The veteran, in other words, merits care in a way that the non-veteran does not.

It is perhaps worth exploring why a veteran might merit special treatment. 'Our' veterans are military personnel who place themselves in danger in order to protect our country and values; therefore, a medico-military criterion, based on merit to protect our country, may be sufficient to gain preferential access to healthcare resources. There is some evidence of public support for this idea. For example, the UK public showed support for British citizenship rights for retired Ghurkas, with a notion that something was owed to the soldiers in return for the risks they exposed to on the behalf of UK.[8] This refers to the principle of reciprocity, in which justice seems to demand those who have been exposed to exceptional risks, be entitled to commensurate consideration.

If this is the case, we then need to consider how extensive this obligation is. Veterans may be injured because they were placed in undue circumstances of risk, but not all veterans have been active in the theatre of war. For example, should those who work in information technology far from the frontline be entitled to prioritised medical care? If two veterans have the same injury, one in a car accident at home out of service, and another as a result of combat in war, should both, as veterans, have equal access to accelerated health services? What if the injury resulted in a deliberate choice not to follow procedure? For example, head injuries from Vietnam War occurred when soldiers did not wear helmets because they were too hot and uncomfortable.[9] Similarly, in Iraq, some soldiers did not wear goggles.[10] Are head and eye injuries resulting from a personal choice not to wear protective clothing less worthy of care? The answer to these questions may simply be that if we accept that healthcare is a basic human right, then the answer is no, we cannot distinguish based either on circumstance or behavioural choices, and treatment must always be given according to medical need. Military service therefore should not add to or detract from an individual's right to healthcare.

If however we accept that veterans ought to receive priority care based on their service to the country, then we also need to ask whether priority treatment ought to be given to other service members who serve their nation in some way, for example, fire, police and paramedic personnel. However, such a benefit is not extended to others who might be injured in the course of their work in the public sector. It also generates a set of ethical duties around how to treat people who perceived themselves as entitled to care that is better in some way because of their status.

There is also another dimension to this debate. Over the last decade, increasing numbers of active service personnel, veterans and families of those killed in war have questioned whether inadequate resources put soldiers at unnecessary risk. With possibilities of depleted resources following a 15% reduction in defence spending (2010–2016),[11] there is risk that serving personnel may be at increased risk in harm and injury. It might be argued that the right to life (as entrenched within the covenant) has been breached, and the government should be accountable for harms caused resulting from inadequate equipment. On the one hand, the covenant provides the soldier with a clause of 'unlimited liability', and on the contrary places the worth of equipment beyond the scope of this morally binding protection. It seems, therefore, that concepts within the covenant are flexible, or in the least, open to political interpretation. A Supreme Court ruling in 2013 established three key principles that the Ministry of Defence (MOD) could be sued for negligence that Human Rights legislation is applicable in military and operational areas, and the interpretation of the combat immunity was narrowed, leading to concerns that the ruling may lead to litigation, affecting training and equipment.[12] If this is the case, it could be argued that soldiers, whose injuries have been sustained as a result of inadequate resources (argued as a form of employer's negligence) ought to receive prioritised healthcare.

VETERANS MAY HAVE DISTINCTIVE NEEDS AND VULNERABILITIES

Possibly from popularised media reporting, there is an assumption that the veteran population in the UK is vulnerable to mental health issues, higher rates of homelessness, alcohol misuse, domestic violence, relationship breakdown and criminal activity.[13] This may be the case, but it could be conversely argued that all persons who experience change are equally as susceptible to such health concerns. However, in transition from the military to civilian communities, differences between civilian and veteran healthcare needs may stem from the unique nature of the military culture. Through processes of basic training, military personnel are socialised to adhere to military cultural norms, including acceptance of regimentation, hierarchy and depersonalisation in favour of the collective, and it is this reproduction of a very specific view of the social world that radically differs from the civilian social world.[14] For some veterans, the move from active military service to civilian life is a major change in culture, leading to problems in independently gaining housing and employment, and to adjust to civilian cultural norms.[15] Cohen defines this as a 'cultural gap' in which differences in the norms, values and culture between the military and civilian spheres exist, leading to a 'connectivity gap' and diminishing contact between the Armed Forces and society.[16] In relation to the UK, Cohen concludes that these lead to a 'respect-value' gap, characterised by citizens respecting but placing little value on the sacrifice of those placed in harm's way to serve the state.

The extent to how this is played out in contemporary healthcare provision for veterans needs further enquiry and understanding.[17] One cannot therefore assume that veterans will have health needs that differ from the civilian population, but must recognise that unique needs that may stem from military service. It may indeed be that the potential vulnerability that results from being or having been active service personnel is unique and distinct from the civilian population. That potential vulnerability creates a distinct duty – that it should not be over-looked by primary care professionals.

CARING FOR VETERANS IN THE PRIMARY CARE SECTOR

The onus of deciding whether medical need is service-related lies with the primary care profes-sional. In primary care in the UK, general practitioners (GPs) are expected, when referring a patient, to state that in their clinical opinion, the condition may be related to military service. Where secondary clinicians agree that the veteran's condition is likely to be service related, they are expected to prioritise veterans over other patients with the same level of clinical need. This does not necessarily mean veterans should be given priority over other patients with more urgent, or greater, clinical need. However, it is therefore dependent upon the primary care professional to recognise whether the patient is a veteran or not. In a survey of 500 GPs, 81% responded that they knew little about priority treatment for veterans, and 85% had not informed secondary care providers of a veteran's entitlement to priority treatment within the prior year.[18] Research data such as these imply that primary care professionals therefore need to be aware of the covenantal duty to ascertain whether the patient has veteran status, and from this, to determine if the nature of the clinical need is linked to that active service.

SPECIALISED SERVICES FOR VETERANS

There are some examples of veteran-specific service provision in the UK, for example, there is government money for veteran mental healthcare that is ring-fenced from the rest of the NHS budget. There has also been an increase of new third-sector providers alongside more estab-lished brands such as the 'Royal British Legion' and 'Combat Stress', which deliver veteran-specific care and support (e.g. Combat Stress specifically offer treatment for Post traumatic Stress Disorder [PTSD]). However, this has resulted in different approaches, interventions and governance procedures. It is also unclear exactly which of these bodies should properly come under the official regulation of bodies such as the Care Quality Commission (CQC), and where the boundaries of treatment versus support lie.

In the UK currently, specific healthcare provision is limited to prosthetics and mental health. This appears specialised to distinct consequences of combat rather than a simple privilege of veteran status. Therefore, a move towards a specific veteran healthcare system, such as that exists in the United States, seems unlikely but it is useful to consider if this would be a good thing. It is of course important to note the differences between the USA and the UK health and social care provision. The need for separate health and social care provision for veterans in countries where healthcare is unequal is more easily justified because veterans otherwise face a lack of healthcare. In the UK, however, the argument is less straightforward as the NHS has been freely available to anyone who wants to avail themselves of it, including veterans. Another key argument against a system similar to the US Department of Veteran Affairs relates to size. The budget of the US Department of Veteran Affairs for an estimated population of 23 million veterans is roughly equivalent to that of the entire NHS. There are 4.5 million veterans in the UK, and any introduction of a specific system would, out of necessity, need to prioritise who ought to be prioritised, with objections to favouring, for example, those who have been injured in the most recent wars over other older groups.[19] Another related issue is that not all health problems are directly attributable to military service. For example, only 50% PTSD cases in currently serving personnel can be directly attributed to deployment.[20] It is also assumed that veterans may prefer to see clinicians with an understanding of and sensitivity towards military life and culture,[21] and whilst 'Veteran-informed,' or 'Veteran-specific' services may be relevant to some individuals, there are likely to be others who would not want either.[22]

CONCLUSION

This chapter has sought to increase awareness of the veterans in the primary healthcare, and to raise important questions about the nature and scope of the duty to care for veterans. Primary care professionals are expected, when referring a patient that they know to be a veteran for a condition that in their clinical opinion may be related to military service, and to make this clear in the referral. Where secondary clinicians agree that the veteran's condition is likely to be service related, clinicians are expected to prioritise veterans over other patients with the same level of clinical need. This does not mean veterans should be given priority over other patients with more urgent, or greater, clinical need. It is therefore dependent upon the primary care professional to recognise and understand the unique experience of the veteran. It is however not clear how much of an understanding healthcare professionals and workers have about the nature of military experience, or even if the patient is a veteran.

Helping veterans manage health and well-being concerns is important, given the demands placed on military personnel,[23] and to date, the nature of the veteran in the primary care sector is poorly understood and there is minimal research that explores the nature of this experience. Past military contribution does not necessarily always confer prioritised access to health services, but may rather operate as a 'tie breaker' when there are many patients of equal need, and that access to services for veterans and their families may be defensible when services required are related to the injuries during military service, *and* only when no other patient with more urgent medical needs requires attention.

REFERENCES

1. Ministry of Defence. 2011. *The Armed Forces Covenant: Today and Tomorrow*. London: MOD.
2. National Health Services Choices. 2015. *NHS Healthcare for Veterans*. Available at: http://www.nhs.uk/NHSEngland/Militaryhealthcare/veterans-families-reservists/Pages/veterans.aspx [Accessed 14 October 2015].

3. Age UK. 2015. *Later Life in the United Kingdom*. Available at: http://www.ageuk.org.uk/ Documents/ENGB/Factsheets/Later_Life_UK_factsheet.pdf?dtrk=true (accessed August 1, 2017).

4. Fossey, M. and Hacker Hughes, J. 2014. *Traumatic Limb Loss and the Needs of the Family: Current Research: Policy and Practice Implications.* London: Blesma.

5. Castles, S. and Miller, M.J. 1998. *The Age of Migration: International Population Movements in the Modern World.* 2nd ed. New York: Guilford Press.

6. Forster, A. 2012. The military covenant and British Civil Military relations: Letting the genie out of the bottle. *Armed Forces and Society* 38(2), 273–290.

7. McCartney, H. 2009. The military covenant and the changing civilian-military contract in Britain. Paper presented at the Inter-University Armed Forces seminar, Chicago, October 24, p. 11.

8. Ghurka veterans claim victory in court for UK visas. Guardian, 2008. Available at: https:// www.theguardian.com/uk/2008/sep/30/military.immigration [Accessed 01 August 2016].

9. Neel, S. 1991. *Medical Support of the US Army in Vietnam 1965–1970.* Washington, DC: US Department of the Army, p. 55.

10. Gwanda, A. 2004. Casualties of war—Military care for the wounded from Iraq and Afghanistan. *New England Journal of Medicine* 251, 2471–2475.

11. Prognosis for defence spending after Budget 2010. RUSI. Available at: https://rusi.org/ commentary/prognosis-defence-spending-after-budget-2010

12. Hines, L., Gribble, R., Wessely, S., Dandekar, C., and Fear, N. 2015. Are the armed forces understood and supported by the public? A view from the United Kingdom. *Armed Forces and Society* 4(4), 688–713.

13. Woodhead, C., Rona, R.J., Iveron, A., McManus, D., Hotopf, M., Dean, K., McManus, S., et al. 2007. Mental health and health service use among post national service veterans: Results from the 2007 Adult Psychiatric Morbidity Survey in England. *Psychological Medicine* 41, 363–372.

14. Bourdieu, P. 1972. *Outline of a Theory of Practice.* Cambridge: Cambridge University Press, p. 164.

15. Cooper, L., Andrews, S., and Fossey, M. 2016. Educating nurses to care for military veterans in civilian hospitals: An integrative literature review. *Nursing Education Today* 47, 68–73.

16. Cohen, E. 2000. Supreme Command. Anchor Books: NY.

17. Forster, 2012, *op. cit.*

18. MOD. 2008. *The Nation's Commitment: Cross Government Support to Out Armed Forces, Their Families and Veterans.* Cm 7424.

19. MacManus, D. and Weesely, S. 2013. Veteran mental health services in the UK: Are we headed in the right direction? *Journal of Mental Health* 22(4), 301–305.

20. Jones, M., Sundin, J., Goodwin, L., Hull, L., Fear, N.T., and Wessely, S. 2013. What explains post-traumatic stress disorder (PTSD) in UK service personnel: Deployment or something else? *Psychological Medicine* 43(8), 1703–1712.

21. Ben-Zeev, D., Corrigan, P.W., Britt, T.W., and Langford, L. 2012. Stigma of mental illness and service use in the military. *Journal of Mental Health* 21, 264–273.

22. Greenberg, N., Thomas, S., Iversen, A., Unwin, C., Hull, L., and Wessely, S. (2003). Do military peacekeepers want to talk about their experiences? Perceived psychological support of UK military peacekeepers on return from deployment. *Journal of Mental Health* 6, 565–573.

23. Ministry of Defence. 2015. *Armed Forces Covenant.* Available at: www.gov.uk/ government/policies/fulfilling-the-commitments-of-the-armed-forces-covenant/ supporting-pages/armed-forces-community-covenant [Accessed 14 October 2015].

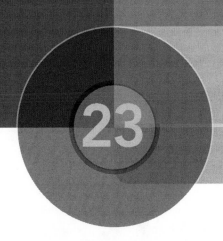

On residential care ethics

23

MICHAEL DUNN

INTRODUCTION

The ethical dimensions of residential care practice have largely been neglected by practical ethicists, meaning that the ethical issues arising in this context are under-explored and poorly articulated. A similar claim has been made about primary care,[1] where it has also been observed that very few of the 'big ticket' concerns in acute or secondary healthcare that have exercised medical ethicists over a number of decades arise. What has been recognised, however, is that ethics – as it is identified, negotiated and managed in residential care – is better understood as being 'everyday' in character.[2]

Importantly, the idea of 'everyday ethics', or the 'ethics of the ordinary' in primary care is now well recognised as capturing something distinctive about the moral character of this sector of healthcare.[1,3] There are important lessons to be learnt from how this concept is correctly articulated between these two care sectors. Partly, these lessons revolve around the ways that ethical issues of particular kinds emerge as problematic in day-to-day care and support interventions, and partly they concern how the interpretation and translation of moral values or principles is correctly thought about when these interventions are enacted.

Residential care is of course a broad church. The only clearly defining feature of these care environments is that care is provided to those 'in residence' of a particular setting. The largest component of residential care, therefore, will be nursing, care or 'group' homes, tracking a significant component of the long-term and social care sector. Not every residential care environment will be long-term, however. Respite care services are an important feature of residential care, where short-term residential placements for individuals are justified on the grounds of the need to give family caregivers a break from their caregiving responsibilities. Equally, not all long-term care settings based within the community are residential; the growing home care sector is not covered by this definition, because in these settings, the individuals receiving care remain resident in their own home.

There will, as I will go on to show, be distinctive ethical features of the residential care setting. This distinctive character will no doubt give rise to differences in the content of the ethical concerns that arise for residential care practitioners in contrast to those working in primary care. There may also be consequent ethical tensions between primary care professionals and their residential care counterparts when they interact in residential care. My aim in this chapter will be to give a fuller account of the ethics of the residential care sector.

I will begin, however, by sketching out the areas of overlap between the kinds of ethical considerations that should be recognised as marking out the shared distinctiveness of the ethics of both residential and primary care practice.

RESIDENTIAL CARE AND PRIMARY CARE: OVERLAPPING ETHICAL CONSIDERATIONS

It is important to clarify whether well-established principles in healthcare can be straightforwardly adopted in the residential care setting. It has been argued that the ethical principles to be applied in residential and other long-term care are different,[4] whilst others have embraced philosophically nuanced readings of the same principles such that they do justice to the particularities of the long-term care environment.[5] One useful way of beginning to settle this question is to make some initial observations about the relational dimensions of caregiving in this setting. Similar to the primary care context, residential care is characterised by a particular and rather unique standpoint towards the relationships that ought to be cultivated between (professional) care provider(s) and care recipient(s).

In British primary care, the care relationship between a general practitioner (GP) and a patient involves recognising that the GP (or other primary care provider) is responsible for ensuring that members of a particular community recognise the local doctor as the 'first port of call' when healthcare needs arise. This is not to imply that GPs, as individuals, will be the sole provider of care in repeated encounters with the patient, but that there is value within primary care to build and maintain such relationships with patients for the longer-term. Similarly, in residential care, the nature of the living environment is such that relationships between caregivers and care recipients are focused on continuous and interpersonal engagement between the two parties, orientated towards ensuring that these individuals' needs can be appropriately identified and met. In nursing homes and other care homes, these relationships transcend public and private space, and are necessarily continuous, often being seen to blur the boundary between family and professional responsibilities and actions.[6,7]

In both primary and residential care, there are clear and distinctive professional ethical obligations that flow directly from these interpersonal caregiving relationships. One important obligation concerns the ways in which the recipient of care is respected as a person, and this obligation will need to be interpreted in ways that do justice to an account of the care relationship that is longer-term and interpersonal. Such respect cannot merely be captured in terms of the 'in-the-moment' obligation to enable and respect the decisions made by a patient about whether to accept a particular kind of intervention. Instead, a more diachronic account of autonomy is required: one that is both backward-looking and forward-looking. This implies a duty of being respectful to the person's changing values with the onset of disability or disadvantage that underpins his/her need for residential support, but that is also focused on promoting choice-making and self-determination into the future through care-planning activities and meaningful forms of engagement with activities.

The value of recognising that *respect* for autonomy here which also extends to include an obligation to *promote* or *create* autonomy[8] is only one of the ways in which autonomy-focused professional duties can be interpreted. A second important feature of the residential care setting is the ways in which it is necessary to interpret personal autonomy in relational terms – an argument that has also been extended to the primary care setting (see Weingarten's contribution in this volume). In residential care, the concept of relational autonomy would require caregivers to pay close attention to the ways in which a person's values are expressed with regards to the concern of others. The onset of chronic conditions, or other such disabilities, that lie behind care recipients' move into a care home setting is disruptive in the sense that it typically involve reconfiguring responsibilities and expectations between individuals and their loved ones. In this regard, it is important to ensure that the principle of respecting the autonomy of those in receipt of long-term care is elucidated in ways that are sensitive to a detailed understanding of the practical ways that people live their everyday lives in such settings.[5]

Nowhere it is this clearer than when light is shone on the ways that decisions concerning the move into residential care, and the content of the care recipient's daily activities in the home, are made. Such decisions commonly involve the person giving due consideration to the interests of friends or family members, rather than being merely self-regarding. Family members are a major presence within residential care settings, visiting regularly, sharing in activities run by the home or even cohabiting with the person so as to maintain valuable connections outside of the private home setting. Respecting the person's values, and the expression of these values through choices made by the person within the home, means recognising that this will likely involve the person foregrounding the interests of others in self-determining the course of his/her own life. Recognising that the obligation to respect the person's autonomy will mean attending to third parties' interests is important, such interests do not contaminate what is owed to the person because these are proper expressions of the person's own interests configured in relational terms.

Importantly, however, the nature of care home provision means that ethical duties towards the person cannot simply be captured by showing appropriate concern to the person's values. Respect for dignity and respect for privacy will also be important. With care and support interventions in nursing and other care homes being continuous, commonly long-term, and particularly invasive, dignity- and privacy-related obligations need to be raised up beyond the level to which they are commonly regarded in medical ethics.

Dignified care will involve attending to the ways in which care recipients are included in interventions into their daily routine, ensuring that they are treated compassionately and humanely at all times. Caregiving in residential care is demanding, time-consuming work. There is often a risk that interventions into people's lives will be justified with regards to the caregivers' own interests, or to manage limited resources and other financial or time pressures in the home, rather than with regards to what is best for the care recipients themselves. Whilst the sustainability of care in a residential setting characterised by finite resources is an ethical challenge in its own right, it is important that care interventions are instigated and justified in ways that remain focused on giving primacy to the interests and dignity of individual persons, and not by recourse to some nebulous sense of communal interests. Equally, the blurring of public and private space in residential care places important duties on caregivers to give due consideration to respecting the privacy of residents. How privacy can be managed will hinge on clarifying the boundaries of private space in the care home, and what respectful engagement with the care recipient requires of caregivers when they are engaged in personal or intimate care work. Respecting privacy will also involve clarifying duties on visitors or other professionals who are not involved in caregiving to limit the spaces of the care home in which they are permitted to intrude, and to ensure that the care recipient is able to give or to refuse permission for circumstances in which caregivers seek to enter his/her private space in the home.

Ethical considerations in residential care extend beyond simply reconfiguring duties relating to respecting persons. Again, similar to primary care, the residential care setting is bounded by a particular community of individuals that it aims to support. In primary care, this is typically a specified geographical region; in residential care, it is a shared home environment. The clearly bounded nature of these two care sectors has important implications for how justice, or the fair treatment of individuals within these communities, is interpreted. Fairness in residential care means recognising that the needs and interests of different recipients of care in the communal spaces of nursing or care home need to be balanced. Certain decisions, particularly those concerning the choice to enter or to leave residential care, will invoke justice-related considerations to other caregivers, most notably family members. In contrast to other healthcare settings, where justice involves making often invisible trade-offs between the health needs of 'statistical' individuals, treating people fairly in residential care will mean balancing the interests of identifiable people in the community setting plus those who might retain some degree of family caregiving responsibilities. Many of these individuals may be vocally expressing why their concerns are more important or pressing than those of other individuals living in the same setting. Providing care in fair ways in the residential home environment means attending to how these interests can be balanced in the most appropriate ways.

'DOING GOOD' IN RESIDENTIAL CARE

Whilst there are overlapping considerations in residential and primary care concerning how to treat people fairly, and to respect care recipients appropriately, there are important differences when attempting to articulate the overarching purposes of these two kinds of care activities. Indeed, in order to establish the ethical obligations of residential caregiving, it is necessary to articulate clearly and compellingly precisely what residential care is *for*, that is to say, what it means to do good in the provision of support in this context, in the broadest sense.

Firstly, it must be acknowledged that the care needs of those receiving support in residential settings are not limited to matters relating to healthcare.[9] The disabilities or impairments most commonly associated with those living in residential care settings (i.e. dementia, intellectual disability or chronic mental health difficulties, often with comorbid physical impairments) require continuous, and often increasing, inputs of personal and social support over time. Crucially, such support does not have as its primary aim the cure or treatment of the underlying disease. Indeed, it is not accurate even to account for residential care in terms of the management of these diseases or impairments – an account that might, instead, be appropriate to define the role of the primary care provider in the residential care setting. Instead, care work in the residential setting is more akin to supporting experiments in daily living under challenging circumstances.[10] How then, ought these experiments to function? Is sustaining human contact the value intrinsic to support of this kind, or can the good life be articulated in a way that is focused entirely on meeting (or maximising) the interests, well-being or flourishing of the recipient of residential care?

One viable route for answering this question convincingly is to draw on the important work that has been carried out recently in capabilities theory (see e.g.[11]). The central idea here is that people may, as a result of disability, impairment or disadvantage, come to lack the real-world opportunities to be and do in ways that they have reason to value. On this account, residential care services (being a site in which such disability, impairment or disadvantage is manifested) ought to act to ensure that such real-world opportunities are safeguarded. Much of the discussion in capability theory in recent years has focused on the question of precisely *what* people have reason to value. Importantly, this account will depart from what people *actually* values, and so capability theory is not founded upon an autonomy-driven or person-centred account of the good life. For Sen,[12] democratic engagement can serve to specify the content of these capabilities in different domains of human activity and welfare; for Nussbaum,[11,13] philosophical reasoning can supply the necessary content, and she identifies 10 central human capabilities: (1) life, (2) bodily health, (3) bodily integrity, (4) senses, imagination and thought, (5) emotions, (6) practical reason, (7) affiliation, (8) contact with other species, (9) play and (10) control over one's environment.

The appeal of this approach for the residential care setting is that the focus on 'beings' and 'doings' closely reflects the everydayness of the interventions that makes up residential care, and that aims to enhance the personal and social functioning of care recipients. This 'functioning' account of care in this setting also connects these capability theory arguments to recent policy formulations about the needs of older adults, and the appropriateness of reconfiguring services to meet the needs of these individuals differently.[14] Clearly, there is much further work to do to specify how core capabilities could be developed in ways that can adequately capture the nature of the interventions that people have reason to value in these different spaces of care. Such work is, I believe, a necessary component of further ethical thinking of residential care practice.

ETHICAL ISSUES IN RESIDENTIAL CARE

The ethical landscape of residential care differs from other care environments in terms of the ethical issues that arise, as well as in terms of the ethical values and principles that underpin good practice in this context. Part of the reason that different ethical issues arise in residential care concerns the particularities of the care work involved, and part of the reason concerns the ways in which the different articulation of values and principles leads to different conflicts between competing obligations. The terrain of these issues has been drawn largely from ethical analyses of dementia, with residential and nursing home care extending to both professional and family caregiving settings,[2,15–19] and these analyses provide a useful springboard for summarising the relevant ethical issues.

RESPECT FOR PERSONS AND RISK MANAGEMENT

One category of ethical issues relates to person-orientated considerations. There is a well-recognised tension in residential care between preventing a person from coming to harm and taking steps to minimise risks in ways that compromise quality of life.[20] Risk of harm comes in many forms: there are risks associated with wandering off and being vulnerable to road traffic or hypothermia, risks from misusing appliances within the home or from other obstacles or risks that arise from eating inappropriately stored food. To reduce risk, caregivers may judge it to be necessary to restrict care recipients' freedoms: preventing them from leaving the home, from moving from a particular place in the home or from accessing certain rooms in the home.

This same kind of issue emerges particularly when caregivers are considering whether to make use of assistive technologies. Such technologies include fall detectors, GPS tracking devices and real-time audio and/or video recording of the home. These technologies have the potential to make substantial improvements to the lives of care recipients, and it has been argued that such technologies are a way of avoiding the dilemma highlighted in the section above. Tracking devices can reduce the dangers from getting lost. Video surveillance methods (telecare) may enable caregivers to respond more quickly in case of need. However, both these uses of technology raise questions of invasion of privacy, and the availability of telecare also raises concerns that the possibility of such remote 'care' will undermine the maintenance of the interpersonal relationships that lie at the heart of residential care practice.[21,22]

BALANCING THE PERSON'S PREVIOUS WISHES AND VALUES WITH THEIR CURRENT INTERESTS

A different kind of issue arises when the care recipient may lose the capacity to make decisions. A dilemma can arise when people have values, or made decisions, that seem at odds with what they currently enjoy and appear to value.[23,24] For example, should a care staff change the television channel if a person who identified himself as being an atheist prior to the onset of dementia is enjoying singing along with the hymns broadcast within a religious affairs programme, when doing so would it cause him or her significant distress?[2] Subsequent questions that arise here relate to the process through which such decisions are made. Who should be involved, and why? How should disagreements between parties be resolved?

TRUTH-TELLING AND DECEPTION

It is widely recognised that respecting a person's dignity and autonomy means that we should not tell lies to them, or engage in other deceptive practices. What should carers do when, because of cognitive impairment, telling the truth causes distress to an individual?.[25] A common concern here arises when people with dementia living in a nursing home keep forgetting that their spouse has died. If every time they ask where they are and are told that their spouse is dead, they may mourn each time anew. Even when relatives believe that it might be right to tell a 'white lie' to prevent distress, some find it very difficult to do so because it is at odds with the history of their relationship,[15] and it is likely that a common intuition might prevail in professional caregiving environments as well.

FREEDOM OF ACTION VERSUS THE INTERESTS OF OTHERS

Other ethical issues emerge out of the fact that in residential care, the person is often receiving support in a communal living environment. Dilemmas about acting in line with the interests of one person can become complex when other individuals might be at risk from the person's behaviour, or when acting in line with these compromises the possibility of acting in line with the interests of other care recipients in the same setting. Within a nursing home, for example, one person's unfettered behaviour may interfere with the freedoms, or enjoyment, of other residents.[19] When should staff intervene to restrict the freedom of one resident for the sake of other residents?

MANAGING SEXUAL RELATIONSHIPS

The lack of privacy that is so often a feature of residential care means that it can be difficult to foster sexual relationships within these environments. However, even in ideal circumstances, there are ethical issues in managing these relationships, some of which will be significantly affected by cultural expectations and religious values.

It is not uncommon in care homes for two residents to form a close relationship with at least some physical intimacy.[26] Care home staff may take a dim view of this behaviour, or be instructed by a spouse or other family to prevent such intimacy. This raises questions of the person's well-being, their likely previous wishes, the interests of the family, the role of the family in decision-making and society's position on what sexual relationships citizens should be allowed to continue.

CONCLUSIONS

Ethical analyses of residential care settings are still in their infancy. In this chapter, I have tried to slowly advance ethical thinking about residential care by showing how the ethical duties on professional caregivers need to depart in important ways from how such duties have been fleshed about in other health care settings. I have also argued that much ethical progress can also be made by getting clear on what it means to do good (i.e. to act beneficently) for those in receipt of residential care, and that – again – this account will be significantly different from accounts of good care that are commonly articulated in health care. I have also shone light on the terrain of ethical issues that can arise in residential care.

Further progress can, I believe, be made in each of these three areas, with advancement in each potentially recalibrating the thinking in the others. For example, examining the fundamental purpose of providing support to people living in residential care opens up the possibility of reconfiguring care services in ways that are sensitive to the moral positioning of different individuals who stand in relation to those with long-term conditions, moving beyond the common but myopic approach of conceiving of the various stakeholders – people with dementia, family carers, care professionals and the state – as parties with different interests that often come in to conflict.

There are also important secondary questions about ethics education, training and support in the residential care sector. The different professional structures and cultures in residential care imply, again, that translating approaches adopted in healthcare ethics will be inadequate. Instead, aligning educational and training initiatives with the induction and workplace-based support mechanisms open to residential care staff is likely to have more success. There is important intellectual and practical progress to be made in residential care ethics, and the growing numbers of those living in these settings should only help to move residential care ethics higher up the agenda in the forthcoming years.

REFERENCES

1. Papanikitas, A., de Zulueta, P., Spicer, J., Knight, R., Toon, P. and Misselbrook, D. 2011. Ethics of the ordinary: A meeting run by the Royal Society of Medicine with the Royal College of General Practitioners. *London Journal of Primary Care*, 4, 69–71.
2. Hope, T. and Dunn, M. 2014. The ethics of long-term care practice: A global call to arms. In A. Akabayashi (ed.). *Towards bioethics in 2050: International dialogues* (pp. 628–643). Oxford: Oxford University Press.
3. Papanikitas, A. and Toon, P. 2011. Primary care ethics: A body of literature and a community of scholars? *Journal of the Royal Society of Medicine*, 104, 94–96.
4. Kuczewski, M.G. 1999. Ethics in long-term care: Are the principles different? *Theoretical Medicine and Bioethics*, 20(1), 15–29.

5. Agich, G.J. 2003. *Dependence and autonomy in old age.* Cambridge: Cambridge University Press.

6. Peace, S. and Holland, C. 2001. Homely residential care: A contradiction in terms? *Journal of Social Policy,* 30(3), 393–410.

7. Dunn, M., Clare, I. and Holland, A. 2010. Living 'a life like ours': Support workers' accounts of substitute decision-making in residential care homes for adults with intellectual disabilities. *Journal of Intellectual Disability Research,* 54(2), 144–160.

8. Seedhouse, D. 1998. *Ethics: The heart of healthcare.* 2nd ed. Chichester: Wiley.

9. Prince, M.J., Acosta, D., Castro-Costa, E., Jackson, J. and Shaji, K.S. 2009. Packages of care for dementia in low- and middle-income countries. *PLoS Medicine,* 6(11), e1000176.

10. Dunn, M. 2014. Dementia: An ethical overview. In C. Foster, J. Herring, and I. Doron (eds.). *The law and ethics of dementia* (pp. 121–134). Oxford: Hart.

11. Nussbaum, M. 2000. *Women and human development: The capabilities approach.* New York: Cambridge University Press.

12. Sen, A. 2005. Human rights and capabilities. *Journal of Human Development,* 6, 151–166.

13. Nussbaum, M. 2003. Capabilities as fundamental entitlements: Sen and social justice. *Feminist Economics,* 9, 33–59.

14. WHO. 2015. *World report on ageing and health.* Geneva: World Health Organisation.

15. Baldwin, C., Hope, T., Hughes, J., Jacoby, R. and Ziebland, S. 2005. *Making difficult decisions: The experience of caring for someone with dementia.* London: Alzheimer's Society.

16. Hughes, J. and Baldwin, C. 2006. *Ethical issues in dementia care: Making difficult decisions.* London: Jessica Kingsley.

17. Kane, R.A. and Caplan, A.L. 1990. *Everyday ethics: Resolving dilemmas in nursing home life.* New York: Springer.

18. Lindemann, H. 2007. Care in families. In R.E. Ascroft, A. Dawson, H. Draper, and J.R. McMillan (eds.). *Principles of health care ethics,* 2nd ed. Chichester: John Wiley & Sons (pp. 351–357).

19. Powers, B.A. 2001. *Nursing home ethics: Everyday issues affecting residents with dementia.* New York: Springer.

20. Nuffield Council on Bioethics. 2009. *Dementia: Ethical issues.* London: Nuffield Council on Bioethics.

21. Ganyo, M., Dunn, M. and Hope, T. 2011. Ethical issues in the use of fall detectors. *Ageing and Society,* 31(8), 1350–1367.

22. Pols, J. 2010. The heart of the matter: About good nursing and telecare. *Health Care Analysis,* 18(4), 389–410.

23. Holm, S. 2001. Autonomy, authenticity, or best interests: Everyday decision-making and persons with dementia, *Medicine, Health Care and Philosophy,* 4: 153-159.

24. Hope, T., Slowther, A. and Eccles, J. 2009. Best interests, dementia, and the Mental Capacity Act (2005), *Journal of Medical Ethics,* 35: 733-738.

25. Schermer, M. 2007. Nothing but the truth? On truth and deception in dementia care, *Bioethics,* 21: 13-22.

26. Dickenson, D., Huxtable, R. and Parker, M. 2010. *The Cambridge Medical Ethics Workbook.* Cambridge: Cambridge University Press.

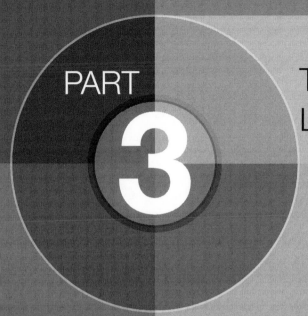

PART 3

TEACHING AND LEARNING

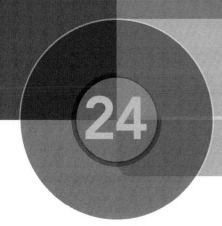

Ethics and the professional identity of a general practitioner in twenty-first century Britain

24

JOHN GILLIES

INTRODUCTION

Professional identity in the twenty-first century is a rather elusive concept. This may be especially true of general practice where professional identity is predicated neither on specialising in one particular organ system, as in many medical sub-specialties, nor on a high degree of technical skill, as in most surgical specialties, but is based on a generalist approach and centred on the doctor–patient relationship. British general practice is offered here as a case study, illustrating the connections between professional identity and practitioner ethics. For the sake of brevity, both general practice and general practitioner are abbreviated as GP (which one is meant should be clear from the text) and 'GPs' refers to general practitioners.

People step into the same waters, and different waters flow onto them.[1]

Another reason for that elusiveness of concept is change. As Heraclitus reminds us from 520 BCE, everything flows and changes: rivers, people, times, ideas, concepts, technology and culture. It is therefore worth asking: What other factors might be contributing to changing ideas about professional identity over the past 20 years?

In the final section, I consider what ethics has to offer and consider developments in a school of ethics that sits intuitively with concepts of professional identity, the virtues.

GENERALISM AND PROFESSIONAL IDENTITY

Twenty years ago, McWhinney asserted that general practice is different from other medical specialities.[2] He described the following core features of general practice:

- It defines itself in terms of relationships, especially the doctor–patient relationship.
- GPs tend to think in terms of individual patients, not abstract concepts of disease.
- It is based on an organismic rather than a mechanistic metaphor of biology.
- It transcends the Cartesian dualism between mind and body.

These differences are significant; it is through such claims to distinctiveness that a profession claims status and rewards for its members. He concluded that 'the importance of being different is that we can lead the way'. While his understanding of professional identity has been profoundly influential, it is debatable whether general practice has 'led the way' over the ensuing 20 years. While GP and primary care are now acknowledged as central to the functioning of health systems,[3] the steadily falling share of NHS resource spent on general practice over the past decade across the UK rather gloomily suggests the reverse.[4] However, following McWhinney's delineation, a great deal of academic work has been done on defining generalism, now regarded as being at the centre of professional identity for GP. Here is one definition of what a generalist is and does:

> We conceptualise generalists as exhibiting compassion, tolerance, trust, empathy and respect (virtues). They reflect carefully on each clinical interaction, recognise its complexity, and acknowledge their prejudices (E.g., towards obesity, unsafe sex practices, single parenthood, substance misuse, poverty, violence, religion). By acknowledging and dealing with their feelings (being reflexive), generalists can begin to fully engage with each patient. The generalists spend time gathering information from the biopsychosocial and cultural domains, rather than focusing solely on physical symptoms and signs.[5]

Mangin et al.[6] subsequently suggested that the continuing rise of multimorbidity, a major characteristic of the work of modern general practice, cannot be addressed by a specialist model of care and single disease guidelines, but requires a well-trained generalist workforce, building on the findings of Starfield et al.[3] The importance of multimorbidity, encompassing both psychiatric and physical morbidities, as a defining feature of modern primary care is well illustrated by a landmark study of 1.8 million Scottish GP records.[7] There is a global consensus that being a generalist is central to the professional identity of GPs, and that simplistic concepts of evidence-based medicine may be inappropriate or insufficient to deal with growing levels of multimorbidity and complexity. As our population of elderly patients with complex morbidity soars, a generalist approach is required to minimise polypharmacy based on unsophisticated ideas of evidence for single diseases.

DOCTORS ARE CHANGING

Generation Y, those born between 1980 and 1999, also referred to in the literature as 'millennials' or 'nexters', and are considered to be technologically savvy, process information rapidly and are reported to embrace change quickly and to become frustrated with uncreative environments with less flexible rules. This generation has been deemed to have a high degree of self-value, to expect respect and to emphasise social interaction and teamwork, with positive interpersonal relationships in the workplace being extremely important to them.[8–12]

These characteristics are reflected in a study of GP trainees in Scotland that further confirmed the significant attachment by generation Y doctors to the inclusive nature of their training environment, respect, feeling valued, support and teamwork[13]. More recently, the importance of feeling valued, and the undermining effect of not feeling valued, has again been reflected in the narrative used by junior doctors when discussing their dispute over the new contract offered by NHS England.

Other studies of doctors have demonstrated the importance that generation Y doctors attach to life–work balance with monetary reward alone being of a lesser importance. For example, a study by Jones and Green[14] on GPs found that early-career GPs were highly satisfied with their job when their career offered a balance between career and family and a range of job experiences which maintained intellectual challenge. They particularly valued the development of relationships with patients. Similarly, good training conditions, opportunities for one's partner and desirable location were important characteristics of attractive training position for trainee doctors in the UK.[15]

However, it is important to remember that the GP workforce is comprised of a mix of baby-boomers, generation X and generation Y.[16,17] There are obviously ample opportunities for value conflicts between these very different age groups! It is also important to note that those in positions of power and influence within the profession are the older age groups. However, we are seeing a gradual shift of power as time and retirement alter the characteristics of the workforce, including a gender shift to a majority female workforce. The embodiment of professionalism may differ between generations; for example, a newly qualified GP in the UK may consider it unusual and even unprofessional to live in the community where he or she practices, while a GP in the 1950s might have considered this a part of the job and possibly even have consulted from the front room of his or her home (note also the change of gender).

THE INTERNET HAS REVOLUTIONISED ACCESS TO MEDICAL KNOWLEDGE

The most widely consulted doctor in today's world is 'Dr Google'. While this trend is sometimes derided by health professionals, it can also be seen as an example of the democratisation of medical knowledge.[18]

Most GPs will be able to give some examples of how Google has helped individuals reach a correct diagnosis. However, the information from Google or any search engine on the internet is of course not always reliable. It seems to be inevitable that some patients will be inappropriately worried, seriously misled or financially exploited by unscrupulous online businesses. Google is taking steps to address this, but it is hard to escape the conclusion that it is almost impossible to police to prevent exploitation on the Internet.[19] Dr Google has no professional qualifications, is not a member of a Royal College and is not subject to registration, jurisdiction or the fitness to practice procedures of the UK's General Medical Council (GMC). The GP is now a guide to reliable medical information, rather then the sole keeper of it. Indeed, there is now too much knowledge for any one human brain – GPs themselves may use internet search engines to locate advice, educational materials and check areas in which they lack intellectual confidence. Attempts to 'know it all' may be a form of hubris and represent poor practice. Knowledge appraisal skills have therefore replaced 'mastery' of a field.

THE AGE OF REGULATION: PROFESSIONAL AND PRACTITIONER VULNERABILITY

The shocking affair of Dr Shipman, the British GP who, during his career, killed over 200 patients, led to major changes in the regulation of medicines and doctors, prompted by Dame Janet Smith's Shipman inquiry in 2000.[20] The inquiry led to changes in death registration, controlled drug storage and record-keeping, better training for coroners and more intensive monitoring and regulation of doctors. In particular, the inquiry also stated that the GMC of that period was an organisation designed to look after the interests of doctors rather than patients. Major changes have followed, and the GMC has substantially more powers to deal with concerns about doctors and take appropriate action. Recently, concern has been expressed about high rates of suicide by doctors being investigated under the GMC's fitness to practise procedures.[21] It came as a surprise to many doctors that the GMC had no senior medical officer overseeing cases where the health of a doctor was of concern. This is being corrected and, at the time of writing, a further review by Professor Louse Appleby is currently helping the GMC review and improve its fitness to practise procedures.[20] While an ethical duty of self-care (to ensure that they are able to care well for their patients) is central to the professional identity of doctors, dealing with mental health problems can pose a particular challenge in this area and needs to be sympathetically addressed. Perhaps the significant thing about these recent events is that some doctors have interpreted them as indicating that, to date, the mental health of doctors was then of low priority for the regulator.[22,23]

GPs' premises and practices have also been regulated and inspected in England by the Care Quality Commission[24] since 2009. It is likely that this process is reassuring for patients and the public. However, concerns have been expressed by the Royal College of GPs (RCGP) that it is onerous, expensive for practices and the NHS, as well as a distraction from the business of providing general medical services for patients.[25] There is also a lack of evidence nationally and internationally that such inspection regimes actually improve quality and prevent harm.

It is certain that these regulatory changes have impacted on professional identity and behaviour. We cannot be sure that the impact has always been one that has been positive for patients, as well as for doctors. This will be explored below. There is a concern that regulation may foster a culture of compliance, which can replace but may diminish cultures of professional judgment.[26]

CHRONIC UNDERINVESTMENT IN GENERAL PRACTICE

Research by RCGP has shown that over the past 8 years, the share of NHS expenditure spent on general practice has fallen by over 2%, from 10.8% to 8.6%. The exact figures vary across the four UK countries but the direction of travel is the same.[27]

This underinvestment in general practice has led to increasing difficulties in meeting the needs of patients, well documented in increased waiting times, problems of decreased continuity, increased stress among GPs and difficulties in recruiting trainees and GPs across the UK, summarised in a recent BMJ editorial.[28] In this sobering assessment, the authors suggest that if general practice fails, the whole NHS fails. Underinvestment seems to be leading not just to a GP crisis but also to an existential crisis for the NHS as a whole across the UK. When doctors like these editorialists, who have both contributed constructively to the development of general practice and to the NHS for decades are speaking in terms like these, we need to consider not just the direct threat to general practice but also the implications for the profes-sional identity of GPs.

This chronic underinvestment suggests an undervaluing of the professional identity of GP. In the UK, GPs have the ability to do a number of clinical roles more cost-effectively than in specialist settings. These include responding to demographic change, complexity and multimorbidity with a generalist approach. That generalism, an adaptive approach to the patient, is undervalued reflects the continuing fallacy of lower professional status attached to GP, despite conspicuous, evidence-based success in delivering quality and cost-effectiveness.[29]

Underinvestment can be considered as a component of a 'conceptual emergency' as set out below.

KEEPING THE ESSENCE OF GENERAL PRACTICE IN THE FACE OF A CONCEPTUAL EMERGENCY

In a 2009 paper on the essence of general practice,[30] it is suggested that to meet the future suc-cessfully, GPs and their professional organisations needed to:

> look critically at current developments, explore ideas, and suggest possible ways
> forward for general practice that both provide continuity with past traditions and
> engage constructively with the rapidly changing worlds of evidence, technology, and
> contemporary culture. In doing so, it was hoped that some characteristics of the essence of
> general practice would be defined.

In the same paper, some aspects of the essence are defined: the qualities, future key roles of GPs and the advantages of a securely financed general practice model for the UK NHS in the future.

Since 2009, the International Futures Forum, a global organisation based in Scotland, has suggested that we have entered a time of 'conceptual emergency', defined thus:

> We are experiencing a step change where complex human systems now operate within
> other complex systems, often with modes of thinking and practice developed in simpler
> days. This is a new world, raising fundamental questions about our competence in key
> areas of governance, economy, sustainability and consciousness. We are struggling as
> professionals and in our private lives to meet the demands it is placing on traditional
> models of organisation, understanding and action. The anchors of identity, morality,
> cultural coherence and social stability are unravelling and we are losing our bearings.
> This is a conceptual emergency.[31]

One can argue that this represents an overly apocalyptic view of the present, and by implica-tion, the future. Another view is that it accurately reflects the world that GPs and their patients live in, reflected both in GPs' lives and the complexities that their patients bring into their surgeries every day. It is important to consider that this is not a despairing view, but a non-pejorative accurate assessment of where we are. If GPs wish to be useful to patients in this world, perhaps we need to adopt a flexibility of professional identity, while at the same time keeping a focus on caring for the individual before us. As suggested in the essence paper, we should not abandon our traditions and values but continually examine and re-examine them in the light of our rapidly changing, culturally incoherent and complex society.

So, to return to Heraclitus, it is clear that the river that we are stepping into every day as GPs is flowing faster and more turbulently than ever before. It is also clear that the new GPs who are stepping into that river have very different ideas and expectations of their work and lives. Is it the work of ethics to help us through that turbulence and avoid us being swept off our feet?

WHAT ETHICS HAS TO OFFER

Much discourse on medical ethics since the Second World War has been based on the principlist approach.[32,33]

The focus on the four principles of medical ethics, respect for autonomy, beneficence, non-maleficence and justice, has served to introduce generations of medical students and post-graduate trainees to an ordered way of considering ethical problems and identifying a way forward. Respect for autonomy is generally considered to be 'primus inter pares' of the principles. Gillon asserts the centrality of the principle of respect for autonomy within the four principles framework.

The development of principlist thinking through successive editions of Beauchamp and Childress's textbook over many years illustrates the success of this approach. It is likely that the emphasis on respect for autonomy grew at least partially out of the appalling research carried out in concentration camps by Nazi doctors, which violated the autonomy of participants already imprisoned in degrading and inhuman conditions.[34] It is important that in considering ethics for professional identity in primary care, we do not ignore or forget these events.

Respect for autonomy, while important in all areas of medicine, may be of prime importance in general practice because of the nature of our professional identity outlined in the first section. As argued by McWhinney, GPs deal with individual patients who have agency, not abstract concepts of disease. The doctor–patient relationship is also central to the speciality of general practice. Respecting autonomy in practice through this relationship, by being respectful and maintaining privacy and confidentiality, is therefore of great significance. Breaches of confidentiality can cause serious problems with trust in the relationship. The difficulties over the past 3 years in NHS England of rolling out the *care data* system of extracting information from GP patient records to support policy and planning, while maintaining the right of the individual patient to privacy of their data, illustrate the challenge of maintaining trust in an age of big data.[35]

This is a major issue in itself, of course, but a central feature of this continuing debate is that the issue of ensuring and maintaining trust may be developing into a discourse not just about GPs maintaining the trust of patients, but also about which institutions, including those of the state, can considered trustworthy when some of those data are shared.[36] Can GPs be both repositories of personal information gained through a trusting doctor–patient relationship and agents of the state in assisting in the collation of some of that information for policy and planning? The answer to this question seems to be still open at the time of writing.

This focus on the individual agent (and patient) is also reflected in the work of Gaita[37] whose conception of good and evil is founded on the preciousness of each individual human life. This, of course, is paramount in all areas of medicine. The centrality in general practice of an 'unconditional regard' for patients[38] is essentially a reflection that each human life is precious, both to that individual and to those who have relationships of kinship and love with them. Our professional identity, as set out above, is based on being a generalist. Generalism integrates biotechnical and biographical perspectives, and the subject of this generalist approach is the unique and precious subject of that biography.[39]

Benatar also argues forcibly that each human life, regardless of place of birth, continent, gender or wealth, has the same moral value, an argument which is not currently given much significance or importance in neoliberal economics.[40] So, while respect for autonomy is a complex concept, it is inextricably tied to notions of individual preciousness in Gaita's thinking, and the intrinsic common moral value of every human being in Benatar's. We should therefore hesitate before disregarding the principlist approach, to which the primacy of respect for autonomy is central.

However, over the past 30 years, as well as the principlist approach, 'there have also been developments in virtue ethics, hermeneutics and phenomenology. Somehow, all these will need to be reconciled and put into some rational order and relationship with each other'.[40]

It is that 'somehow' that Singer et al. see as a problem. However, I am not convinced that it is possible, desirable or practical to try to reconcile irreconcilable ethical theories or approaches. The major change that we have seen is of that of a shift to different approaches based on virtue ethics. These, and their relevance for professional identity, will be discussed below.

AFTER MACINTYRE

Alasdair MacIntyre's book[41] was published in 1981 with the nostalgic title *After Virtue*, and is an analysis of what he sees as the moral fragmentation of our post-enlightenment world. MacIntyre's argument is that people are clinging to superficial fragments of ethics and morality, sometimes paying lip service to ideals while ignoring them in action. This is because the deeper understanding and internalisation of morality have been lost. Despite being a complex, difficult and not altogether cheerful work, it has been very influential in moral theory and in shaping thinking about how we should create communities and professional identities in many fields.

MacIntyre's thesis is that we should develop our virtues – human qualities such as courage, compassion and integrity – to help us to achieve internal goods which are central to leading a flourishing human life, or what Aristotle described as 'eudaimonia'.[42]

Moving closer to professional identity in primary care, I discuss below two authors who have very significant things to say on this.

THE REGULATIVE IDEAL

The most searching and rigorous articulation of a virtue approach to professional roles is probably that of Oakley and Cocking,[43] whose idea of virtue is that of a regulative ideal, defined thus:

> they have internalized a certain conception of correctness or excellence in such a way that they are able to adjust their motivation and conduct is such a way that it conforms or least does not conflict with that standard. (p. 25).

So, in medicine, the good or virtuous doctor will have the requisite skills and competences, will be up to date, compassionate and conscientious, and will exercise judgment carefully when needed, not because of a set of rules or diktats from a regulator, but because he or she has assimilated from study, experience, reflection and role modelling what a good doctor should be. This process, and probably this result, is described by McDowell as 'ethics from the inside out, not the outside in'.[44]

This is not to say that external regulation by the GMC or the Care Quality Commission is redundant or superfluous, but to suggest that it represents ethics applied 'from the outside in' to use McDowell's phrase. It is certainly likely that the GMC rules or duties of a doctor[45] form part of the material that the good doctor will have studied and assimilated, but in deciding what to do in conditions of considerable uncertainty (which are very common in GP), he or she will also rely on his or her internalised understanding of what in this particular case is good clinical practice.

FLOURISHING

Peter Toon has made a considerable contribution to the philosophy of general practice over 21 years with the publication of two RCGP occasional papers on a virtue-based approach to the philosophy of general practice,[46,47] His new book *A Flourishing Practice?* takes the virtue ethics analysis a step further.[48] Toon has been profoundly influenced by MacIntyre and in his latest work, applies MacIntyrean analysis to our current healthcare system in the UK. He suggests that it is characterised by moral fragmentation – in ethical thinking, in legal analysis and in managerial, market-driven and consumerist thinking. The resultant confusion makes dysfunctionality of the system inevitable.

MacIntyre's answer to this dysfunctionality, in general societal terms, is that virtues are developed and exercised within 'practices'. These are varieties of coherent, organised and cooperative human activity to realise internal goods. The internal goods arise from the activities and contribute to the flourishing of the individuals involved and to that of their communities and wider society. These are different to external goods such as the remuneration achieved and the acquisitions – houses, cars and holidays, acquired with these goods, for example.[49]

Toon argues that general practice should be considered to be a MacIntyrean practice with internal goods, founded on the virtues. For GPs, their roles include relieving the suffering of patients and helping them manage, understand and interpret their illnesses or unwellness, thereby helping them lead flourishing lives in an Aristotelian sense. This requires the exercise of certain virtues by GPs: compassion, humility, conscientiousness and an emphasis on relationships, collaboration, reciprocal roles and mutual benefits.[50] He suggests that the current emphasis on deontological frameworks, such as the GMC's good medical practice[44] would be better recast as framework of virtues rather than duties. Toon's focus on virtues is attractive for a profession that has emphasised throughout its history a vocational element to practice, and a focus on role modelling those seen as exemplars of good behaviour and practice. It is also a good fit with Generation Y's focus on being valued, relationships, flat hierarchies and teamwork.[14]

Oakley and Cocking's internalising of a conception of virtues and excellence underpinning the professional role also reflects the history of British GPs and fits well with a serious idea of what a GP should be, as well as what he or she should do.

There is also much in Toon's view of moral fragmentation that reflects the International Futures Forum assertion that we are in 'a conceptual emergency'; his arguments set out firmly the way in which we should address that emergency.

Questions remain, however. Are the 'moral fragments' that MacIntyre and Toon describe not also aspects of a tolerant and pluralistic society that we should strive to maintain and develop at a time when tolerance and pluralism are under attack? Is twenty-first-century democracy characterised by an ability to not only argue forcibly but also to agree to disagree, rather than by a lack of virtue? Can Toon's model really represent a way of maintaining continuity with past tradition,[51] a major feature of MacIntyre's nostalgic view, and deal with the torrent of change in Heraclitus's river? This includes Dr Google, generational shift, quasi-oppressive regulation, underinvestment and the political hostility which GP faces. Is it Procrustean or even Utopian to try to fit general practice into this model?

CONCLUSION: THE CENTRAL PLACE OF *PHRONESIS*

So how do we move forward in a conceptual emergency? A 'somehow' is needed, through which these different approaches will 'be reconciled and put into some rational order and relationship with each other'.[40]

I suggest that rather than struggle to reconcile irreconcilables, we accept that in a time of great clinical, organisational and conceptual complexity, we look towards a conception of rationality that underpins both the principlist and the virtue-based approaches. This is one based on practical wisdom or *phronesis,* and deriving from that, one of perceptual capacity.[52] I suggest this not as an ethical escape clause, but as a way forward that acknowledges and embraces our conceptual emergency: the complexity and the unremitting, accelerating change of the twenty-first century.

Practical wisdom, the usual translation of the Greek *phronesis*, is the virtue of being able to deliberate well. 'The man who is able to deliberate well is he who is able to aim in accordance with calculation at the best for man of things attainable in action'.[53]

Allowing for the sexism of the fourth century BC, this encapsulates much relevant to today: *aim* (look at where you wish to go, but be aware that you may not get to precisely this point), using *calculation* (applying the evidence base) and *attainable in action* (in practice, even general practice, and therefore not just in theory).

What the principlist approach often leaves us with is an understanding of several different ways of looking at a difficult ethical situations viewed through the lenses of the principles, but sometimes no clear way forward, even with the addition of 'scope' to principlist discourse.[54]

Deliberating well may provide a way of using all the different lenses to give us a coherent vision which then enables us to make the correct decision. We should not abandon principles but recognise that we need phronesis to use them effectively in general practice.

Oakley and Cocking, in a discussion of their regulative ideal, suggest that while a 'virtuous person's motivational structure is governed by a particular regulative ideal, appropriate to a particular virtue', the general regulative ideal, involving an understanding of the general good for us all, is phronesis or practical wisdom.[55]

In his account of flourishing professionals, Toon also suggests that phronesis encapsulates the qualities of, among others, technical competence, sound judgment, openness and honesty. It is therefore also central to the development of the virtues necessary for MacIntyrean practice in Toon's conception.

Putting this argument in the context of generalism as the core of the professional identity of GP, Reeve's definition[56] is crucial:

> Generalism describes a philosophy of practice which is person, not disease centred; continuous, not episodic; integrates biotechnical and biographical perspectives; and views health as a resource for living and not an end in itself.

There is a complexity here which underpins the need for phronesis. The good GP understands the patient as well as the disease or illness. She sees the biomedical aspects as a feature of the patient's life. She uses a non-Utopian, functional definition of health as a guide.

There is, of course, the persistent niggling argument that relying on phronesis for making decisions leaves us with a 'black box' of judgment which we cannot penetrate.[57]

Essentially, however, that is the nature of judgment. It is where the processes of reasoning, deliberation and discussion take us to in complex situations such as clinical decision-making in a generalist discipline. In depth, explorations of this can be found in Occasional Paper 86 and later discussions on perceptual capacity.[51,58]

GPs rely on perceptual capacity as a central part of professional identity, especially in consulting with patients. This is founded on *phronesis*, and is the ability to read or assess a situation correctly, in depth and breadth. Wiggins[57] called this *'aithesis'* or 'situational appreciation', and Nussbaum 'some sort of complex responsiveness to the salient features of one's situation'.[59] It is based on sound clinical knowledge, the exercise of empathy and compassion and the judicious use of imagination and finely tuned emotional responses. To achieve this, professionals should 'aim' as Nussbaum suggests, to become 'a person on whom nothing is lost'.[59] It is this capability that is at the heart of both the regulative ideal and the internal goods of general practice. It is the foundation of professional identity as general practitioners.

ACKNOWLEDGEMENT

I would like to acknowledge the contribution of Dr Sharon Wiener-Ogilvie, General Practice training unit, NHS Education Scotland, to the discussion on baby boomers and Generations X and Y. Also, Dr Mark Sheehan, Oxford Biomedical Research Centre Ethics Fellow, for past significant conversations on philosophy and ethics.

REFERENCES

1. Brunschwig J, Lloyd G. (Eds.). *Greek thought: A guide to classical knowledge.* Cambridge, MA: The Belknap Press of Harvard University Press; 2000, p. 633.
2. McWhinney I. The importance of being different. William Pickles lecture 1996. *Brit J Gen Pract* 1996; 46: 433–436.
3. Starfield B, Shi L, Macinko J. Contribution of primary care to health systems and health. *Millbank Q* 2005; 83(3): 457–502.
4. Royal College of GPs 'Put patients first: Back general practice'. http://www.rcgp.org.uk/campaign-home.aspx (accessed 31 March 2016).
5. Gunn J, Palmer V, Naccarella L, et al. The promises and pitfalls of generalism in achieving the Alma-Ata vision of vision of health for all. *Med J Aust* 2008; 189(2): 110–112.
6. Mangin D, Heath I, Jamoulle M. Beyond diagnosis: Rising to the multimorbidity challenge. *BMJ* 2012; 344: e3526.
7. Barnett K, Mercer S, Norbury M, et al. Epidemiology of multimorbidity and implications for health care, research and medical education. *Lancet* 2012; 380: 37.
8. Hewlett SA. How Gen Y & Boomers will reshape your agenda. *Harv Bus Rev* 2009; 87(7–8): 71–76, 153.
9. Borges NJ, Manuel RS, Elam CL, Jones BJ. Differences in motives between Millennial and Generation x medical students. *Medical Educ* 2010; 44(6): 570–576.
10. Lavoie-Tremblay M, Paquet M, Duchesne M-A, et al. Retaining nurses and other hospital workers: An intergenerational perspective of the work climate. *J Nurs Scholarsh* 2010; 42(4): 414–422.
11. Cubit KA, Ryan B. Tailoring a graduate nurse program to meet the needs of our next generation nurses. *Nurse Educ Today* 2011; 31(1): 65–71.

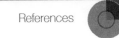

12. Laurence CO, Williamson V, Sumner KE, Fleming J. 'Latte rural': The tangible and intangible factors important in the choice of a rural practice by recent GP graduates. *Rural Remote Health* 2010; 10(2): 1316.

13. Wiener-Ogilvie S, Bennison J, Smith V. The general practice training environment and its impact on preparedness. *Educ Prim Care* 2014; 25: 8–17.

14. Jones L, Green J. Shifting discourses of professionalism: A case study of general practitioners in the United Kingdom. *Sociol Health Illn* 2006; 28(7): 927–950.

15. Cleland J, Johnston P, Watson V, et al. What do UK doctors in training value in a post? A discrete choice experiment. *Med Educ* 2016; 50(2): 189–202.

16. Howe N, Strauss W. *The fourth turning.* New York: Broadway Books; 1997.

17. Ahluwalia S, Tavabie A. *General practice specialty training; Making it happen.* London: RCGP Publications; 2016.

18. Slack B. *Dr Google will see you now.* http://www.newstatesman.com/2015/11/dr-google-will-see-you-now (accessed 29 March 2016).

19. Sifferlin A. *Here's what 6 doctors think of Dr Google.* http://time.com/4025756/google-health-issues-doctor/ (accessed 29 March 2016).

20. Smith J. *The Shipman inquiry reports.* http://webarchive.nationalarchives.gov.uk/20090808154959/http:/www.the-shipman-inquiry.org.uk/reports.asp (accessed 29 March 2016).

21. Horsfall S. *Doctors who commit suicide while under GMC fitness to practice investigation.* http://www.gmc-uk.org/Internal_review_into_suicide_in_FTP_processes.pdf_59088696.pdf (accessed 29 March 2016).

22. GMC Press release 3rd December 2015. *GMC appoints former mental health tsar to improve its support for vulnerable doctors.* http://www.gmc-uk.org/news/28380.asp?AcceptCookie=true (accessed 29 March 2016).

23. *The fitness to practice process may do more harm than good. Pulse News,* 2 February 2015. http://www.pulsetoday.co.uk/your-practice/regulation/the-fitness-to-practise-process-may-do-more-harm-than-good/20009091.fullarticle (accessed 29 March 2016).

24. Care Quality Commission. *For GP surgeries and out of hours services.* http://www.cqc.org.uk/content/gp-practices-and-out-hours-service-providers (accessed 29 March 2016).

25. RCGP Press release 15th October 2015. *Response to care quality commission report on the state of health and social care in England 2014–15.* http://www.rcgp.org.uk/news/2015/october/rcgp-response-to-care-quality-commission-report-on-the-state-of-health-and-social-care-in-england-2014-2015.aspx (accessed 29 March 2015).

26. O'Neill O. A Question of Trust: the Reith lectures 2002. p.89.Cambridge University Press Cambridge.

27. *RCGP policy brief: Put patients first.* http://www.rcgp.org.uk/policy/~/media/Files/PPF/Put-patients-first-campaign-brief.ashx (accessed 29 March 2016).

28. Roland M, Everington S. Tackling the crisis in general practice. *BMJ* 2016; 352: i942

29. Starfield et al., 2005, *op. cit.*

30. Gillies J, Mercer S, Lyon A, et al. Distilling the essence of general practice: A learning journey in progress. *Brit J Gen Pract* 2009; 59(562): e167–176.

31. International Futures Forum. *Conceptual emergency: Make space for confusion as the context.* http://www.internationalfuturesforum.com/conceptual-emergency (accessed 30 March 2016).

32. Gillon R. *Philosophical medical ethics.* London: Wiley; 1986.

33. Beauchamp T, Childress J. *Principles of biomedical ethics.* 7th edition. Oxford: Oxford University Press; 2012.

34. United States Holocaust Museum. *Nazi medical experiments.* https://www.ushmm.org/wlc/en/article.php?ModuleId=10005168 (accessed 31 March 2016).

35. NHS England. *The care data programme; collecting information for the health of the nation.* https://www.england.nhs.uk/ourwork/tsd/care-data/ (accessed 30 March 2016).

36. O'Neill Baroness O. *Which comes first: Trust or trustworthiness?* http://www.bbc.co.uk/news/magazine-20627410 (accessed 30 March 2016).

37. Gaita R. *Good and evil: An absolute conception.* London: Routledge; 2004, p. 95.

38. Mathers N. *The Tao of family medicine: James Mackenzie lecture 2013.* https://www.sheffield.ac.uk/polopoly_fs/1.403203!/file/The_James_Mackenzie_Lecture_2014_by_Professor_Nigel_Mathers.pdf (accessed 30 March 2016).

39. Benatar S. Moral Imagination: The missing component in global health. *PLOS Med* 2005; 2(12): e400. DOI: 10.1371/journal.pmed.0020400.

40. Singer PA, Pellegrino E, Siegler M. Clinical Ethics revisited. *BMC Med Ethics* 2001; 2: 1. DOI: 10.1186/1472-6939-2-1.

41. MacIntyre A. *After virtue; a study in moral theory.* 3rd edition. London: Duckworth; first published 1981; 2007.

42. Aristotle. Brown L (Ed.), Ross D (transl.). *The Nicomachean ethics.* Oxford: Oxford World Classics; 2009.

43. Oakley J, Cocking D. *Virtue ethics and professional roles.* Cambridge: Cambridge University Press; 2006.

44. McDowell J. Virtue and reason. In McDowell J (Ed.), *Mind, value and reality.* Cambridge: Harvard University Press; 1998, pp. 50–73.

45. General Medical Council. *Duties of a doctor.* London: GMC; 2013.

46. Toon P. What is good general practice? A philosophical study of the concept of high quality medical care. *Occ Paper R Coll Gen Pract* 1994; 65: 1–55.

47. Toon P. *Towards a philosophy of general practice; A study of the virtuous practitioner.* Occ. Paper no 78. London: RCGP Publications.

48. Toon P. *A flourishing practice?* London: RCGP Publications; 2014.

49. MacIntyre, 2007, *op. cit.,* 187–189.

50. Toon, 2014, *op. cit.,* 79.

51. Gillies et al., 2009, *op. cit.*

52. Gillies J. *Getting it right in the consultation: Hippocrates problem; Aristotle's answer.* Occasional paper no.86. London: RCGP Publications; 2005.

53. Aristotle, 2009, *op. cit.,* NE1141b 12-14.

54. Gillon R. Medical Ethics: Four principles plus attention to scope. *BMJ* 1994; 309: 184. DOI: 10.1136/bmj.309.6948.184.

55. Oakley, Cocking, 2006, *op. cit.,* 29–30.

56. Reeve J. Protecting generalism: Moving on from evidence-based medicine. *Brit J Gen Pract* 2010; 60: 521–523.

57. Wiggins D. Deliberation and practical reason. In Wiggins D (Ed.), *Needs, value, truth.* 3rd edition. Oxford: Clarendon Press; 2002, pp. 215–237.

58. Gillies J, Sheehan M. Perceptual capacity: Invisible yet indispensable for quality of care. *Brit J Gen Pract* 2005; 55(521): 974–977.

59. Nussbaum M. The discernment of perception; an Aristotelean conception of private and public rationality. In Sherman N (Ed.), *Aristotle's ethics: Critical essays.* Lanham: Rowman and Littlefield Publishers; 1999, pp. 145–181.

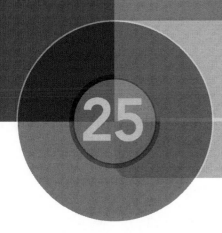

25

Teaching and learning ethics in primary healthcare

ANDREW PAPANIKITAS AND JOHN SPICER

INTRODUCTION

Much has been written about the content of ethics in terms of primary healthcare. Arguments for the importance of a nuanced ethics education have been advanced in terms of the nature of the clinician–patient relationship outside the hospital setting as well as the sheer volume of patient–clinician contacts in primary healthcare. Many such ideas inform the scope of this volume. There is relatively little written about ethics education in the context of primary care *per se* – and this is largely confined to descriptions and justifications of syllabus and pedagogic approach for teaching ethics to general practitioners.[1–4] We would like to propose a broader account of ethics education. Just as healthcare might aim to focus on the needs of patients and populations, education similarly has those who commission and purchase it, those who receive the education and those who receive the benefits of the education. These various stakeholders might attach different value to different content and different modes of education. In this chapter, we will consider what might be taught, why it might be taught and finally offer some concrete examples of where it is or could be taught in the context of British general practice (as just one example of primary healthcare). This chapter focusses on medical ethics education in the UK context but borrows unashamedly from other disciplinary perspectives. We will not dwell on legal and statutory aspects of medical ethics education because these will vary depending on the country and the profession, and because it is addressed elsewhere.[5] The aim of the authors is that this should be used as a case study that may inform any healthcare professional involved in teaching and learning ethics in the primary care setting.

TEACHING AND LEARNING ETHICS 'IN', 'OF' AND/OR 'FOR' PRIMARY HEALTHCARE

Considering ethics education 'in', 'of' and 'for' primary healthcare adapts an approach by Draper and Ives to consider the 'content' of ethics education in relation to primary care.[6]

Ethics 'in' primary care, for example, might be attractive in the undergraduate medical education setting. Medical students can see everyday principles such as consent and confidentiality in action (and ways in which these are tested) when, for example, someone agrees to have a routine blood test, or where many family members are looked after by the same clinician. Patients are generally more likely to be well enough to assert their rights and expectations,[7] and clinicians such as general practitioners may espouse a holistic rather than a more narrowly biotechnical approach to treatment.[8–10] This ethics in primary care may be important for students, trainees and trainees who are 'only passing through' as learners – the learning in primary care can, we suggest, enhance clinical interactions in other settings. The idea of ethics 'in' primary care relies on the idea that primary care is a good learning environment for ethics education and that clinicians are good teachers.[11] Even the facts that so much of healthcare is community-based and office-based rather than hospital-based or that many patient healthcare narratives begin in the primary care setting might imply that ethics ought to be taught and learnt in the these contexts. This approach makes no claims that there is a particular academic–intellectual blend of ethics in primary care, only that this is a context qualitatively or quantitatively rich in ethical experience and therefore potential learning.

"GPs are sometimes a bit smug about medical ethics. We are the ones trained in ethics, communication skills, and patient-centred medicine — we just are the good guys. Also we don't go around turning off life support machines, deciding who gets the transplant, or fiddling with stem cells, so if biomedicine makes mistakes it won't be our fault."[12]

Ethics 'of' primary care implies that there is a particular species (or blend) of ethical scholarship that has emerged from and is possibly distinctive to the primary care setting. This might imply simply that ethics is experienced in a particular way in the primary care setting that is not usual in other settings. It might imply that particular skills are needed or that a particular approach (Virtue ethics has been a conspicuous offering[13]) might be better for practitioners' and patients' ability to flourish. However, the ethics 'of' primary care implies learning about what ethical practices and understandings exist as well what they ought to be. Ethics 'of' primary care implies that primary care is an area that might be researched and studied including by non-clinicians as a source of scholarship. An ethics of primary care might incorporate elements such as 'inter-professional' ethics or the 'ethics of the ordinary.' We see this less as 'What ethics can be taught in primary care?' as 'What ethics can primary care teach?'

Ethics 'for' primary care implies that there are forms of ethics education (in terms of syllabus and/or pedagogy) which can enhance primary care practice. Greenhalgh (for example) argues that primary care is an applied, problem-orientated discipline drawing on a range of other theoretical and applied disciplines.[14] Most (of many) definitions include first-contact care, undifferentiated care, continuity over time, coordinated within and across sectors and a focus on the individual and the population or community.[15] She identifies core values for good primary care, which are as follows:

1. *Holistic:* Embraces the complexities and interactions of bodily systems, mental responses, family community and sociocultural context. It also seeks continuity of care through time.
2. *Balanced:* Seeks a middle ground between breadth and depth of knowledge, between lay and medical models of illness and distress between intervention and leaving well alone.
3. *Patient-centred:* Sees each patient as an individual and seeks to offer personalised rather than standardised packages of care.
4. *Rigorous:* Primary care seeks to draw judiciously on multiple sources of evidence (patient's unique predicament, relevant research literature and wider family and social context) when considering the action to take in relation to a particular problem.

5. *Equitable:* Takes responsibility for social justice in the allocation of scarce resources, hence works proactively with, and plays an advocacy role for, the disempowered, inarticulate and socially excluded. This may include challenging the educated, worried well when they seek a disproportionate share of healthcare resources.

6. *Reflective:* It is practiced in conditions of ignorance and/or uncertainty. Requires a questioning attitude, willingness to revise provisional diagnoses in light of emerging findings and the humility to defer to higher authority (specialist, parent, patient) when appropriate.[15]

FIVE BASIC ORIENTATIONS FOR ETHICS EDUCATION: FROM 'WHAT' TO 'WHY'

Having considered what ethics might be taught in the context of primary healthcare, it is worth considering the purpose of ethics education related to the context of primary care. To do this, we consider ethics education through the ways in which education is broadly orientated. Eisner argued (based on a wealth of educational theory and insights from empirical studies) that there are five basic and important orientations to a curriculum. Awareness of these orientations allows the educator to see behind the immediate issues affecting educational programmes and to make vivid the major ways in which those programmes are conceived. Eisner refers to cognitive processes, academic rationalism, personal relevance, social adaptation and social reconstruction and curriculum as technology.[16] All these orientations have a bearing on ethics education.

An orientation towards the development of cognitive processes emphasises the belief that curriculum and teaching strategy should foster the student's ability to think and reason. The focus is on helping the learner to learn, to use and strengthen their intellectual faculties. Implicit is the idea that facts and theories change, whilst there is eternal currency in critical thinking skills and the ability to make a good argument and recognise logical flaws and fallacies. This orientation may prioritise content that is meaningful to the learner and problems that are intellectually challenging. It requires the ability to raise the kinds of questions that direct learners' attention to levels of analysis that they would not have been likely to use without the aid of a teacher.

Academic rationalism is one of the most recognisably traditional orientations in education. It argues that the function of education is to foster the intellectual growth of students in those subject matters most worthy of study. This might be expressed in our context in two key ways: Firstly, ethics is one of those worthy subjects – critical to reflexive practice (though we note that reflection is an educational method, it is also critical to ethics education) and professional citizenship. Secondly, the content of ethics education is prescribed in the form of worthy texts – for example, the works of Aristotle, Thomas Aquinas or Peter Singer. As an example of the recommendation of worthy content for UK general practice education, see Knight, who argues that the four principles of Beauchamp and Childress ought not to replace the first principles of deontology, consequentialism and the virtues.[17] Because many human problems have been addressed by great minds over the generations, we are invited to stand on the shoulders of those giants and select the very best of them to learn from. Academic rationalism leads to two key difficulties in ethics education; as we have alluded to the above, there is much debate over the right content for a syllabus. Furthermore, the selection of the syllabus and correct pedagogical methods and academic language with which to master it fosters academic specialisation.

This is problematic because jargon and highly developed argumentation may render some work in scholarly journals unintelligible to non-experts. Primary healthcare workers need to be able to access the intellectual content of education if it is to be meaningful in practice.

Personal relevance emphasises the primacy of personal meaning and the educator's responsibility to make such meaning possible. In practical terms, this might mean developing education with student involvement. This orientation is founded on the respect for learners as persons. This might be proactive in terms of ethics education – asking students to identify those issues that are important to them or more indirect/post hoc in the forms of a sincere approach to the involvement of students in educational design or feedback. A difficulty that may arise here lies in the heterogeneity of learner in terms of background, perceived and actual learning needs and place in a healthcare hierarchy among other sources of diversity. McAuliffe, for example, points out that higher education has been traditionally focussed on discipline-specific ethics education, making interprofessional ethics education more problematic.[18] 'Personal relevance' approaches may also have a distorting effect on ethics education, when students see its role as granting the ability to win arguments and justify prejudices or to steer clear of criticism only.

Social adaptation and social reconstruction collectively are an orientation that derives its aims and content from an analysis of the society that education is designed to serve. It might be said that the mission of educators is to locate and be sensitive to social needs in providing their programmes, clearly a socially adaptive or reconstructive approach. This is very evident in historical accounts of the origins of the bioethics movement in medicine and the biosciences more generally, where unethical behaviour (mainly by doctors) is implicated in humanitarian atrocities committed in the furthering of medical knowledge[19] and other abuses of medical knowledge and status.[20] More cynically, however, a social adaptation orientation might identify with an institutional purchaser of education in response to the needs of the institution – for example, if a healthcare provider noticed that complaints against its staff were on the rise and accordingly commissioned ethics education. By contrast, social reconstruction is aimed at developing levels of critical consciousness – the aim of such programmes is not so much to help students to adapt to a society that is in need of fundamental change but to help them recognise the real problems and do something about them. Ethics education may aim at social adaptation. This is reflected in the recent court case where the British Association of Physicians of Asian and Indian Origin unsuccessfully sued the Royal College of General Practitioners for having an examination that discriminated against non-white international medical graduates. The court determined that more efforts were needed to enable the acculturation of such candidates for practice in Britain.[21] It can also aim at 'increasing the good in the world' by providing learners with the tools for activism and societal change. This is evident in much of the educational content of global ethics, and the ethics of procurement. Most recently, some writers have examined the vulnerability of healthcare workers to moral distress, emotional burnout and political disenfranchisement (see chapters on Commissioning, Global Ethics and Self-care in this volume).

Curriculum as technology is an orientation that conceives of curriculum planning as a technical undertaking, relating means to ends that have already been formulated. These ends are made operational through statements that are referenced to observable behaviour. This approach favours the systematic mapping of educational objectives to observable objective measures. Expectations seen in industry are transferred into education with efficiency and effectiveness procedures applied to the product (learning). Not only are the students graded according to preset criteria but teachers are also evaluated on their ability to educate the students. This orientation should be very familiar to medical educators in the UK and elsewhere.[22] An issue for ethics education may be difficulty in seeing the outputs or payoffs that are measurable in the same way as teaching a clinical procedure such as performing venesection. The danger here for learners is that in a curriculum as technology orientation, goals that cannot easily be measured or quantified may fall by the wayside. The emphasis on behaviour neglects the substance and rationale so that the learner may 'do' without a good understanding of 'why.' Correct procedure may be overemphasised at the cost of understanding and reflection. This is noted in RCGP curricular materials for trainee GPs in the UK, with the caution that unless a trainee is able to reflect on the ethics of their actions, they risk falling into unethical practice.[23]

Orientations as described by Eisner are models for parallel conceptions of educational virtue. Whilst it seems unlikely that any one orientation would be encountered in a pure form, it is possible that one might predominate. Dominance of any particular orientation has consequences for the practical operation of learning and teaching. Each orientation serves to both legitimise certain practices and discriminate against others. A seminar in ethics for trainees on a medical speciality programme may well have a different orientational 'flavour' to an online module for a Masters' level degree in evidence-based healthcare, to a professional education session offered at a medical conference or to a postgraduate diploma in philosophy and ethics aimed at all healthcare professionals. These and many other settings will be influenced by not only the commissioner of education and the learner but also the teacher (and the academy which influences the curriculum). Where any particular orientation predominates, there may be twin concerns that ethics education is not unjustly deprioritised (or indeed that it eclipses other necessary learning), or reduced to a series of thoughtless actions or statements aimed at satisfying a test criterion. Awareness of curricular orientation is therefore of use to all who have a stake in the education, whether as a tool for reflection or for analysing the actions of others.

Next, we will consider some specific medical contexts for teaching and learning ethics in primary healthcare. This is because the medical context is what we as teachers happen to be familiar with. That is not to argue that others do not have teaching expertise and learning needs that are relevant. Indeed, we invite colleagues in other medical disciplines and other healthcare professions to construct analogous schemata.

ETHICS EDUCATION ALONG A PROFESSIONAL LIFE COURSE

Medical students and immediately qualified doctors in the global West are pluripotential. They have yet to begin the specialising process, though they may, even at entry into medical school have particular career aspirations. Ethics education provided in medical school is largely aimed at creating virtuous doctors and doctors who are capable of recognising duties and reconciling conflicts.[22] In the previous section, we have discussed ethics 'in' primary care. Ethics curricula, such as the UK Institute of Medical Ethics (IME) consensus statement on what an ethics curriculum should contain, aim to show medical students knowledge, skills and attitudes required for practice as a junior doctor.[24] This is a blend of general ethical principles including major troublesome yet everyday concepts such as confidentiality and global citizenship concepts such as justice. Given that juniors are less professionally autonomous, the ability to ration does not seem immediately relevant until we factor in the possibility that junior doctors may sometimes be less ideally supported in time-critical decision-making.

General practitioners, in the UK and elsewhere are encouraged to adopt a holistic approach towards patients' and families' bio-psycho-social needs. Such an approach is naturally appropriate to those who work in primary care, sharing as they do the key attributes of primary care work. Elsewhere in this book, Spicer discusses the 'Oughts' of generalist practice. Ethics for and ethics of primary care may predominate here. General practice trainees in the UK and other countries may also lack some of the moral conveniences of good hospital settings (they are far from guaranteed either in hospital or community), such as a supportive hierarchy, functioning interdisciplinary teamwork, a fixed and easily accessible geographical space for discussion (the doctors' mess or common room) and education (the postgraduate education centre). Accordingly, ethics education should not only address key predicted issues, such as confidentiality in the family setting, but also prepare trainees to be more proactive in use of learning opportunities available. Some may be provided, such as a session on vocational training, or readings in dedicated training materials. Some may need to be accessed independently, such as books and papers in both general healthcare and bioethical literatures, a website or an educational course.

Ethics education may be seen as instrumental to a variety of purposes, such as leadership, management, and teaching and commissioning. Cox and Papanikitas, for example, outline an ethical approach to commissioning in this book. Leadership training may have an overt orientation towards social reconstruction (recognising the need for and leading change).

Fully qualified and experienced professionals are unlikely to cease to have learning needs. Some of these needs, however, are not about taking on an enhanced role but survival and flourishing as a practitioner. Elsewhere in this book, McKenzie-Edwards discusses ethics as necessary for surviving and flourishing. General practitioners and their equivalents, for example, need an equitable way of managing workload, because in many settings, the demand far exceeds both the supply and the available means to resource it. Having language with which to discuss moral conflicts, and spaces where discussion is relatively safe, may offer a potential antidote to both overt moral distress and ways of recognising the ethical issues.

CONCLUSION

In this chapter, we have eschewed the temptation to systematically list, in the manner of a syllabus, a collation of ethical content or skills that a primary care professional could and should possess, whether they are medical or other types of practitioner. The literature such as it is majors on the medical though our consistent opinion is that it is transferable between types. Instead, we have used a variety of prepositions to dissect the various educational themes that seem to be important to the learning and teaching of ethics as a primary care endeavour. Essentially, ethics education should follow the patient, and as most care takes place in the community, it follows that the learning and teaching about ethics as about other curricular objectives should follow too. However, realist education should also account for the fact that clinicians are not 'Platonic gentlemen'[25] but people who are engaged in an often difficult, emotionally rewarding and taxing endeavour. Ethics education that does not take account of the complex relationship between profession, civil society and state[26] risks being a source of burnout or honoured in word only. We suggest that Eisner's model[15] has much to offer as a structure for consideration of primary care ethics education, and bears comparison with the other aspects of education theory relevant to its practice. We further suggest that diversity of providers and the holistic elements of practice can mean that primary healthcare has much to contribute to ethics education for healthcare in general.

REFERENCES

1. Boyd K. Teaching medical ethics to medical students and GP trainees. *J Med Ethics* 1987; **13**: 132–3.
2. Molyneux D. Teaching ethics to GP registrars on the day-release course: An evaluation. *Educ Prim Care* 2001; **12**: 379–86.

3. Knight R. Tools for teaching medical ethics to specialty registrars. *Educ Prim Care* 2007; **18**: 749–53.

4. Gillies J. Ethics in primary care: Theory and practice. *InnovAiT* 2009; **2**: 183–90.

5. Slowther A, Spicer J. Ethical and legal issues. In: Carter Y, Jackson N, eds. *Medical education and training – From theory to delivery.* Oxford: Oxford University Press; 2009: 339–50.

6. Draper H, Ives J. An empirical approach to bioethics: Social science 'of', 'for' and 'in' bioethics research. *Cogn Brain Behav* 2007; **11**(2): 319–30.

7. Brody H. The physician–patient relationship. In: *The healer's power.* New Haven, CT: Yale University Press; 1992: 44–66.

8. Reeve J. Protecting generalism: Moving on from evidence-based medicine? *Br J Gen Pract* 2010; **60**(576): 521–3.

9. Reeve J. Interpretive medicine: Supporting generalism in a changing primary care world. *Occas Pap R Coll Gen Pract* 2010; (88): 1–20, v.

10. Reeve J, Irving G, Dowrick CF. Can generalism help revive the primary healthcare vision? *J R Soc Med* 2011; **104**(10): 395–400.

11. Hafferty FW, Franks R. The hidden curriculum, ethics teaching, and the structure of medical education. *Acad Med* 1994; **69**(11): 861–71.

12. Misselbrook D. The BJGP is open for ethics. *Br J Gen Pract* 2012; **62**(596): 122.

13. Toon PD, Towards an understanding of the flourishing practitioner. *Postgraduate Medical Journal,* 2009; **85**: 399–403.

14. Greenhalgh T. The 'ologies' (underpinning academic disciplines) of primary health care. In: *Primary health care: Theory and practice.* Oxford: Blackwell; 2007: 23–6.

15. Greenhalgh T. Introduction. In: *Primary health care: Theory and practice.* Oxford: Blackwell; 2007: 1–22.

16. Eisner EW. Five basic orientations to the curriculum. In: Eisner E, ed. *The educational imagination: On the design and evaluation of the school programs.* New York: Macmillan Publishing; 1985: 61–86.

17. Knight, 2007, *op. cit.*

18. McAuliffe D. Introduction. In: *Interprofessional ethics: Collaboration in the social health and human services.* Victoria: Cambridge University Press; 2014: 1–5.

19. Wilson D. Criticising club regulation and 'the birth of bioethics'? In: *The making of British bioethics.* Manchester: Manchester University Press; 2014: 43–50.

20. Wilson D. 'Who's for bioethics?' Ian Kennedy, oversight and accountability in the 1980s. In: *The making of British bioethics.* Manchester: Manchester University Press; 2014: 105–39.

21. HCT. *The Queen on the application of Bapio Action Ltd (Claimant) v Royal College of General Practitioners (First Defendant) and General Medical Council (Second Defendant). EWHC 1416 (Admin)* 2014.

22. Eckles RE, Meslin EM, Gaffney M, Helft PR. Medical ethics education: Where are we? Where should we be going? A review. *Acad Med* 2005; **80**(12): 1143–52.

23. Riley B, Haynes J, Field S. Essential feature 2 – Attitudinal aspects. In: *The condensed curriculum guide for GP training and the new MRCGP.* London: RCGP; 2007: 114–5.

24. Stirrat GM, Johnston C, Gillon R, Boyd K; Medical Education Working Group of Institute of Medical Ethics, associated signatories. Medical ethics and law for doctors of tomorrow: The 1998 Consensus Statement updated. *J Med Ethics* 2010; **36**(1): 55–60.

25. Toon P. General practice as a business and patients as consumers. In: Perreira-Gray D, ed. *What is good general practice?* London: Royal College of General Practitioners; 1994: 37–41.

26. Salter B, Who rules? The new politics of medical regulation, Social Science and Medicine, 2001; 52: 871–883.

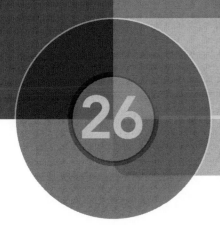

26

Interprofessional ethics in the primary care setting

HILARY ENGWARD

INTRODUCTION

Interprofessional care is the process in which different professional groups work together to deliver healthcare, its underpinning premise being to promote the well-being of the patient.

Generally, it is assumed that interprofessional working leads to enhanced patient care, although literature suggests that interprofessional working may not always have a positive impact on patient care. Issues around poor communication and a limited understanding of others roles/responsibilities lead to conflicts across in patient care.[1] While there is wide discussion of interprofessional working in the literature, most relates to the acute sector.[2] It is therefore important that interprofessional working and the ethics inherent in those working in the primary care sector are better understood.

Ethics is the study of what is right or wrong, which includes the values and principles that govern individual, organisational and political conduct. If focus is primarily given to 'shared values' or 'individual personal qualities', we risk ignoring the more complicated interplay between people, policy, political ambitions and health outcomes – such phenomena inform how people act and set limitations on possible courses of action and outcomes.[3] As such, understanding ethics in interprofessional working in primary care needs to consider the individual encounter, the organisation within which that encounter occurs and the politics within which that practice is contained.

The purpose of this chapter is therefore twofold; firstly, we consider how we might better understand interprofessional working in the primary care sector, and secondly, we consider ethics in interprofessional working in primary care. To do this, it is argued that interprofessional ethics ought to be considered at team and organisational levels. Using examples, interprofessional and organisational differences between how ethics can be understood are identified. Conclusions suggest means of developing ethics in primary interprofessional care.

CLARIFYING 'INTERPROFESSIONAL WORKING'

Prior to exploring the ethical dimensions of interprofessional working, the term itself needs to be clarified. Leathard[4] uses the term to refer to 'interactions between professionals involved, albeit from different backgrounds, but who have the same joint goals in working together'. This includes communication and decision-making, accountability, coordination, equality of resources, open communication, cooperation, assertiveness, autonomy and mutual trust and respect. As such, interprofessional working is about team effectiveness, in which members of the team value each other's roles as important to the team's functionality.

Three different team approaches are distinguished and described to judge the quality of teamwork and team performance in healthcare: multi-, inter- and trans-disciplinarity. 'Multi-' refers to different professions/disciplines each working on their own goals in a rather autonomous way, 'inter-' refers to them working closer together on a common goal and sharing a team identity and 'trans-' refers to the disciplines or professions sharing competencies and therefore being able to takeover tasks from other team members.[5] Inter- and transdisciplinary teamwork have been associated with enhanced team functioning and higher treatment quality,[6] better clinical outcomes,[7] and improved patient safety[8] and higher job satisfaction,[9] and organisationally, increased cost savings and reduced turnover.[10]

Whilst effective team working is a valuable pursuit in its own right, it may be, however, that the prerequisites of effective team functionality may bring about ethical challenges within that functioning. For teams to function effectively, there needs the requirement of open communication, autonomy and equity of resources across professional groups. This however requires shared understandings about the purpose of each disciplines' function, and understanding as to how the individual within the disciplines in the teams values each-other's role in the team. This may bring about disagreement as to how to best manage care. As such, the focus of ethics in interprofessional working needs to be at the team level, and is more an ethics of teamwork. To think about ethics of teamwork therefore means we have to shift our focus away from the patient, and instead focus on the team.[11]

ETHICS IN PRIMARY CARE AND
INTERPROFESSIONAL WORKING

Clark et al., argue that teams learn to negotiate and understand in three distinct but inter-related elements: (1) principles (guidelines for behaviour), (2) structures (established forms of knowledge and patterns of behaviour) and (3) processes (how things are done). These are considered in further detail as follows:

Firstly, principles act as guidelines for behaviour. In healthcare, ethical issues are conceptualised in terms of codes of ethics. Most codes call for their professionals to work collaboratively with other professions, and most practitioners would ascribe to this as being a good thing. Ethical standards are often developed under the assumption that care would be provided in uniprofessional settings, and most codes apply to all members of that profession in all contexts. This is important because ethical standards are independent of context and are not specific to primary care. However, the primary care professional is likely to encounter situations that fall outside their uniprofessional expertise, which can result in differences in priorities between members of the team. Being deontological in focus, codes specify duties and moral obligations of the professions, but how the tenets of duties and obligations interplay between the professions has received limited attention, and how ethical concepts are understood and used by the professions in the team may differ; the concept of confidentiality may have different emphasis between professions, leading to a nuanced application by professionals, for example, between the general practitioner (GP), genito-urinary practitioner and social worker, where focus may be on the individual and/or the family unit, where the individual needs and family needs may differ and be difficult to navigate, where the issue of 'who' is being treated is relevant and may differ in relation to the purpose of the discipline in that team.

Codes that are confined to 'disciplinary silos'[12] risk of uniprofessional collegiality, in which professions pursue their own goals at the exclusion of other professions.[13] Dynamics between professions can be influential in how the team works together, for example, Mitchelle[14] found that nurses experience conflict in the interprofessional relationship due to different discourses between the professional–patient relationship, leading to a lack in coherence between what the nurse feels they ought to do and what they actually do. This could be experienced by any member of the interprofessional team, but maybe more opaque in the primary care sector due to the diversity between the professions and the geographical vastness the interprofessional team is likely to cover.

The large volume of care provided in primary care settings across diverse geographical locations means that ethically challenging situations may occur at a higher frequency than in acute settings, even if the situations are not unique to primary care. Although the codes of ethics offer some clarity and congruence regarding aspects of care, they do not fully address the complexities of practice in primary care, where ethical norms are not easily transferrable across care contexts. A useful example here is consent. Consent, broadly, is the communication between the patient and the professional that results in an agreement to undergo specific medical interventions. Consent taking in primary care is not necessarily a one-time event, but is an ongoing, thoughtful and purposeful process. For example, it is more likely that consent to treatment may occur over several visits rather than at one single point in time. This is especially relevant to primary care, where the patient may not fully understand that they could be engaging in conversations with different members of the team that could result in an assessment, diagnosis, treatment or change of treatment, of which the patient may not be aware of. Conventional methods of consent-taking at one point in time are not necessarily realistic to the pace of primary care, and patients need a better understanding of what is involved in their care and reviewing their records/history. Further, good practice might suggest that patients should be provided with verbal discussions/printed materials to ensure understanding of what is being agreed to, and they should understand that their information will be documented in their medical records and may be viewed by many different professionals in the delivery of their care. The ultimate goal of teamwork is enhanced patient care. However, what this enhanced care might be does not exist within in a vacuum, but is subject to various professional-specific principles that can be influential in how care is delivered in the interprofessional team. This does not mean all disciplines need to agree with one another's approach to their practice, but rather that the differences should be clearly understood and used to increase the effectiveness of the care provided across the teams.

An important element often associated with types of care that are provided in the primary sector is the covenantal nature of care relationship with the person and persons in the community. This care relationship may continue irrespective of whether a person chooses to accept the care provided or not. This contrasts to care where, if intervention is refused, or consent is withdrawn, the care interaction often ends (a form of relationship often associated with secondary care. In the primary care context, however, this relationship is ongoing. For example, an alcohol-dependant person may refuse support services, but the care and supporting relationships between the professionals and their patients and communities may continue indefinitely. With increasing numbers of people living longer with multiple morbidities, and patients living longer with more complex health and social needs, integrated service processes need to work together to provide a cohesive care approach within interprofessional working.

Secondly, in the Clark et al. model is structures, such as established forms of knowledge and patterns of behaviour. Here, a socio-historical perspective is useful to consider how professions have been socialised. Looking at the development of the professions, Friedson[15] describes a profession as 'an occupation which has assumed a dominate position on a division of labour, so that it gains control over the determination of the substance of its own work'. How professions have historically evolved can indicate how professions worked together, which in turn informs how they currently work. For example, nursing was associated as a female occupation and viewed as less important than medicine, and as such, paid less. Research by van der Lee et al.[16] explored the historical development of the collaboration between obstetricians and midwives in Dutch maternity care and found that interaction between the professions could be characterised as competitive rather than collaborative, where both professions used unidisciplinary protocols, strived to preserve autonomy in professional practice; although both professions shared the same patient population and pursued the same goal, that is, good maternity care,[17] there was no evidence of 'interprofessional governance' and 'shared goals and vision'. What is important here is that there may be historically and culturally embedded perceptions about power between differing professions, where those in subordinate groups are socialised to be dependant to the needs of the dominant group.

To explore this further, Friend and Cook[18] suggest that collaboration involves parity, mutual goals, shared accountability, shared resources and voluntariness. Here, collaboration is neither top-down or bottom-up, but rather acknowledges that each individual brings unique knowledge and skills that benefits the decision-making process. The establishment of mutual goals for collaborative action is identified as the hallmark of collaboration where goals must be acceptable to all involved. This entails some form of 'formalisation' and 'internalisation' of acceptable processes and limitations of practice; however, whilst parity across the team is desired, it may be difficult to attain. For example, van der Lee et al.[16] identified that the formalisation of collaboration between the midwives and obstetricians entailed the introduction of regulations restricting midwifery practice to the physiological processes of pregnancy and delivery, without any usage of instruments or medication. Whilst this division gives obstetricians a dominant position over the midwives, it may unhelpfully restrict the experience of midwives to physiological pregnancy and doctors to pathological pregnancy in ways that ultimately disadvantage patients.

Thirdly, in the Clark et al. model is processes, or how things are done. As previously identified, the primary care team is however dispersed across a wide geographical community and consists of differing disciplines, but also may have differing employers, contracts and differing professional agendas. The space where ethical decisions are made and enacted in primary care may be virtual or via a telephone, and members of the team may never meet one another, therefore, it is difficult to understand each member's role and responsibilities in the team. An unclear or incomplete understanding of one's own role and other professionals' roles in the collaboration is known to have a negative effect on a person's attitude towards collaboration and to inhibit collaboration skills.[19] A study within the practices of GPs showed that the extent of GPs' collaboration with and patient referral to allied health professionals was negatively influenced by the GPs' limited understanding of the roles and capabilities of those allied professionals.[20]

A lack of understanding of each other's roles and responsibilities can lead to decision-making that serves the interests of the discipline as opposed to the patient. King[21] uses a case study of a patient who requires wound dressing more often than the community can provide, and therefore has to access services at the local emergency department (ED). Simplistically viewed, the community team may have a moral duty, but not the resources. The ED team possibly have the resource (this too is debatable) but whose primary duties are to a different population. Whilst changes in service provision and process may make internal sense, the patient is powerless to change or challenge the change, and may suffer harm as a result.

Internal processes therefore can be delivered in isolation without awareness of the consequences on other service provision and service users. Another useful example here is to consider how professional resources are deployed and consequences on the interprofessional team working and patient care. For example, in community mental health service provision, there may be a reliance on locum psychiatrists, leading to inconsistent care planning, with inconsistency in the care prescribed, where the community psychiatric nurse needs to negotiate differences between the locum psychiatrist's decisions in order to support the patient in the community. Akin to this may be difficulty in accessing in patient acute psychiatric beds for patients in crises. This compromises the purpose of primary care services, that being to care for persons, whether they are ill or not.

CONCLUSION

The contemporary context of primary care makes this anthology timely. Ethics is the study of what is right or wrong, of moral duty and obligation, and to develop and extend ethical debate in relation to how teams can work interprofessionally to enhance patient care fits with primary healthcare arrangements in both Europe and other global settings. This includes better understanding the values and principles of conduct of individuals who work in teams, although this latter part is perhaps not explicitly discussed. Applying a framework such as that used by Clark et al. enables us to see and explore different structures that influence interprofessional team working, centralising the wider principles, processes and structures the interprofessional team works within. In this context, for ethics to be its most useful, we need to ask questions about how care is able to be done within organisations, teams, and how individuals in teams become intrinsically ethical in their approach to their work. This is not saying that individual is not important, but we rather forward it is of equal importance to understand ethics as socio-culturally located, in order to understand how interprofessional work ought to be.

As such, for a more nuanced understanding of ethics in interprofessional working in primary care, some translational work is needed. By this we mean that a better empirically based understanding is needed to explore working realities of interprofessional working in primary care, but we also need to re-explore what we already know of healthcare ethics in relation to the context of primary care. Here the 'ideal theory' may be useful. The ideal theory sets aside 'real world' complications, what the ideal 'ought' to be like. This book is setting the scene to explore the ought of primary care, and our job is to explicate what the relationship between healthcare ethics as a theoretical activity, means in relation to the actual doing of healthcare practice in the primary care context. The challenge therefore, to ask what ethics in interprofessional working ought to be, how the ethics of interprofessional working is, and how the relationship between the two can be better understood.

REFERENCES

1. Indepdent Policy Complaints Committee. 2009. *Report into contact between Fiona Pilkington and Leicester constabulary 2004–2007.* Available at: https://www.ipc.gov.uk. (accessed August 1, 2017).
2. Bowman, D., & Spicer, J. (eds.). 2007. *Primary care ethics.* Oxford: Radcliffe.
3. Wintrup, J. 2015. The changing landscape of care: Does ethics education have a new role to play in health practice. *BMC Medical Ethics*, 16, 22.
4. Leathard, A. (ed.). 2003. *Interprofessional collaboration: From policy to practice in health and social care.* London: Routledge.
5. Reeves, S., Lewin, S., Espin, S., & Zwarenstein, M. 2010. *Interprofessional teamwork for health and social care.* Chichester, West Sussex: Blackwell.
6. O'Leary, K. J., Sehgal, N. L., Terrell, G., & Williams, M. V. 2012. Interdisciplinary team-work in hospitals: A review and practical recommendations for improvement. *Journal of Hospital Medicine*, 7, 48–54.
7. Xyrichis, A., & Lowton, K. 2008. What fosters or prevents interprofessional teamwork-ing in primary and community care? A literature review. *International Journal of Nursing Studies*, 45, 140–153.
8. Salas, E., Gregory, M. E., & King, H. B. 2011. Team training can enhance patient safety – The data, the challenge ahead. *Joint Commission Journal on Quality and Patient Safety/Joint Commission Resources*, 37, 339–340.
9. Körner, M. 2010. Interprofessional teamwork in medical rehabilitation: A comparison of multidisciplinary and interdisciplinary team approach. *Clinical Rehabilitation*, 24, 745–755.
10. Zwarenstein, M., Goldman, J., & Reeves, S. 2009 Jul 8;(3):CD000072. doi: 10.1002/14651858.CD000072.pub2. Interprofessional collaboration: Effects of prac-tice-based interventions on professional practice and healthcare outcomes. *Cochrane Database System Review*, 3.
11. Clark, P., Cott, C., & Drinka, T. 2007. Theory and practice in interprofessional eth-ics: A framework for understanding ethical issues in healthcare teams. *Journal of Interprofessional Care*, 21(6), 591–603.
12. Long, T., Dann, S., Wolff, M. L., & Brienze, R. S. 2014. Moving from silos to team-work: Integration of interprofessional trainees into a medical home model. *Journal of Interprofessional Care*, 28, 473–474.
13. Hall, P. 2005. Interprofessional teamwork: Professional cultures as barriers. *Journal of Interprofessional Care*, 19, 188–196.
14. Mitchelle, C. 1982. Integrity in interprofessional relationships. In: G. Agida, ed. *Responsibility in healthcare.* Dordrecht, The Netherlands: Kluwer.
15. Friedson, E. 1998. Professions of medicine: A study of the sociology of applied knowl-edge. In: L. Mackay, ed. *Classic texts in healthcare.* Oxford: Butterworth–Heinnemann.
16. Van der Lee, N., Driessen, E. W., Houwaart, E. S., Caccia, N. C., & Scheele, F. 2014. An examination of the historical context of interprofessional collaboration in Dutch obstet-rical care. *Journal of Interprofessional Care*, 28, 123–127.
17. De Vries, R. G. 2004. *A pleasing birth: Midwives and maternity care in the Netherlands.* Philadelphia, PA: Temple University Press.
18. Friend, M., & Cook, K. 1990. Collaboration as a prediction for success in school reform. *Journal of Education and Psychological Consultation*, 1, 69–86.

19. van der Lee, N., Fokkema, J. P., Westerman, M., Driessen, E. W., van der Vleuten, C. P., Scherpbier, A. J. J. A., & Scheele, F. 2013. The CanMEDS framework: Relevant but not quite the whole story. *Medical Teacher*, 35, 949–955.
20. Baker, L., Egan-Lee, E., Martimianakis, M. A., & Reeves, S. 2011. Relationships of power: Implications for interprofessional education. *Journal of Interprofessional Care*, 25, 98–104.
21. King, A. 2007. Interprofessional team working: A moral endeavour? An exploration of clinical practice using Seedhouses's ethical grid. In: D. Bowman and J. Spicer, eds. *Primary care ethics.* Abingdon: Radcliffe.

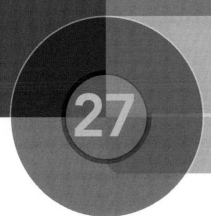

27

The ethics of teaching and learning in primary care

JOHN SPICER AND ANDREW PAPANIKITAS

INTRODUCTION

Just as every clinical interaction between a healthcare professional (HCP) and patient will have a professional, ethical and legal component, it can be said that every learning interaction should be viewed similarly. If that is so, then those learning interactions merit some analysis, argument and even an evidence base.[1] The benefits for patients participating in healthcare education are often indirect or intangible, often less than the predicted costs or harms. Accordingly, writers have even drawn comparisons between the ethics of research and the ethics of education, suggesting and understanding of the former could usefully inform the latter.[2]

Contextually, the history of clinical education does not emphasise primary and community care as it does secondary care. The medical schools of Europe are historically founded in the hospitals for the poor. Writers such as Foucault have highlighted the influence of this historical trend on the biomedical 'gaze' that sees patients as holders of anatomy, physiology and pathology rather than as a whole person.[3] This gaze may limit the appreciation of patients' full personhood, especially after clinicians' induction into scientific medicine. The involvement of general practice and other community HCPs in healthcare education and training has, until the later part of the twentieth century, been largely confined to apprenticeships. The extension of gaze beyond the biotechnical is a distinctive feature of generalist primary care such as general practice or family medicine. It arguably enhances the practice of both those students and trainees who are passing through primary healthcare and those destined to remain.

Clearly, we should differentiate education for the practice of primary care from the wider issue of using primary care as a learning environment for all disciplines at earlier professional stages, wherever they may eventually practice. In each situation, teaching and learning in the community require a cadre of appropriately trained teachers, across the disciplines, as well as all the other curricular and support mechanisms in place.[4] An immediate ethical dichotomy that arises from this is the difference between 'student' and 'trainee'. For our purposes, here the emphasis for a student is on learning, with supervised involvement in patient care and little if any clinical autonomy. The trainee by contrast is a service provider and a learner – the priority given to learning, and the level of supervision decreasing with career progression.

In general terms, the list of ethical issues in education is frighteningly long and includes conflicts of interest, justice issues and balancing benefits and harms.[5] In nursing, for example, Fowler and Davis subdivide issues into those concerning: faculty, students, faculty-student roles and interaction, academic and scientific integrity, educational administration and 'Profession, society and global relations'.[6] For the purposes of this chapter, we will reflect on the patient in the primary healthcare setting, with particular focus in consent and the ethical distortions of task focus and observation on the learner consultation. We discuss the Hippocratic duty to teach and ethical issues relating to the needs of learners. We also look at more systemic concerns such as curricula and workforce development as well as how professional diversity and the dispersed nature of primary healthcare may have ethical import. We have illustrated this chapter with cases – these are hypothetical with one exception that is adapted from a qualitative study. We invite the reader to reflect on them and consider the issues in the reader's context (whether or not it differs from the case).

THE PATIENT IN PRIMARY HEALTHCARE

If, as we would argue, experiential learning is the better way to acquire clinical skills, then access to patients is a *sine qua non*. It is now without serious contest accepted that patients should consent prior to their involvement in primary care education, as elsewhere.[7,8] As such, a consent may be regarded as a 'flak jacket,' protecting the educator from accusation that patients' rights have been violated, though the underlying issues bear examination.[9] There are often (in high-income countries at least) differences in the quality of the healthcare encounter. For example, patients' ability to consent to be seen by a student may be influenced by their long-standing relationship with a general practitioner – in short, they might for various reasons find it hard to say no. The most powerful of these reasons could actually be the long-standing relationship between doctor and patient, mirrored in other primary care disciplines. Where both parties know each other well, over time, it might be that patients feel obliged in some way to be party to an education session they might rather not be part of. Familiarity might be said to breed consent in a long-standing clinical relationship, but it may also breed coercion, unless the educator is careful.[10,11] The benefits of a purely educational encounter for the patient may relate to the satisfaction of improving the overall quality of local healthcare. This may be more evident in a primary care setting where the learners may remain in practice and the patients may themselves reap the benefits of a more experienced clinician at a later date. For students and itinerant trainees, this benefit may be paid forward – patients benefit from others' generosity in a manner analogous to herd immunity from vaccination. There may also be tangible gains such as a financial honorarium or enhanced access to healthcare for patients who participate.

Medical students and trainees (and other HCPs in training) learn *inter alia* about disease by obtaining data from patients (taking a history) and then presenting the data back to their teachers. However, as they progress towards independent practice, taking a history should become more shaped by the patient's values and agenda, on the basis that the doctor is there to help the patient.[12] When medical learners forget this and prioritise the task (history-taking) over the broader aims of talking to the patient, this hinders a humane discourse between the student or trainee and the patient. The following scenario is adapted from a recent qualitative study in ethics education.[13]

CASE 1

Nawal, an experienced GP educator, is supervising Joe, a medical student who has just started his clinical attachment in general practice. Nawal warns Joe that the next patient has agreed to see a student but is suffering with a number of psychological problems. He asks Joe to be sensitive to this. Joe has studied a summary of the information that a good psychiatric history requires, and attempts to ask a series of questions in the order that they appear on his summary. The patient starts to cry and gets up to leave.

'Taking a history' can become an end in itself rather than a means to finding out what is ailing the patient. An approach that is too focussed on obtaining the pieces of information that the learner considers to be important can fail to elicit what patient's relevant ideas, concerns and expectations are.

Techniques such as filming or otherwise recording consultations can pose consent issues. Where the patient views the content of the consultation as uncontroversial, consent may be readily forthcoming to use a recording for education and even assessment purposes.

This does not solve the problem of those consultations that are characterised by major emotional content, extreme disagreement or a perceived stigma that is not dissipated.

Problems of positive bias and patient consent are less of an issue – video recording is now generally used in the UK for educational purposes and workplace-based assessment only.[14] As the stakes are lower, the temptation to hide deficiency is less, though not completely absent.

THE DUTY TO TEACH

CASE 2

Phil, a general practitioner, attends a meeting of the practice partners at the healthcare centre where he works.

They are discussing how many medical students they can host – a local, independent psychotherapist would like to hire a room in the centre for private practice and this would mean reducing the number of students.

They are also concerned about access targets for numbers of appointments set by the local healthcare commissioners. GPs in the surgery who are supervising a student or trainee have some time set aside in each clinic so that they can teach, answer questions and check what the relevant learner has done. It is proposed that these 'catch-up slots' are removed. Teaching sessions are marked separately in the appointments calendar and patients are asked if they would be happy to see a student or a trainee. If patients are not happy to see a student trainee, they are offered an appointment at another time. It is proposed that this is inconvenient for patients, so if the patient does not wish to participate in training, the student or trainee should be asked to step outside for the consultation.

If, as we also suggest, there may be a duty on behalf of patients to be involved in clinician education, then it is appropriate to ask whether a comparative duty exists on behalf of primary care clinicians to teach, especially in virtue of the relative historical lack of teaching in these environments. In a UK context, clinicians in secondary care are assumed to be capable teachers simply by their place of work, though primary care clinicians must professionalise their teaching skills in addition to their clinical skills by the formal attainment of a qualification. This is not a universal description but is common enough to suggest that the teaching role is a right for those working in a hospital, but a privilege for those in a community clinic. This is odd, and without obvious ethical justification.

Followers of the Hippocratic Oath held that all doctors, at least, were under a duty to teach their craft to their juniors (those who were the children of their colleagues at least). The duty to teach our juniors is a view we can extend to all HCPs in the modern age, and not only those who are junior. It is fraught with problems however. Despite the transferable skills between clinical practice and teaching, it is by no means clear that all clinicians have the motivation or competence to teach, as opposed to practice.[15] So, any notional Hippocratic duty to teach is at once undermined. Furthermore, as a subset of motivation, the nature of teaching as a moral enterprise bears examination; under this header lie the character attributes normally held to be virtuous in any teacher – integrity, authenticity and good example.[16,17]

Generally, the motivation of primary care clinicians to teach is not in question, as much research has demonstrated, even in high workload contexts that generally primary care clinicians are keen to teach.[18]

CASE 3

Two friends, Omar and Phil, are chatting over drink in the pub. Omar is a hospital physician and Phil is a GP. Phil is an enthusiastic teacher of young doctors in training – it keeps him on the ball, he feels. Omar is irritated at his teaching responsibilities, which his Medical Director requires him to do on top of his clinical workload. Omar's point is that he feels he's no good at it, dislikes having learners around and he's better occupied looking after his patients in the intensive care unit.

LEARNERS' ISSUES

Whether or not Omar (above) is any good as a teacher is as much subjective as objective, and the assessment of his skills is beyond the scope of this chapter, but if we accord him a duty to teach, it is possible he may not do it very well. Phil seems to thrive on teaching, though his primary care location is accidental in this example, and may thus enthuse his learners as a result. It is even possible Phil will help his learners cope with some of the pressures of clinical education, such as assessment overload, poor learner–patient relationships or overwork among qualified learners.[19,20]

Dealing with learners' issues, described largely, could be said to be part of the teacher's lot: whether they are progression problems, pastoral difficulties or any other variation.[21] In primary care, by virtue of its distributed nature, it is likely that teachers' ability to support learners in difficulty is more difficult to achieve: there is a less clearly defined faculty, less access to continuing professional development (CPD) as a teacher and less kudos for teaching. One of the largest challenges for any postgraduate learner is dealing with the balance between rendering a service to the patient (from whom he or she is learning, by doing this) and keeping a space for learning.[22] This is a difficult ethical conundrum to resolve. Teachers must arrange suitable working weeks that allow learning to take place in a supported manner,[23] but graduate them to make their learners ready for the realities of clinical working life. It is unlikely that healthcare resourcing will ever allow clinical practice to be undemanding, much as we may wish it thus. Whilst there is insufficient space in this chapter to consider fundamental differences of values between teachers and learners, many of their sources are covered in this book including conscience, intergenerational difference and the distinction between self-care and selfishness.

LEARNING ENVIRONMENTS

A distinctive characteristic of patient care in the community is the distributed nature of its organisation. Whilst hospitals are discrete, bounded entities, loosely identifiable within a geographical setting and possessing of support services and educational infrastructure, community care may have little of this. Instead, any given community might have a number of venues, purposes and staffs, managerially unrelated. It is not necessarily a coherent faculty within which to deliver teaching and learning, and thus requires a higher level of organisation to achieve this task.

This distributed network may be of value as it might generate diversity, innovation and flexibility of educational approach. In our chapter on teaching ethics, we reflect on the need for better interprofessional ethics in response to the diversity and plurality of primary healthcare providers and their infrastructures. A moral approach to healthcare education includes an ethical approach to hierarchy both within and across professions. Notions of equality and diversity may be useful in respecting and addressing the concerns of learners, colleagues and patients by giving them a voice. The reverse is testimonial injustice, where a group of people are unjustly denied a voice because of some aspect of their identity: being junior, an ancillary profession, female, etc.

Even the residence of the patient may, conceptually, be considered to be a learning environment for primary care clinicians; there is no doubt that teaching and learning takes place in such a place, and arguably the more challenging the venue, the greater the learning that might ensue, though it may be difficult to maintain resource standards. There may also be enhanced ethical tensions between education and care – for example, when inexperienced HCPs travel to geographical areas of high healthcare need and inadequate provision – a phenomenon seen in medical electives in low- and middle-income countries.

CASE 4

Bill, a student nurse, accompanies his supervisor, Reena, to a home visit at a long-standing patient's residence. The house is cold, untidy and full of assorted junk collected over many years. The patient, Edna, appears happy in this situation. She receives meals via a charity each day, and has little need of cooking facilities. Reena observes Bill conducting a full community nursing assessment of Edna and her needs. Later they debrief on the assessment. Reena is impressed at Bill's skills, but wonders if it was in fact safe to take a learner to such a venue.

More generally of course, the learning environments of primary care are practices, family planning clinics, child health centres and much else. They are notable by their variety and situation in the heart of the communities they serve. They are situated and perhaps even embodied in their patients.

CURRICULAR ISSUES

We will espouse the wider meaning of the curriculum here, encompassing as it does the entire learner journey from curriculum design to evaluation. Each stage manifests its own ethical conundrums.

At an academic council meeting, Dora and Fakole are discussing community nurse placements for their university's undergraduate nursing programme. They disagree quite heatedly, as Fakole is arguing for a significant expansion in the time devoted to community placements. She believes that the university has a duty to expose their students to as wide a variety of placements as possible, and as future healthcare will be increasingly shifting out of hospital, their students' learning must shift too. Dora does not want to disturb the status quo, where students in hospital placements can be easily supervised and brought back for formal teaching. She also worries about the quality and number of supervisors available locally outside hospital.

Fakole is onto something here. Whilst the story above may concern, on its face, the convenience of faculty, it is important to recognise that one of the strongest influences on career choice is the venue of placements undertaken at a pre-licensing phase of learning. So, it is right by inference to place learners in the places of work (and learning) that are needed for the future delivery of healthcare. Curricular design of this type can determine not only career choice but also professional identity evolution, collaborative practice competences and even support diverse clinical care. It matters, and has moral weight.[24]

When designing a curriculum, or more realistically a syllabus, it is important to ask how the content of a clinical course is arrived. Other than the primacy of ethics content, which the present authors would argue powerfully for, what else should define content? The greatest influence on clinical curricula is that of official regulators, exemplified in the UK by the General Medical Council, Nursing and Midwifery Council and other regulators.

Their role is quasi-legal, in that they are invested by government with the power to determine curriculum and standards of teaching. At an undergraduate level, traditional power and influence have favoured basic science and research, at least in medicine. The question might be asked as to how is syllabus actually blueprinted against the needs of population and individual health. The 'outcome-based' education methodologies claim to answer this question, linking as they do content and delivery directly to patient care.[25] One example of such a curriculum design, from the Association of Medical Educators of Europe, summarises neatly the role of the physician as doing the right thing, doing the thing right and the right person doing it. Each of these qualifiers clearly refers to right in a moral, as well as educational sense.

However, this is not quite as far as one might argue an ethical or even adequate approach to curricular design.[26] Particularly for primary care, at the point of first access as it is, curricula might be said to need designing utterly on the existence of patients' healthcare needs (those which present and those which are hidden by cultural taboos and inverse care laws).[27] If a healthcare need exists, it needs placing on a curriculum. In a healthcare system of universal coverage where social solidarity is held to be of high value, then this aspect is even more justifiable. It does demand more speed and agility in curricular designers for primary care than is currently the case. However, as things are, the curricula that govern teaching and learning for the disciplines of primary care are set by colleges and regulators, with only a partial regard for the clinical content of primary care.[28] This disjunction is awkward as it does not, in the end, serve patients' needs. We might deduce therefore that there is an ethical imperative to design a curriculum as closely aligned to patient need in their various clinical environments as possible.[29–31]

In a UK context, there is much variation as to the investment in the education of the various disciplines, and historically, medicine has had the greater share. Whether this is fair and equitable can be argued about *ad nauseam*. Suffice to say, in a context where multiprofessional learning is held to be a common good, and workforce requirements indicate a broader skill mix is needed than hitherto, some readjustment may be necessary.

One example of variation between professions in primary care is in access to clinical supervision. Traditionally, non-medical disciplines, and psychiatrists, have valued the supervision process as part of continuing learning for practice, and time is set aside as part of employment contracts to attend supervision groups or similar. Supervision may itself vary in its orientation, for example, whether the focus is on assessment of competence and quality of care or on clinician flourishing more broadly. Evidently, there is an inequity of access between professions, and there are employment or service complications founded on the balance between continuing professional development (CPD) and service delivery.[32] This is particularly an issue in primary and community care due to the relative smallness of clinical provider organisations, rendering access to this form of CPD more difficult. So the Hippocratic duty to maintain skills is that much harder to obey.

Curricula for primary care, given its undifferentiated and diverse nature, should be orientated at patients' needs, designed to be flexible and sponsor-reflective practice in all its various forms. Such curricula derive their moral strength from the adequacy of the educational process involved and the health gain of the population in consequence.[33,34]

WORKFORCE ISSUES

A broader issue concerns the aims of education for primary care. As is argued elsewhere in this book, we believe primary care to be relatively underfunded and undervalued, compared with specialist practice. The trend of learners to select specialist practice, or at least to preferentially avoid primary care, is well documented.[35] There may be many reasons for this: pay rates, professional esteem and historical imperatives to name but a few. In any event, if as we believe primary care is essential to a well-functioning universal health coverage system, then this has obvious implications for the provision of HCPs to staff such a system. It is not only about the nature of the curriculum that future primary HCPs can and should pursue, but also about the numbers, placements and working relationships that these HCPS should be offered. It is fair to say that the science of workforce planning is uncertain at best, but nonetheless, a morally driven healthcare system should necessarily aim to engender a workforce that can offer the population the best health outcomes it can. Though utilitarian in construction, such an aim can claim to be ethical. What follows is how such a laudable end point can be achieved. For example, is it reasonable to leave to a market driven-system, such as obtains in the United States, the commissioning for numbers of doctors and other HCPs needed for universal primary care coverage? It may be thought to be rather haphazard to do so, where the alternative is the imprecise art of workforce planning based upon assumptions of population need.[36] How primary care education responds to wider society is imbued with ethical aspects and the above is but one example. The discussion of whether education is orientated towards the flourishing of individual learners, training or adapting a workforce to do a task well, or equipping a workforce to be proactive citizens and reconstructing society is a live issue in education broadly.[37] Several chapters in this book offer insight into these questions in the context of primary healthcare.

CONCLUSION

This chapter has moved from consideration of individual learners to the bigger picture issues of population health need, and how clinical education should serve it. Although the welfare of the consumer may not be the main concern of a business trying to sell a product at a profit, the welfare of patients is central to good healthcare practice.[38] Ultimately, patients are end users of the various education streams that underlie HCP development, and it is for this reason that healthcare education is a moral enterprise, almost exactly analogous to clinical care in itself. In a more obvious manner than in direct clinical care, patients are also 'means' to the education of HCPs – the personhood of patients must not however be lost in educational settings. We must also not forget that both primary healthcare and education are peopled – the moral agency of teachers and learners is potentially subject to many external pressures and their personhood is also worthy of respect – they too are 'ends' as well as 'means'. As such a robust set of educator values, preferably defined across the primary care professions is to be welcomed and the discourse that leads to it.[39]

REFERENCES

1. Archer J, McManus C, Woolf K, Monrouxe L, Illing J, Bullock A, et al. We can no longer leave research into medical education to chance. *BMJ* 2015; 350; h3445.
2. Jagsi R, Lehmann LS. The ethics of medical education. *BMJ* 2004; 329: 332–334.
3. Foucault M. *The birth of the clinic.* Routledge; 2003 [Originally Naissance de la Clinique 1963 Presses Universitaires de France]. Abingdon.
4. Mohanna K, Tavabie A, Chambers R. The renaissance of generalism. *Education for Primary Care* 2006; 17: 425–431.
5. Campbell E. *The ethical teacher.* Philadelphia, PA: Open University Press; 2003.
6. Fowler MD, Davis AJ. Ethical issues occurring within nursing education. *Nursing Ethics* 2013; 20: 126–141.
7. Torrance C, Mansell I, Wilson C. GMC, NMC and learning objects? Nurse educators' views on using patients for student learning: Ethics and consent. *Education for health* 2012; 25(2): 92–97.
8. Leung GKK, Patil NG. Medical students as observers in theatre: Is an explicit consent necessary? *The Clinical Teacher* 2011; 8: 122–125.
9. Lucas B, Pearson D. Patient perceptions of their role in undergraduate medical education within a primary care teaching practice. *Education for Primary Care* 2012; 23(4): 277–285(9).
10. Bowman D, Spicer J, Iqbal R. *Informed consent: A primer for clinical practice.* Cambridge University Press, Cambridge, 2012.
11. Sturman N. Teaching medical students: Ethical challenges. *Australian Family Physician* 2011; 12: 992–995.
12. Agledahl KM, Forde R, Wifstad A. Clinical essentialising: A qualitative study of doctors' medical and moral practice. *Medical Health Care and Philosophy* 2010; 13: 107–113.
13. Papanikitas A. Caught between the task and the vocation. In *From the classroom to the clinic: Ethics education and general practice.* PhD Thesis, Department of Education and Professional Studies, King's College London, 2013, pp. 315–318. http://ethos.bl.uk/OrderDetails.do?uin=uk.bl.ethos.646972 (accessed 25 August 2016).
14. Burkes M. Workplace-based assessments in the registrar year. In Burkes M, Logan A (eds.), *The good GP training guide.* London: Royal College of General Practitioners; 2014, pp. 188–194.
15. Lake J, Bell J. Medical educators: The rich symbiosis between clinical and teaching roles. *The Clinical Teacher* 2015; 12: 1–5.

16. Powers BW, Navathe AS, Jain SH. Medical education's authenticity problem. *BMJ* 2014; 348: g2651. DOI: 10.1136/bmj.

17. Frank JE. Conscientious refusal in family medicine residency training. *Family Medicine* 2011; 43(5): 330–333.

18. May M, Mand P, Biertz F, Hummers-Pradier E, Kruschinski C. A survey to assess family physicians' motivation to teach undergraduates in their practices. *PLoS One* 2012; 7(9): e45846. DOI: 10.1371/journal.pone.0045846.

19. Devine OP, Harborne AC, McManus AC. Assessment at UK medical schools varies substantially in volume, type and intensity and correlates with postgraduate attainment. *BMC Medical Education* 2015; 15: 146. DOI: 10.1186/s12909-015-0428-9.

20. Manninen K, Henriksson EW, Scheja M, Silén C. Patients' approaches to students' learning at a clinical education ward-an ethnographic study. *BMC Medical Education* 2014; 14: 131. DOI: 10.1186/1472-6920-14-131.

21. Mendel D, Jamieson A, Whiteman J. Remediation. Ed., Walsh K. In *Oxford textbook of medical education.* Oxford University Press, Oxford; 2013. pp. 362–371.

22. Swanwick T. Postgraduate medical education: The same, but different. *Postgraduate Medical Journal* 2015; 91: 179–181. DOI: 10.1136/postgradmedj-2014-132805.

23. Balmer DF, Hirsh DA, Monie D, Weil H, Richards BF. Caring to care: Applying noddings' philosophy to medical education. *Academic Medicine* 2016; 91(12): 1618–1621.

24. Rodriguez C, López-Roig S, Pawlikowska T, Schweyer FX, Bélanger E, Pastor-Mira MA, et al. The influence of academic discourses on medical students identification with the discipline of family medicine. *Academic Medicine* 2015; 90(5): 660–670. DOI: 10.1097/ACM.0000000000000572.

25. *Outcome-based education.* AMEE Medical Education Guide No 14. https://www.amee.org/getattachment/AMEE-Initiatives/ESME-Courses/AMEE-ESME-Face-to-Face-Courses/ESME/ESME-Online-Resources-China-Dec-2015/Guide-14-Outcome-based-education.pdf (accessed November 12, 2016).

26. Samuel O. Curriculum design for primary care physicians. *Postgraduate Medical Journal* 1993; 69: 629–633.

27. Tudor-Hart J. The inverse-care law. *The Lancet* 1971; 297: 405–412.

28. Coulehan J, Williams PC. Vanquishing virtue: The impact of medical education. *Academic Medicine* 2001; 76(6): 598–605.

29. Blythe A, Hancock J. Time for a national undergraduate curriculum for primary care. *British Journal of General Practice* 2011; 61(593): 721. DOI: 10.3399/bjgp11X601406.

30. Littlewood S, Ypinazar V, Margolis SA, Scherpbier A, Spencer J, Dornan T. Early practical experience and the social responsiveness of clinical education—Systematic review. *BMJ* 2005; 331: 387–391.

31. Brienza RS. At a crossroads: The future of primary care education and practice. *Academic Medicine* 2016; 91(5): 621–623. DOI: 10.1097/ACM.

32. Dimond B. Legal aspects of clinical supervision: Employer vs employee. *British Journal of Nursing* 1998; 7(7): 393–395.

33. Fraser SW, Greenhalgh T. Coping with complexity: Educating for capability. *BMJ* 2001; 323: 799–803.

34. Oelke ND, Thurston WE, Arthur N. Intersections between interprofessional practice, cultural competency and primary health care. *Journal of Interprofessional Care* 2013; 27(5): 367–371.

35. McPake B, Squires A, Mahat A, Araujo EC. *The economics of health professional education and careers: Insights from a literature review.* Washington, DC: World Bank Group; 2015.

36. Goodfellow A, Ulloa JG, Dowling PT, Talamantes E, Chheda S, Bone C, et al. Predictors of primary care physician practice location in undeserved urban or rural areas in the US: A systematic literature review. *Academic Medicine* 2016; 91(9): 1313–1321. DOI: 10.1097/ACM00000000000001203.

37. Eisner EW. Five basic orientations to the curriculum. In Eisner EW (ed.), *The educational imagination: On the design and evaluation of the school programs.* New York: Macmillan Publishing; 1985, pp. 61–86.

38. Benn P. Conscience and healthcare ethics. In Ashcroft RE, Dawson A, Draper H, McMillan JR (eds.), *Principles of healthcare ethics,* 2nd ed. Chichester: Wiley; 2007, pp. 345–350.

39. Storch JL, Kenny N. Shared moral work of nurses and physicians. *Nursing Ethics* 2007; 14(4): 478–491.

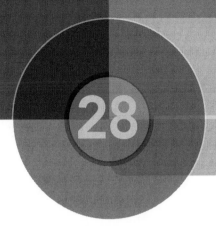

Evidence-based primary care ethics

28

ROGER NEWHAM AND ANDREW PAPANIKITAS

INTRODUCTION

'Evidence-based medicine' is often quoted as 'the conscientious, explicit and judicious use of the current best evidence in making decisions about the medical care of the individual patients'.[1] This has been extrapolated to 'the conscientious and judicious use of the best evidence relevant to the care and prognosis of the patient to promote better informed and better justified ethical decision-making'.[2] The two statements can perhaps be essentially read as saying the same thing. It seems odd that if one is committed to using the best available evidence in the everyday setting, one might not use it in ethically difficult circumstances. Both statements, however, seem to imply that where evidence supports a treatment as the 'best' available, clinicians should favour it, and moreover should not recommend any treatment that the evidence does not support. This simplistic approach trades on leaving the notion of evidence somewhat vague. For example, should the term 'evidence' include both the normative and the empirical, or to put it another way, ethical or moral 'arguments, reasons and values' and 'facts'? In this chapter, we will discuss what might constitute an evidence base for primary care ethics and what might constitute its use for the process of ethical decision-making. We will reflect on the forms of evidence that make up 'ethics' in practice. We will consider some of the ways in which quantitative and qualitative empirical research claims to inform healthcare ethics, two ways of 'systematically' reviewing literature for worthwhile healthcare ethics content and an account that combines the normative and the empirical as a single methodological research approach. We do not propose to solve the problems of disputed ethical language, modes of reasoning and conclusions. However, using a case and examples relevant to primary healthcare, we aim to make the reader aware of those disputes, and to foster a critical and reflexive approach to healthcare ethics.

THE FORMS OF EVIDENCE ON WHICH ETHICAL DECISIONS IN PRACTICE MIGHT DEPEND

The evidence base which appears to be common in the UK primary healthcare education is similar to that which informs undergraduate medical education. We have initially interpreted 'evidence' very broadly here as that on which ethical deliberation and action might depend.

- Philosophies of practice
- Philosophical ethical framework
- Authoritative statements/guidelines/the law
- Empirical work: Surveys, quantitative research, qualitative research, systematic reviews of quantitative studies, systematic reviews of qualitative studies
- Religion and culture
- Political ideology
- Stories of how clinical cases were managed, including personal reflective accounts.

Consider which of these you would count as evidence. One divide may be that normative (knowledge that informs how we ought to act, or moral values) and the empirical (knowledge that tells us what is, or 'facts') are different and distinct. Another division may be that within the empirical, on the type of research which a 'fact' is based and on the quality or rigour of the studies. Or, another division for a possible divide between what counts as evidence could be between practicality and justification.[3] Practicality highlights the need for a focus on actual practice such as influencing the behaviour of actual patients (or broader policy concerns), and justification highlights their legitimisation.

In her book, *Evidence-Based Medicine – A Critical Reader*, Ridsdale[4] addresses medical ethics in general practice by offering two common scenarios, and applying personal experience, communication skills, the law and Beauchamp and Childress' Four Principles method as made popular in the UK by Gillon.[5] She acknowledges the major influence of outcomes-based ethics and duty-based ethics. If we applied her rationale to a hypothetical question raised by one of the author's urban colleagues, it might look like this:

A 24 year old politics, philosophy and economics student attends your GP clinic. He tells you that back home in USA he saw a doctor (speciality unspecified) for concentration problems during his first degree. The doctor diagnosed him with attention deficit hyperactivity disorder, for which he has since purchased methylphenidate by mail order. He would like to be prescribed this medication.

The Ridsdale method invites the reader to ask: How do I ensure good communication? What do I know about my legal liabilities? How do I apply beneficence, non-maleficence, autonomy and justice to analyse the problem?

Ridsdale focuses on the four principles, but in practice, clinicians may be exposed to an *ethical smorgasbord*.

- Medical School: Four principles of autonomy, beneficence, non-maleficence and justice
- Postgraduate education: Virtues (professionalism) and duties (e.g. laws and, professional guidelines such as from the General Medical Council in the UK)
- Politically: A contractarian language of rights and obligations
- Evidence-based medicine and healthcare resource allocation *as often used*: emphasis on utilitarian/consequentialist thinking.

This paints a confusing picture, and different clinicians may favour synthesised principles, one or more grand theories or reject all of the above in favour of combinations of narrative, the law and common sense.

The list below covers the issues on which BMA members have most frequently sought advice from the BMA Ethics Department in 2009–2010:

1. Under what circumstances can confidential health information be disclosed?
2. Who can apply for access to a patient's health records?
3. What should a doctor do when they have child protection concerns about a patient?
4. How much information should patients be given in order for consent to treatment to be valid?
5. What should doctors do if they are asked by a terminally ill patient to write a medical report to go abroad for assisted dying?
6. Do patients have the right to see a medical report written about them?
7. Under the *Mental Capacity Act* 2005, when is a person judged to lack capacity?
8. How and when, can a doctor broach the subject of private treatment with NHS patients?
9. Are general practitioners (GPs) able to register asylum seekers and refused asylum seekers?
10. What is the BMA's position on organ donation?

This list does not however tell us with certainty which issues are common, but those which were the commonest to result in requests for advice to one particular advice service for one undifferentiated profession in one country at one point in time. The list appears to be focussed mainly on issues with medicolegal ramifications. And yet, these issues or concerns are all pertinent to primary care, reflecting the differing and potentially conflicting types of evidence GPs and others in primary healthcare may need to be aware of and use in their differing roles. Such evidence includes empirical facts, underlying or 'hidden' values such as respect for individual patient autonomy, public health aspects of primary care and resource allocation involved in commissioning.[6] The many types of evidence need to be combined with the normative moral philosophical analysis.[7]

EMPIRICAL ETHICS

Empirical ethics may be defined as

> … research strategies in ethics that aims to combine the collection and analysis of empirical data with moral philosophical analysis. These research strategies are generally undertaken to shed light on issues in practical ethics: that is, the endeavour to make normative claims about practical situations.[8]

Sociologists in particular have offered a critique of empirical ethics or bioethics: (where bioethics is understood as being concerned with issues in applied ethics such as practical issues in primary healthcare but with philosophical analysis being in some sense primary).[9]

- Philosophical bioethics lacks a sense of context, as evidenced by unrealistic thought experiments and complex jargon.
- Sociologists are better than philosophers at identifying injustice and understanding the imperfections of the real world.
- Ethics is just another way in which those who are in power oppress those who are not.[10]

For their part, moral philosophers have offered critiques of empirical methods for ethics by distinguishing facts from values or for drawing normative conclusions from non-normative premises (alone).[11] The fact–value distinction is well discussed in medical ethics.[12]

Thus, both philosophical normative evidence and empirical evidence must be critically considered when considering evidence-based medicine and its use in evidence-based ethics.

EVIDENCE-BASED MEDICINE AND ETHICS

Traditionally, evidence-based medicine has been taught in terms of a hierarchy of evidence. In this hierarchy, systematic reviews [which assess the quality of available randomised and controlled trials (RCTs)] and meta-analyses (which combine the data from multiple RCTs) are the best kind of evidence being 'maximally informed and minimally biased'.[13] By contrast, case reports and personal experience are the lowest form of evidence. If there is a clear population, intervention, comparison and outcome (PICO), then an RCT may well be appropriate. Indeed, there have been calls for government policy to make more use of PICO and RCTs in testing new and existing policies. This may challenge untested political ideology as a source for policy if that policy does not work or is shown to cause harm.[14] If the ideal of best evidence consists of RCTs or other quantitative research methodology, then for the most part, explicit use of values and moral values is limited with the ideal perhaps being value-free (at least with regards to justification), the focus being on physiological outcomes of or as treatment effects. However, the evidence base as empirical research can and perhaps should come from other disciplines, for example, from the social sciences of psychology, sociology and anthropology, which (like the non-empirical as law, religion and moral philosophy understood as practical ethics) need applying to the particular case.

The inclusion of other, non-RCT, types of empirical research as evidence is especially relevant for evidence-based ethics in primary care because patients often present (at least in the first instance) with 'non-specific symptoms that may be related to complex social and psychological factors as well as physical pathology'.[15] Such social and psychological factors lead to another important 'outcome' of medicine or healthcare that of quality of care. Quality may include patient satisfaction with treatment or care, leading to patients and those around them flourishing more generally; hence, the importance of qualitative methods as evidence, particularly when patients present to their GP with problems around coping with their conditions (ibid.). Primary care disciplines such as general practice (and its worldwide equivalents) involve both the science and art in an especially integrated fashion with some claiming anecdote, patient stories and personal experience, though classified as 'lower levels' of evidence having an equally valid contribution to make to decision-making.[16]

In a sense, the use of RCTs and meta-analysis does have an ethical underpinning when thinking about (physical) benefits and harms to patients and the need to avoid bias in deciding what these are or the risk of them. However, as mentioned above, perhaps especially in primary care, the external validity of such trials may often be problematic. However, there is a growing body of literature suggesting that systematic reviews of non-empirical research are required as evidence in evidence-based ethics to help GPs and policymakers avoid ethical bias.[17,18]

McCullough et al. proposed that a systematic review of clinical ethics literature should address a PICO like regular systematic reviews. Unlike regular systematic reviews, they should end with a moral outcome rather than a physical one. For example, such a question might sound like, 'In university students who claim to have a prior diagnosis of attention-deficit hyperactivity disorder, is prescription by a general practitioner of drugs which may also be used as cognitive enhancers, rather than referral to a psychiatric specialist, ethically justifiable?'

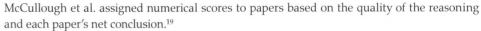

McCullough et al. assigned numerical scores to papers based on the quality of the reasoning and each paper's net conclusion.[19]

Sofaer and Strech proposed that a systematic review of reasons addresses the empirical question of what reasons have been given for the ethical question and has conceptual analysis applied post review.[20] This might generate a different kind of question. 'What are the reasons for and against the prescription of cognitive-enhancing medications to university students by general practitioners?' They suggest searching multiple types of database and coding (grouping under a descriptive heading) the eligible literature in terms of reasons mentioned in passages of text and reason types. Reasons that occur in multiple publications are thematically 'stronger' but this does not necessitate what ought to be done, merely what the more usual reasons considered in the literature are. Their approach appears in essence to be a form of thematic analysis of reasons. They add that a table of characteristics of included publications allows reviewers to assess the state of the field and identify gaps. The rationale for such reviews is to make reasons available to policymakers and decision-makers and this plausibly will include academics, educators and practitioners in primary care in order to improve decision-making.

So what amongst the many empirical methods (as well as non-empirical, political or theological approaches) is to be counted as evidence and why it should be so counted have been and remain contested. It has been suggested that until this is clarified, then the very idea of evidence-based ethics ought to be put on hold, especially since the evidence in ethics is often of a qualitative nature thus compounding problems about quality.[21] Others have also claimed that evidence-based ethics ought to be put on hold for the reason that it is actually incompatible with a (bio)ethics normative mandate.[22] However, two forms of evidence have recently offered promise: systematic reviews of reasons and development of a 'narrow' account of fully integrated empirical ethics.

RECENT EVIDENCE

Empirical disciplines do not explicitly claim to justify how people ought to behave or what people ought to do ethically speaking. This is traditionally the province of philosophical ethics which seeks justification of the particular practices via authority as binding universally independently of any particular standpoint or context, although this account of ethics is often seen as contentious in sociological research[23] and in some philosophical literature.[24–26] If there were agreement as to what counts as evidence or 'best' evidence for primary care ethics, for which there currently is not, a further and related issue is the use that is made of it. How is the philosophical theoretical account of normativity 'combined' with the empirical and other types of evidence for evidence-based *ethics* or empirical ethics?

Evidence-based ethics has largely focussed on empirical bioethics, though 'reason-based reviews' are also developing, in the sense that the evidence is a synthesis of facts that 'inform' moral decision-making, thus seemingly, leaving the answer quite vague. Empirical evidence (and some form of 'mother wit' or intelligence) has always informed ethical deliberation, but unless the empirical determines the ethical, the problem of the integration between the empirical and the ethically normative for evidence-based ethics remains.[27,28]

Two types of strategies seem common. Davies et al. carried out a systematic review of methodologies that used both empirical research and philosophical analysis that aimed at drawing normative conclusions, not just descriptions of data to support factual premises or just philosophical analysis regarding moral authority but an 'integrative' approach. The results found two broad poles, 'dialogical' and 'consultative'. Roughly, the dialogical approach involves getting a shared understanding and normative *consensus* on a discrete problem. The consultative approach uses an external thinker who analyses the data and then independently develops normative conclusions based on theoretical coherence. Others recommend similar approaches as 'pragmatic', where evidence is thought to be neutral in regards to people's explicit values which, in our multi-cultural and liberal democratic times, seems to afford a way of consensus.[29] A dialogical approach in the case of our example might ask how the ethics of treating students with cognitive-enhancing medications emerges from qualitative research involving clinicians and patients. A consultative approach might gather relevant qualitative and quantitative data and pass them to a philosopher who would produce a reasoned judgement on the ethics of treating students with cognitive-enhancing medications.

This still raises three important questions as to the use of evidence in evidence-based (bio) ethics for normative justification, which are as follows: (1) The justificatory question as to how moral justification can be found through coherence or consensus, (2) The analytic process used; notably where the priority should lie between the thinker, theory or stakeholders and (3) The kind of conclusion that is sought; general or particular.[30]

The second strategy is more radical than the rest in that it attempts to combine empirical findings ('is' data) with normative ('ought' arguments) as 'new methodological practices', rather than coherence between two separate research methods.[31] Briefly, Dunn et al. claim that the empirical research ought to inform normative argument and that the normative arguments ought to influence research to shape (for instance) individuals' attitudes and experiences. This is not meant to be the method of wide reflective equilibrium[32] or other coherentist accounts that are cyclical.[33] These, they claim, are problematic as accounts of how such integration is achieved in research. Rather, they suggest new strategies aimed to be *practically convincing* and based on similarity to social scientific research for *methodological* development in empirical ethics (seen as synonymous to evidence-based medical ethics). It is different from social scientific methods in its integration of normative philosophical theory. It differs from more contextualised and from pragmatic approaches that call for meta-ethical revision – for example, about the importance of general features of agents for moral authority. They call for a new generation of ethicists skilled in both empirical and philosophical methods.

CONCLUSION

Primary healthcare offers a rich testing ground for evidence-based ethics, partly because evidence-based medicine is already nuanced in this context – a hierarchy of evidence with an RCT at the top does not adequately answer the questions that need answering. Practice in primary healthcare is not exclusively technology or even physiology dependent and many decisions and interventions defy statistical analysis. Extrapolating from Sackett's seminal definition of evidence-based medicine, evidence-based ethics is the conscientious and judicious use of the best evidence concerning the care and prognosis of the individual patient in making ethical decisions.[34] The key issue is the ethical responsibility of a healthcare professional to make use of good 'evidence' in ethical decision-making. What is to count as evidence is usually understood as an empirical matter both quantitative and qualitative, though other sorts of 'evidence' may need to be somehow included. Concerns have arisen as to the quality of such evidence, especially of a non-RCT type though the claim that only those things which may be counted (such as in an RCT) are 'true' has been hotly debated. 'Empirical' evidence-based ethics seems to imply that it has straddled the divide between the seemingly distinct empirical facts and normative philosophical ethics and moral values. Again the literature is characterised by debate. Perhaps the best that can be offered in terms of justification and academic consensus in terms of 'evidence' is the offering of 'is' data and well-curated 'ought' arguments, as in Sofaer and Strech's systematic review of reasons. We do not present these questions as unsettled to unleash a form of postmodern ethical existentialism but to make some simple points: a reflexive practitioner or policymaker may consider how a good decision is made.

REFERENCES

1. Sackett DL, Rosenberg WM, Gray JA, Haynes RB, Richardson WS. (1996). Evidence based medicine: What it is and what it isn't. *British Medical Journal* 312: 71–72.
2. Major-Kincade TL, Tyson JE, Kennedy KA. (1998). Training paediatric house staff in evidence-based ethics. *Journal of Perinatology* 21: 161–166.
3. Dunn M, Sheehan M, Hope T, Parker M. (2012). Toward methodological innovation in empirical ethics research. *Cambridge Quarterly of Healthcare Ethics* 21: 466–480.
4. Ridsdale L. (1995). *Evidence Based General Practice: A Critical Reader.* Saunders/Baillierre Tindall, London.
5. Beauchamp TL, Childress JF. (2001). *Principles of Biomedical Ethics.* Oxford University Press, New York, NY; 2001.
6. Slowther A, Ford S, Schofield T. (2004). Ethics of evidence based medicine in the primary care setting. *Journal of Medical Ethics* 30(2): 151–155.
7. Dunn et al., 2012, *op. cit.*
7. Ibid.
8. Ibid.
9. Hayry M, Takala T. (2003). *Scratching the Surface of Bioethics.* Rodopi, New York.
10. Hoeyer K. (2006). 'Ethics wars': Reflections on the antagonism between bioethicists and social science observers of biomedicine. *Human Studies* 29: 203–227.
11. Pigden C. (2013). The is-ought gap. *The International Encyclopedia of Ethics.* DOI: 10.1002/9781444367072.wbiee078.
12. Fulford KWM. (1989). *Moral Theory and Medical Practice.* Cambridge University Press, Cambridge.
13. Slowther et al., 2004, *op. cit.*
14. Haynes L, Service O, Goldacre B, Togerson D. (2012). *Test, Learn, Adapt: Developing Public Policy with Randomised Controlled Trials (Policy Paper).* Cabinet Office Behavioural Insights Team, London.
15. Slowther et al., 2004, *op. cit.*
16. Jacobson L, Edwards A, Granier S, Butler C. (1997). Evidence based medicine and general practice. *British Journal of General Practice* 47: 449–452.
17. Sofaer N, Strech D. (2012). The need for systematic reviews of reasons. *Bioethics* 26(6): 315–328.
18. McCullough L, Coverdale J, Chervenak F. (2007). Constructing a systematic review for argument-based clinical ethics literature: The example of concealed medications. *Journal of Medical Philosophy* 32: 65–76.
19. Ibid.
20. Sofaer and Strech, 2012, *op. cit.*
21. Stretch D. (2008). Evidence based ethics-what it should be and what it shouldn't? *BMC Medical Ethics* 9: 16. DOI: 10.1186/1472-6939-9-16.
22. Sofaer and Strech, 2012, *op. cit.*
23. Hayry and Takala, 2003, *op. cit.*

24. Ibid.
25. Williams B. (1985). *Ethics and the Limits of Philosophy.* Harvard University Press, Cambridge.
26. Hooker B, Little M. (2000). *Moral Particularism.* Oxford University Press, Oxford.
27. Salloch S, Schildmann J, Vollman J. (2012). Empirical research in medical ethics: How conceptual accounts on normative-empirical collaboration may improve research practice. *BMC Medical Ethics* 13: 5.
28. Goldenberg M. (2005). Evidence based ethics? On evidence based practice and the 'empirical turn' from normative ethics. *BMC Medical Ethics* 6: 11.
29. Davies R, Ives J, Dunn M. (2015). A systematic review of empirical bioethics methodologies. *BMC Medical Ethics* 16: 15. DOI: 10.1186/s12910-015-0010-3.
30. Dunn et al., 2012, *op. cit.*
31. Ibid.
32. Daniels N. (1979). Wide reflective equilibrium and theory acceptance in ethics. *The Journal of Philosophy* 76(5): 256–282.
33. McMilan J, Hope T. (2008). The possibility of empirical psychiatric ethics, in Widdershoven G, McMillan J, Hope T, and van der Scheer L (eds.). *Empirical Ethics in Psychiatry.* Oxford University Press, Oxford. pp. 9–22.
34. Major-Kincade et al., *op. cit.*

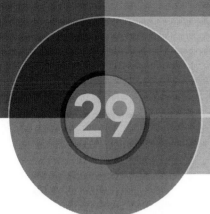

Narrative ethics and primary care

29

JOHN LAUNER

INTRODUCTION

Over the last 50 years, a wide range of academic and practical disciplines have undergone what has generally been called a 'narrative turn'. In its broadest characterisation, one could describe this as a move from asking the question 'what is *really* going on here?' to asking 'what kinds of accounts or *stories* are people telling about it?'. The origins of this intellectual shift lie with many different influences, including social constructionism and postmodernism, together with gender and cultural studies. Narrative studies or 'narratology' has now diversified into many different streams, but all are united by the view expressed by philosopher Charles Taylor: 'We understand ourselves inescapably in narrative',[1] and the psychologist Jerome Bruner, who has written: 'To be in a culture is to be bound in a set of connecting stories'.[2] Story-telling, according to such thinkers, is the way we as humans experience, communicate and indeed create ourselves. It is the way we try to influence others and are in turn influenced by them. Such ideas are now central in the social sciences and humanities, and have affected almost every area of academic study, including medicine and law. (In common with most writers nowadays, I use the words 'narrative' and 'story' interchangeably.)

The narrative turn has had its critics.[3] Some have pointed out – with justice – that the term 'narrative' is now used by different writers to describe everything from short spoken utterances to so called 'grand narratives' like Marxism or neoliberalism. Others have drawn attention to the tendency of narrative scholars to place an emphasis on Western middle-class constructions in place of culturally diverse ones,[4] on long-term instead of episodic experience,[5] on good stories in preference to deceitful or manipulative ones[6] and on language at the expense of other forms of expression.[7] In spite of this, narrative theorists have, by and large, been able to hold on to their positions through accommodating to these critiques, and by promoting the strengths of their defining stance, rather than trying to defend specific articles of faith.

NARRATIVE MEDICINE

Narrative ideas entered medicine on both sides of the Atlantic as a result of cross-disciplinary dialogue in many different centres.[8] Around the turn of this century, an identifiable 'narrative medicine movement' coalesced around the publication of two influential books. One was a collection of essays published in the United Kingdom, edited by Greenhalgh and Hurwitz.[9] The other was a monograph by the New York physician Rita Charon.[10] These books described, and provided further stimulus to, a wide range of educational and research activities around the world, involving doctors, health professionals and students.[11] This has included:

- Studying literary works, and looking at how these can heighten empathy and professionalism
- Studying stories about personal illness, written by historical or contemporary patients, or by clinicians who have also been patients
- Encouraging practitioners and students to write stories and poems or keep reflective diaries
- Carrying out research into how patients describe their illnesses when talking to doctors or to each other
- Examining the way that doctors talk to each other about their work and how they 'construct' medical knowledge in this way
- Examining the way that patients and clinicians negotiate between their different accounts of illness
- Training doctors and other professionals to be more attentive to patients' stories and to collaborate with them in creating more satisfactory ones.

In spite of its protean nature, there are two concepts that appear to distinguish narrative medicine and hold it together coherently in all its different forms. One is the way that it claims legitimacy for individual stories as a *counterpoise to evidence-based medicine,* and as an essential complement to evidence. The other unifying concern of narrative medicine is with what Rita Charon describes as 'narrative competence'. This encompasses skills for listening and expression, but most of all for empathic interaction through language. Narrative-based primary care, active mainly in the United Kingdom but with adherents in Scandinavia and elsewhere, has attempted to impart these skills for general practitioners (GPs) and those working alongside them in the community.[12] It has also placed an emphasis on the need for professionals to share narratives with each other in the context of peer supervision.[13]

NARRATIVE ETHICS

From the outset, narrative medicine has been as much an ethical enterprise as a clinical and educational one. In an early book, edited with her colleague Martha Montello, Rita Charon wrote:

> Narrative approaches to ethics recognize that the singular case emerges only in the act of narrating it and that duties are incurred in the act of hearing it. How the patient tells of illness, how the doctor or ethicist represents it in words, who listens as the intern presents at rounds, what the audience is being moved to feel or think—all these narrative dimensions of health care are of profound and defining importance in ethics and patient care ....[14]

A more recent volume on narrative ethics has combined the thinking of contemporary bioethicists with essays from some of the earlier pioneers of the narrative medicine movement, including the physician Howard Brody and the sociologist Arthur Frank. In their contribution to the book, Brody and his colleague Mark Clark describe how narrative ethics has the capacity to bring together moral case reasoning (casuistry), principlism and virtue ethics.

Stories can combine the strengths of all three approaches and do so in especially vivid and compelling ways. The cases that casuistry presents us with are already in narrative form. We can decide what to do by looking carefully at the 'facts' of the case, but we also decide what to do by comparing stories with other stories… Finally, stories are a superb vehicle for demonstrating to us how the sorts of persons we are determine how we will act in specific situations and how specific situations call forth and shape our enduring moral character, blurring any useful distinction between 'situation ethics' and virtue ethics.[15]

Similarly, the bioethicist Jodi Halpern writes:

A listener's power to influence a speaker's possibilities is at once deeply mysterious and a very familiar experience in our daily life. How someone listens to us does not just affirm our story after the fact; it builds a scaffold for our thinking and telling, making it possible to imagine a wider or more constricted range of options. Yet the ethical implications of the role of the listener have not been sufficiently attended to in normative ethics, including bioethics. Narrative ethics, with its emphasis on the power of the story for guiding our moral lives, has a special responsibility to attend to the interpersonal context in which ethically significant narratives emerge.[16]

All these writers, along with their fellow contributors, regard narrative not as something static on a written page, nor recorded once and for all on an audio file, but as an act of ethical creativity. Many GPs and primary care professionals will recognise this as something they engage in everyday – or certainly aspire to – even though they may have been unaware of the intellectual framework that underpins this.

PRIMARY CARE

Practitioners in primary care occasionally deal with some of the headline issues of bioethics, such as end-of-life decision-making, or the dilemmas associated with assisted reproduction. More often, primary care is more mundane. In some ways, this makes it ethically more challenging for its practitioners, rather than less. Firstly, we are more likely to be conscious of the ethical dimension of every moment in our working lives, and know that apparently trivial encounters can expose underlying existential questions. Secondly, we may be acutely aware of how little guidance we have in order to make the necessary ethical decisions from moment to moment, apart from our own moral compass, our generic training in professionalism and communication skills, and intuition. Because of this, narrative ethics may be more applicable to primary care than anywhere else. Consider, for example, these two alternative versions of the same consultation.[17]

Version A:

Patient: I've come about the spots on my face.
Doctor: How long have they been there?
Patient: I've had them since I was a teenager. But they've really broken out badly in the last few months.

Doctor: Have you tried anything for them?

Patient: I've bought a few things at the pharmacist but nothing seems to work.

Doctor: Well, let's have a look then …

Version B:

Patient: I've come about the spots on my face.

Doctor: How long have they been there?

Patient: I've had them since I was a teenager. But they've really broken out badly in the last few months.

Doctor: you have any idea why?

Patient: I'm not sure. Could it be stress?

Doctor: Why do you ask?

Patient: Well I lost my job about six months ago, and then my boyfriend left me in the summer and I've been pretty low generally and … (starts to cry).

Although the opening of the consultation is the same in both versions, the doctor guides it in two entirely different directions. In the first version, the doctor either fails to hear that the young woman's spots have broken out badly 'in the last few months', or he studiously chooses to ignore it. (I am assuming a male doctor and female patient here for clarity.) The reasons for his inattention may be multiple: pressure of time, or perhaps a lack of affection for this patient, is among the likeliest. In the second version, the doctor not only hears the cue but also offers the patient a chance to extend her story into what is commonly called the 'lifeworld'.[18] Through the use of two simple, open questions, each responsive to the patient's exact words, he has offered to take on the role of an active collaborator in helping the patient take her narrative where it needs to go. For both the patient and the doctor, what happens from now on will be unpredictable, indeterminate and involve risks on both sides. Paradoxically, it is also more likely to lead in the end to the best decision about treatment for her spots.

There are many ethical frameworks one might use for understanding this kind of encounter, including a traditional, 'principlist' one,[19] conversational ethics[20] or virtue ethics.[21] These different frameworks are neither exclusive nor contradictory. Yet, the framework of narrative ethics offers something unique here. It enables us to view every juncture in a conversation as presenting an ethical choice, allowing the clinician either to exert power through imposition of a professional model, or to share power by tracking the patient's story and creating opportunities for it to progress.

Seeing ethics in terms of narrative-making rather than decision-making has many advantages. Patients can direct professionals towards what matters, and decisions about treatment, if needed, can emerge through evolution, rather than being mechanically introduced at the end. Patient choice therefore becomes embedded in every moment of the consultation. If narrative medical ethics has one defining characteristic, it is that decisions are actively co-constructed through conversation, with a conscious wish on the part of the clinician to reach an account of matters that has both coherence and practical utility for the patient.

ETHICS AND PRAGMATICS

While primary care professionals deal with the mundane, we deal with far more serious matters too, where we have to be active listeners in two senses: not simply facilitating good conversations, but paying attention to risk and possibly major pathology as well. The following account describes a consultation I held some time ago, although I wrote down an extended record of it very soon afterwards.[22] It represents an attempt to apply the principles of narrative practice and ethics, while also attending to my role as a trained physician. I have altered it in many respects, for anonymity.

I was approaching the end of my morning surgery, having already seen fourteen patients, with two more to go. I checked my computer screen and saw that the next patient was someone who had just registered that morning and had never been seen at the practice before. I went into the waiting room and called her in: she was a black woman in her early 40s, somewhat overweight and with a sad and distracted expression. She came into the room and told me that she had hurt her bottom the previous day. Simultaneously, she took out of her handbag a number of packets and bottles of medications to show me what she was currently taking.

I asked her how she had hurt her bottom and she told me that she had fallen. I enquired how this happened, and she said that her partner had pushed her. When I questioned her further about this, she said they had been arguing in a car, she had got out, but he had followed her and pushed her over on the pavement. I asked if this happened a lot and she said yes it did, mainly because of her drinking. She had been an alcoholic for some time but was now trying to give up. I asked if she was getting any help for her alcohol problem and she said no, but she was a mental patient and had been getting help with her mental problems until recently when she moved away into our area.

I asked her to tell me something about her mental problems and she said she got hallucinations, hearing and seeing things that were not there. I enquired if she had ever been admitted to hospital because of these. She said no but she had been in hospital for a few weeks during the summer for another problem. When I questioned her about this, she told me that she had a tumour. I enquired where the tumour was, and she said it was in her brain.

At this point I thought that the tumour might be a delusion, so I asked her if she could show me the scar. She showed me a fresh but well-healed scar behind her right ear that was entirely consistent with recent brain surgery. She then told me that it had been a 'Meningi-something', and when I suggested the word 'Meningioma', she said yes that was it. She told me the name of the consultant she was seeing for this. At the same time, I was examining the packets of medication she had laid out on my desk, and some of these were anti-epileptic pills. (The other ones were a type of sleeping tablet, and beta-blockers which might have been for anxiety, or for raised blood pressure or migraine).

I said to her that it sounded as if her life was very difficult, and I wondered if there was anyone at home who was looking after her. She said that her partner did not live with her, but her children were at home. I asked her how many children she had and she started to cry, saying that she had had five children but only three were alive now. When I asked her how this came about, she told me that her first child had died soon after birth, having been born very prematurely. However, her main cause of grief was the death of her eldest son from a drug overdose two years previously. I expressed my sympathy, and then asked her how old her surviving children were. She explained that they were 15, 7 and 1 year old, respectively.

I suggested at this point that we should attend to the problem she had originally brought to me, namely her painful bottom. I examined her briefly, reassured her that she had only been bruised, and at her request prescribed some painkillers that would not interact with her other medication. I suggested that she should make a follow-up appointment in a few days with the GP in the practice she would be registering with. (I was only working part-time in the practice). I also suggested that I should book her in to see the community mental health nurse. She agreed with both suggestions, and I gave her a written slip to hand in at the desk to fix this up. The consultation record-keeping and communication took, in all, about seventeen minutes.

Almost every GP and primary care clinician will recognise much that is familiar about this consultation. There is the unfolding succession of losses and tragedies that at times beggars belief, and yet is only too real. Any one of these might require, from a medical point of view, separate attention and analysis that could potentially take up the entire time allotted for this consultation, if not more. At the same time, the overall narrative invites a completely different stance from the clinician: the ability to bear witness, to remain empathic and to allow the story to go in the directions that have personal meaning and weight for the patient. Perhaps the most difficult task in primary care is to conduct a complex consultation like this, so that it meets both the narrative requirements and what one might call 'normative' ones, namely the conventional biomedical tasks that clinicians are right expected to perform, and to do so within a realistic time frame. Thus, the professional's task goes far beyond so-called 'patient-centred' medicine. It means recognising the legitimacy of the patient's need for self-expression, along with one's own needs to achieve pattern recognition, action and closure.

Primary care practitioners face such dilemmas every day. Narrative ethics, I would suggest, offers a way to manage these. It invites us to abandon the rigid inquiries that prevent professionals from hearing patients' stories with any degree of fullness, and instead to use other techniques: tracking language, following feedback, using responsive questions and being transparent about the constraints of time and clinical risk. It involves a willingness to reconceptualise the primary care consultation as a therapeutic encounter during which, in however limited a way, patients have the opportunity to tell their stories directed by their own preoccupations and evolving sense of self, and applying the conceptual framework of the clinician as a secondary rather than primary driver for the conversation. Paradoxically, as both the examples in this chapter show, paying attention to the narrative, and according it primacy in the consultation, may in the end lead to a more complete disclosure of what really matters, and hence to better technical as well as ethical care.

REFERENCES

1. Taylor C. *Sources of the self: The making of the modern identity.* Cambridge: Cambridge University Press; 1989.
2. Bruner J. *Acts of meaning.* Cambridge, MA: Harvard University Press; 1990.
3. Woods A. The limits of narrative: Provocations for the medical humanities. *Medical Humanities* 2011; 37: 73–78.
4. Saville-Troike M. *The ethnography of communication: An introduction.* 2nd ed. Oxford: Blackwell; 1989.
5. Strawson G. Against narrativity. *Ratio* 2004; 17: 428–452.
6. Gabriel Y. The voice of experience and the voice of the expert – Can they speak to each other? In: Hurwitz B, Greenhalgh T, Skultans V (eds.). *Narrative research in health and illness.* London: Blackwell; 2004. pp. 168–186.
7. Sartwell C. *End of Story: Towards an annihilation of language and history.* Albany, NY: State University of New York Press; 2000.
8. Jones EM, Tansey EM (eds.). The development of narrative practices in medicine c.1960–c.2000. In: *Wellcome witnesses to contemporary medicine,* vol. 52. London: Queen Mary University of London; 2015.
9. Greenhalgh T, Hurwitz B. (eds.). *Narrative-based medicine: Dialogue and discourse in clinical practice.* London: BMJ Books; 1998.

10. Charon R. *Narrative medicine: Honoring the stories of illness.* Oxford: Oxford University Press; 2006.

11. Kalitzkus V, Matthiessen P. Narrative-based medicine: Potential, practice and pitfalls. *The Permanente Journal* 2009; 13: 80–86.

12. Launer J. *Narrative-based primary care: A practical guide.* Abingdon: Radcliffe Medical Press; 2002.

13. Launer J. Narrative-based supervision. In: LS Sommers and J Launer (eds.). *Clinical uncertainty in primary care: The challenge of collaborative engagement.* New York: Springer; 2013. pp. 147–161.

14. Charon R. Introduction. In: Charon R, Montello M (eds.). *Stories matter: The role of narrative in medical ethics.* New York: Routledge; 2002. p. x.

15. Brody H, Clark M. Narrative ethics: A narrative. Narrative ethics: The role of stories in bioethics, special report. *Hastings Center Report* 2014; 44: S7–11.

16. Halpern J. Narratives hold open the future. *Narrative Ethics: The role of stories in bioethics, special report, Hastings Center Report* 2014; 44: S25–27.

17. Launer J. Taking a narrative stance in the consultation. *Primary Care Mental Health* 2003; 1: 111–112.

18. Mishler EG, Clark A, Ingelfinger J, Simon, M. The language of attentive patient care: A comparison of two medical interviews. *Journal of General Internal Medicine* 1989; 4: 325–335.

19. McCarthy J. Principlism or narrative ethics: Must we choose between them? *Journal of Medical Ethics: Medical Humanities* 2003; 29: 65–71.

20. Parker M. A conversational approach to the ethics of genetic testing. In: R Ashcroft, Lucassen A, M Parker, Verkerk M, Widdershoven G. (eds.) *Case analysis in clinical ethics.* Cambridge: Cambridge University Press; 2005. pp. 149–164.

21. Toon PD. *Towards a philosophy of general practice: A study of the virtuous practitioner.* Occasional Paper 78. London: Royal College of General Practitioners; 1999.

22. Launer J. New stories for old: Narrative-based primary care in Great Britain. *Families, Systems, Health* 2006; 24: 336–344.

Learning from the assessment of ethics in UK general practice

30

DAVID MOLYNEUX

INTRODUCTION

In this chapter, I outline the rationale and methods used in the assessment of ethical practice in primary care. This chapter is divided into three parts: In the first part of the chapter, I clarify some of the terms used in assessment and describe some problems with ethical assessment in primary care.

In the middle part of the chapter, I describe the methods used to assess UK general practitioners (GPs) both as part of their training and when they are independent practitioners. Finally, I reflect on the strengths and weaknesses of the ethical assessment of UK GPs and discuss how these problems might impact on the training of other primary healthcare professionals.

WHAT IS ASSESSMENT?

Assessment is 'any process that is used to estimate learning for whatever purpose'. The term is derived from the Latin *ad sedere* – 'to sit down beside'.[1]

The UK General Medical Council (GMC) definition described in *Tomorrow's Doctors*[2] is useful and will be used throughout this chapter:

> [Assessment is] … all activity aimed at judging students' attainment of curriculum outcomes, whether for summative purposes (determining progress) or formative purposes.

Assessment can thus be *formative* or *summative*. Formative assessment is a type of assessment where the aim is to provide feedback to learners or practitioners to help them to learn (and to help teachers to find ways to help learners). Summative assessment, by contrast, is a type of assessment that provides evidence of the achievement of learners, by attaching a value or score to learning.

Assessment can also be formal or informal. Formal assessment is that assessment which is conducted in a structured or organised way, often in relation to pre-set criteria (criterion-referencing) or in relationship to other learners (norm-referencing). Informal assessment, by contrast is the assessment which occurs in a non-structured or ad hoc way, as part of day-to-day educational or clinical activity.

Assessment can be knowledge based, skill based or attitude based. *Knowledge*-based ethical assessment measures a learner's recollection of ethics and law-based facts. This type of assessment can best be achieved using simple recall tests, typically multiple-choice questions (MCQs). Ethical *skills* can be assessed by more complex assessments, such as objective structured clinical examinations (OSCEs) and extended essay questions. *Attitudes* are very hard to assess – they need time and complex interactions between assessor and those being assessed. Ethical attitudes can be assessed (albeit partially), for example, by such measures as self-completed questionnaires, scenario-based cases, observations of behaviour and oral examinations. The generic difficulty in measuring attitudes is particularly important when assessing overall ethical competency – because of the overriding importance of attitudes in the ethical development of students and practitioners. I will come back to this point in the final section.

Another taxonomy that has some similarities to the knowledge/skills/attitude taxonomy is Miller's triangle (pyramid).[3] This is shown in the diagram below. The whole triangle represents a hierarchy of competences. Each 'slice' of the triangle represents a particular competence that can be assessed, with the most 'basic' competences at the base of the triangle, and more complex competences above the base. The most complex competence is at the apex of the triangle (Figure 30.1).

Each 'slice' of Miller's triangle can be individuated for the particular type of assessment one is doing – so if one was doing an ethical assessment, the base layer would be 'Knows ethically' and the apex layer would be 'Manages complex ethical dilemmas in practice'. Another important consideration is that each layer of the triangle will 'contain' layers below it – for example, to be able to manage a patient who refuses a life-saving treatment in practice, one would need to know the 'facts' about consent and treatment refusal ('Knows') and be able to demonstrate this in a tutorial or examination ('Shows how').

It is important to note that though the triangle is a hierarchy of competences, it is also a hierarchy of assessment methods. For example, 'knowledge' would be typically assessed by

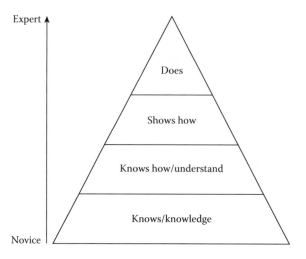

Figure 30.1 Miller's pyramid.

fact-based assessment tools such as MCQs, whereas 'Shows how' would need to be assessed by some form of practical clinical examination such as an OSCE, and 'Does' would have to be assessed in day-to-day practice.

There is no equivalent of 'Attitudes' in Miller's pyramid. This is a particular problem in ethical assessment as the ethical attitude of a learner can remain 'opaque' to the assessor.

CURRICULUM LINKAGE

It is important that assessment is linked to the knowledge skills and attitudes that the practitioners are expected to develop. In other words, the assessment should be 'curriculum-aligned'. Until relatively recently, this would be have been difficult to achieve in primary care as there was no agreed curriculum available. Over the last decade, the Royal College of GPs (RCGP) has developed a widely accepted curriculum which is divided into professional and clinical components.[4] In addition, there is now a core curriculum for teaching of medical ethics to students.[5] Learning outcomes can be derived from the curriculum, and these learning outcomes can then be linked to assessment methods.[6]

HOW GOOD IS OUR ASSESSMENT?

Because so much hangs on to assessment (see later), it is vital that we know we are doing the assessment well. So how can we be sure that our ethical assessment is of a high standard?

Two measures are important – validity and reliability. Assessment can be valid and/or reliable (or neither). A valid assessment measures what it sets out to measure. If an assessment purports to be measuring (for example) knowledge about GMC guidance, or ethical sensitivity or ethical decision-making, then it is valid if it actually measures these things – rather than related things or different things altogether. A reliable assessment is one which gives consistent and repeatable results when measuring a particular practitioner (intra-personal reliability) or group of practitioners (inter-personal reliability).

In addition, assessments should normally focus on a higher rather than a lower level on Miller's pyramid. This will ensure that ethical assessment reflects ethical decision-making in real-life situations.

Finally, assessments should be achievable – either in terms of the resources of the assessors or the cost of the assessment process.

To summarise, therefore, a perfect assessment tool would:

- Have a high level of validity
- Have a high level of reliability
- Measure 'high' competences on Miller's triangle
- Be realistic and achievable.

WHY ASSESS?

It is important to be clear on the purpose of assessment. Assessment is important for the learner or practitioner – it fosters motivation to learn or motivation to develop and hone clinical and other skills. Besides motivation, it provides valuable feedback on how a skill or knowledge set is progressing. Finally, assessment provides information to teachers and clinical supervisors/trainers – that the practitioner is progressing in the right way (or not) and, if there are problems, what those problems might be. This would be true of all assessment – but end-of-training and fitness-for-practice assessment have the additional role of providing external bodies such as the RCGP and the GMC (and ultimately the public) with the evidence that a practitioner is safe and capable of independent practice.

TYPES OF ASSESSMENT

Just as there are different aims of assessment and different reasons for assessment, there are also different *methods* of assessment. Below is a reasonably comprehensive list of assessment measures. Interestingly, not all these methods are used for the assessment of GPs, and even fewer of these methods are used for the *ethical* assessment of GPs.

Type of assessment	Used in the assessment of GP ethical competence?
Multiple-choice questions	Yes
Essay questions	No (used in past)
Oral examinations	No (used in past)
Audit	Yes
Reflective log	Yes
Significant event analysis	Yes
Consultation review	No (used in past)
Patient satisfaction questionnaire	Yes
Colleague feedback	Yes
Practical clinical examination	Yes
Video submission	Yes
Dissertation/thesis	No
Course work	No

ASSESSMENT IN THE PRIMARY CARE SETTING – WHAT ACTUALLY HAPPENS?

Having outlined some theoretical and definitional principles of assessment, I will now discuss what actually is done in practice. This description relates to assessment of GPs – but many of these assessments apply to other practitioners too, and I discuss generic features of primary care assessment in Section 3.

Assessment for primary care physicians can be divided into three phases:

1. Assessment *before* a primary care career
2. Assessment *at entry* into primary care career
3. Assessment *after* qualifying as a primary care physician.

The first phase will be discussed for completeness, but only briefly.

ASSESSMENT BEFORE ENTRY

An increasing number of assessments occur *prior* to the embarking on a career in primary care. These include:

- University finals
- Selection centre MCQ

- Selection centre situational judgement test
- Selection centre clinical examination
- Selection centre written paper
- Subspeciality exams such as Diploma of the Royal College of Obstetricians and Gynaecologists.

ASSESSMENT AT THE PROCESS OF ENTRY INTO A PRIMARY CARE CAREER

When I became a GP (some 30 years ago), assessment was minimal – one had to complete four junior hospital doctor posts and then 1 year in a supervised (training) practice. No exams or formal assessments were required, though keen GPs could attempt the Membership of the RCGPs (MRCGP) examination which was at that time entirely optional. (This consisted of an MCQ exam, a written paper and two oral examinations, one of which was on a submission of cases seen in primary care.)

Subsequently, assessment became much more rigorous, evolving via the process of summative assessment (video consultation submission + audit submission) into a compulsory MRCGP examination, which has become the licensing examination for entry to the profession.

Currently, assessment within GP training has three components:

- The applied knowledge test (AKT)
- The clinical skills assessment (CSA)
- Workplace-based assessment (WPBA).

THE APPLIED KNOWLEDGE TEST (AKT)

This is a computer-based multiple-choice assessment based on (and linked to) the GP curriculum. The great majority of this examination (80%) is clinical in nature – but 10% of the exam deals with critical appraisal and 10% deals with practice management. Within the practice management section, there is a section on medical ethics. Assuming that ethics-based questions are one in five of the practice management section (this is probably an over estimate), then this means that knowledge-based assessment of medical ethics is very minimal. Perhaps this is not a bad thing – arguably, the AKT-type question format is a poor way of assessing ethical competence, and in any case, fact-based assessment such as the AKT will only assess the lower areas of Miller's pyramid, such as 'Knows' or possibly 'Knows How'.

The AKT assessment group of the RCGP has produced a useful AKT content guide which lists the subjects that will be tested in the AKT.[7] For ethical topics, these are:

- Beginning of life issues including termination, adoptions surrogacy and antenatal diagnosis
- Capacity (includes power for attorney and Advanced decision to refuse treatment)
- Chaperones
- Children
- Consent and dissent
- End-of-life care
- Ethics of genetic testing
- Medical management and working with colleagues
- Probity (e.g. gifts, conflict of interests, financial, payment by results)

- Raising and acting on concerns
- Referral to other healthcare practitioners including self-referral
- Research ethics
- Safeguarding (includes children, elderly and those vulnerable to domestic violence)
- Welfare of practitioners.

Most of the questions in the AKT examination are single best answer (SBA) questions, but the following types of questions are also present, though in lesser numbers.

- SBA
- Extended matching questions
- Table/algorithm
- Picture/video format
- Drag and drop
- Data interpretation
- Free text
- Rank ordering

A typical question might be:

Consent for disclosure of medical information

Which two of the following statements are the most appropriate considerations when providing information to third parties such as insurers? Select two options only:

A. Disclose all information written in the medical record
B. Do not disclose the content of the report to your patient
C. Ensure the patient has sufficient information about the likely consequences of disclosure
D. Relevant information can be withheld under certain circumstances
E. Use the pro-forma provided by the third party
F. Patient consent can be automatically assumed by receipt of the insurer's request

(Answer C and D)

Strengths and weaknesses of the AKT assessment method

The AKT exam is reliable and repeatable, provided the questions are written to avoid ambiguity and there is truly only one correct answer per question. The test is computer marked and very cheap to run. And, in terms of validity, the test performs well on most statistical measures of validity – it really does measure knowledge and this includes ethical knowledge. However, the test operates at the very lowest level of Miller's pyramid, and is inappropriate for assessing more complex skills. Importantly, because of the range of material to be examined, the amount of specifically *ethical* material is minimal and at best it can only cover a tiny fraction of any ethical curriculum.

THE CLINICAL SKILLS ASSESSMENT (CSA)

The clinical skills examination is a practical test of consultations skills. The candidate attends a national assessment centre and is assessed on his/her management of 13 carefully written cases where the patient is played by a trained role player. Each candidate is therefore assessed by 13 different assessors. Each 'consultation' lasts for 10 minutes with a 2 minute gap between cases. Each case is marked in three domains:

Data collection (the ability to take a clear history of a presenting problem from the role player)
Clinical management (the ability to correctly diagnose and manage the patient's problem with a safe and up-to-date management plan)
Interpersonal skills (the ability to develop a rapport with the patient, show empathy, assess the reason for attendance and involve the patient in the diagnostic process and management plan)

The cases are all linked to the GP curriculum, and there is a rigorous procedure to make sure that the assessment 'samples' a wide range of the curriculum.

Ethical competence can be assessed in these cases in two main ways (though there is an overlap between the two sorts of methods).

Firstly, there are specific 'ethics' cases where the key issue in the case is an ethical issue, and the assessment process focuses on the way the candidate deals with this specific issue. Examples of these sorts of cases might be:

- A relative ringing for information from their doctor (ethical issue – confidentiality)
- A patient who refuses treatment (ethical issue – treatment without consent)
- A patient with a learning disability (ethical issues – assessing capacity, treatment with respect)
- A patient at the end of their life (ethical issues – end-of-life care, refusal of treatment, assisted suicide)
- A patient with a new diagnosis of an illness with a very poor prognosis (ethical issue – truth telling)
- A patient who demands a particularly expensive treatment when cheaper alternatives are available (ethical issues – rationing and dealing with patient demands).

Secondly, there are ethical components to most clinical cases, even when the nub of the case is not obviously ethical. Such ethical components might include:

- Empathy
- Respect for persons
- Obtaining consent to examine patients
- Ethics of requesting (or not) a chaperone.

Such an assessment measures attributes at a higher level than the AKT – typically at the Miller's pyramid level of 'Shows how' (though as this is an examination, this would not reach the level of 'Does'). The assessment is done by experienced GPs (whose reliability is regularly scrutinised) and the ethical content is explicit and reflected in the marking scheme.

Strengths and weaknesses of the CSA assessment method

The CSA exam is reasonably reliable (though not as much so as the AKT exam). Reliability is enhanced by careful training of examiners and role players, with frequent calibration of examiners and 'rehearsal' of the case with role players each day before the exam starts. Each candidate is assessed by 13 different examiners, thus reducing bias due to naturally occurring variation in the severity of examiner marking styles. The cases are carefully written and 'road tested' and they do seem to assess the ability to manage real-life practical problems associated with ethical challenges and dilemmas, and in terms of Miller's pyramid, assessment seems to genuinely be at the level of 'Shows how'. The assessment is however expensive to run and is intensive on time – 13 examiners and role players, and lots of administrative support are needed to examine 13 candidates, and the examination takes just over 3 hours to run.

WORKPLACE-BASED ASSESSMENT

The UK general practice trainees are assessed throughout their training – the so called 'work-place-based assessment'. This 'on-the-job' assessment assesses at the pinnacle of Miller's pyramid at the level of 'Does'. Over the 3 years of GP training, the trainee is assigned an educational supervisor who meets the learner a minimum of twice a year for an educational review. There is also a clinical supervisor (trainer) who works in the same environment as the learner and reviews the work of the trainee regularly. (Usually, the educational supervisor and the clinical supervisor for the time spent in primary care are the same person).

Over the period of training, there are a number of practical assessments done by the clinical supervisor or the educational supervisor. These are listed in the table below.

Type of assessment	Description
Consultation observation tool (COT)	Assessor watches consultation either directly or on video and assesses the consultation according to explicit criteria.
Case-based discussion (CbD)	Assessor discusses a case brought by the learner and assesses according to explicit criteria.
Self-assessment of learning by trainee	Learner assesses his learning in 13 clinical areas.
Analysis of trainee's self-assessment of learning by educational supervisor	Educational supervisor reviews and assesses trainee's self-assessment of learning.
Out-of-hours review	Educational supervisor reviews learner's reflection on out-of-hours work.
Clinical review	Clinical supervisor reviews a period of clinical activity.

As well as formal assessments done by supervisors, there are also assessable entries about educational events made by the trainee. These are called 'Naturally occurring evidence', and include:

- Tutorials
- Patient encounters
- Professional conversations
- Out-of-hours sessions
- Trainee-initiated learning such as books, articles, e-learning, etc.

All this information is recorded electronically on an e-portfolio.

Such assessments may or may not be about ethical issues. A skilled trainer will make sure that ethical issues are covered in the CbDs and the COTs but an unskilled trainer may not do this, and a trainee who wants to avoid considering his ethical performance might be able to complete this assessment without ethical reflection.

In a section of the e-portfolio called *naturally occurring evidence*, the trainee will need to be able to discuss and share information entered on to the portfolio. This is an effective resource for reflecting on ethical issues but some trainees may be able to avoid discussing ethics if they wish to – as before, a good trainer will be able to identify and discuss the ethical issues raised by the evidence in the portfolio.

The final sign-off of the trainee involves an assessment of 13 areas – one of which is 'Maintaining an ethical approach'. This area of assessment does force both trainee and trainer to consider and assess ethical competence (the trainee can only complete training if all of the 13 areas is graded at 'Competent' or above) – but the assessment may be only based on a few cases, selected by the trainee.

This classifies overall ability in the general practice workplace into one of four standards – *insufficient evidence – needs further development – competent – excellent. Insufficient evidence* is unhelpful and worrying as it suggests that over the assessment period, there is no evidence available that will allow a meaningful discussion of ethical competence. The word pictures for the remaining three assessment conclusions (listed below) are brief and possibly too vague to be very helpful.

Needs further development	Competent	Excellent
Awareness of the professional codes of practice as described in the GMC document 'Good medical practice'.	Demonstrates the application of 'Good medical practice' in their own clinical practice. Reflects on how their values, attitudes and ethics might influence professional behaviour.	Anticipates the potential for conflicts of interests and takes appropriate action to avoid these.
Understands the need to treat everyone with respect for their beliefs, preferences, dignity and rights.	Demonstrates equality, fairness and respect in their day-to-day practice.	Anticipates situations where indirect discriminations might occur. Awareness of current legislation as it applies to clinical work and practice management.
Recognises that people are different and does not discriminate against them because of those differences.	Values and appreciates different cultures and personal attributes both in patients and colleagues.	Actively supports diversity and harnesses differences between people for the benefit of the organisation and patients alike.
Understands that good medical practice requires reference to ethical principles.	Reflects on and discusses moral dilemmas encountered during the course of their work.	Able to analyse ethical issues with reference to specific ethical theory.

Strengths and weaknesses of the WPBA assessment method

The advantage of the assessment is that it assesses at the level of 'does' – at the very top of Miller's pyramid. The assessment is time-consuming for both trainee and trainer, but these time and financial costs are absorbed into the overall cost for the training programme. Unfortunately, the reliability of this method of assessment is poor. There is a large degree of inter-assessor variation – some trainers are 'hawks' and some are 'doves', and unlike in the CSA, there is no mechanism for calibration of assessors. Many trainers naturally develop friendship with their trainee and this can cause their assessment to be biased and unrepresentative of the true ability of the trainee. Validity is also a problem – because the assessment of ethical ability hinges on the self-reported identification and review of perhaps only two or three cases, then the assessment tool may not be measuring what it aims to measure – the ability of trainee GPs to cope with day-to-day ethical cases.

ASSESSMENT WHILST THE GP IS AN INDEPENDENT PRACTITIONER

Once the GP trainee has become accredited as fit for independent practice, the amount of ethical assessment that the new GP undergoes can often decrease and become much more variable in quality. The only *compulsory and formal* ethical assessment is the requirement of all doctors on the 'performers list' to undergo annual appraisal and 5-yearly revalidation. However, there may be some *informal* ethical education and assessment which occur in parallel with the formal process of appraisal/revalidation. I will discuss the appraisal/revalidation process below and then review informal methods of assessment.

In order to continue in independent practice, British GPs must demonstrate that they are up to date and fit to practice. This is achieved by means of the revalidation process, which consists of a yearly appraisal meeting combined with a 5-yearly (paper-based) external review.[8] Over the 5-year period, the GP must demonstrate continuing education with formal requirements for professional development, audit, significant event analysis, patient feedback and colleague feedback. There is also a need to demonstrate a range of educational and reflective activities and, importantly, there must be reference and linkage to GMC guidance. In addition, there is a specific requirement to make a declaration about probity and honesty.

The process is poorly designed to assess ethical competence. It is easily possible to complete the appraisal process with minimal or no reference to ethical understanding or competence. The appraisal process attempts to assess whether continuing learning and reflection about performance and learning are occurring, but (apart from the probity statement above) there is no systematic evaluation of any ethical knowledge, skills or competence. Of course, if a practitioner is *really* determined to talk about ethics in his or her appraisal, it is possible to do so, but the lack of rigour and consistency in the appraisal process is an opportunity missed.

In addition, there may also be a life-long, background, process of *informal*, non-structured, ethical feedback and assessment which offsets the lack of formal ethical review. Unfortunately, this feedback process is dependent on the willingness of the practitioner to listen, and so can vary in impact from life-changing to unnoticed. It certainly lacks reliability and repeatability, though it may be surprisingly valid. It is probably the main way that practitioners learn and develop ethically and have their performance assessed.

This type of ethical 'assessment' may include the following components:

- Listening to patients reflecting on how a consultation has proceeded – either directly or via the medium of the receptionist or practice nurse
- Discussing difficult ethical cases with colleagues and testing whether your ethical take on the case matches the opinion of your colleagues
- Responding to complaints about consultations that did not go well or had unexpectedly bad outcomes (or, occasionally, had good outcomes!)
- Listening to feedback, requested and unrequested, from colleagues about your ethical performance
- Responding to trainees who are sitting in with you who ask difficult and probing questions about your last consultation ('Why did you do that.....?').

CONCLUSION

There is little controversy about the importance of ethics content and ethics understanding in primary care, and this is reflected in the inclusion of ethics content in the general practice curriculum and in most consensus documents about education in general practice. Experienced practitioners all attest to the richness of ethical content in primary care. The centrality of ethics content in clinical practice is true not just for GPs, but also for all practitioners within primary care.

There is less consensus, however, about the *effectiveness* of assessment of ethics competences and capabilities. Assessment of ethical *knowledge* is certainly possible and seems to possess validity and reliability. However, sadly, this misses much of what is important in primary care ethics. Unfortunately, attempts to assess *higher* levels of ethical competence are not satisfactory; they either lack validity or reliability (or both) or are swamped in the learner's or practitioner's mind by the huge amount of other material that has to be assimilated. The hardest assessment task of all seems to be the attempt to assess ethical *attitudes*[9] – the very thing that matters the most in primary care ethical assessment. Not only are the methods to assess ethical attitudes at a basic stage, but also there seems to be a paradox that it is impossible to achieve both reliability and validity – achieve one and you lose the other. And the underlying message seems to be that assessment is not a quick fix – it takes time and effort and will undoubtedly be demanding of resources. However, it matters – not just for GPs, but all members of the primary care team. Ethical education and assessment need to be made central (and given protected time and space) within any primary care curriculum.

REFERENCES

1. Oxford Brooke's University. *Oxford Centre for staff and learning development.* Available at: https://www.brookes.ac.uk/services/ocsld/resources/writing_learning_outcomes.html (accessed 20 May 2016).
2. GMC. *Tomorrow's Doctors: Outcomes and standards for undergraduate medical education.* 1993. Available at: http://www.gmc-uk.org/Tomorrow_s_Doctors_1214.pdf_48905759.pdf (accessed 20 May 2016).
3. Miller G. *Assessment of clinical skills/competence/performance.* 1990. Available at: http://winbev.pbworks.com/f/Assessment.pdf (accessed 20 May 2016).
4. RCGP Curriculum. *Core curriculum statement.* 2016. Available at: http://www.rcgp.org.uk/training-exams/~/media/Files/GP-training-and-exams/Curriculum-2012/RCGP-Curriculum-1-Being-a-GP.ashx (accessed 20 May 2016).
5. Stirrat GM, et al. Medical ethics and law for doctors of tomorrow: The 1998 Consensus Statement updated. *J Med Ethics* 2010;36:55–60.
6. McCulloch M. *University of Glasgow. An introduction to assessment.* 2007. Available at: http://www.gla.ac.uk/media/media_12158_en.pdf (accessed 20 May 2016).
7. *The Applied Knowledge Test Content Guide August 2014.* Available at: http://www.rcgp.org.uk/gp-training-and-exams/mrcgp-exam-overview/~/media/D96EB4E0188E4355BCC9221B55859B08.ashx (accessed 20 May 2016).
8. Caesar S. *RCGP Guide to supporting information for appraisal and revalidation.* 2016. Available at: http://www.rcgp.org.uk/revalidation/~/media/Files/Revalidation-and-CPD/2016/RCGP-Guide-to-Supporting-Information-2016.ashx (accessed 20 May 2016).
9. Martin J, et al. *Professional attitudes. Can they be taught and assessed in general practice?* 2002. Available at: phttp://www.clinmed.rcpjournal.org/content/2/3/217.full.pdf (accessed 20 May 2016).

FURTHER READING

Fenwick A, et al. Institute of Medical Ethics. *Medical ethics and law. A practical guide to the assessment of the core content of learning. A report from the education steering group of the institute of medical ethics.* 2013. Available at http://www.instituteofmedicalethics.org/website/index.php?option=com_jdownloads&Itemid=7&view=finish&cid=86&catid=3 (accessed 20 May 2016).

Singer P and Robb A. *The Ethics OSCE: Standardized patient scenarios for teaching and evaluating bioethics.* 1994. Available at: http://www.spp.utoronto.ca/sites/default/files/resources/ethics_osce.pdf (accessed 20 May 2016).

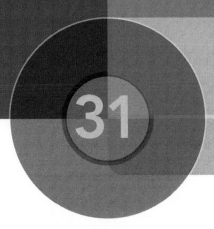

Try this at home: Values-based practice and clinical care

31

BILL (KWM) FULFORD AND ED PEILE

Values-based practice is a decision support tool that as its name suggests is a partner to evidence-based practice. Evidence-based practice provides a process that supports clinical decision-making where complex and conflicting evidence is in play. Values-based practice provides a counterpart process that supports clinical decision-making where complex and conflicting values are in play.

The processes involved are different, of course. Where evidence-based practice relies on meta-analyses and other technical process elements, values-based practice relies primarily on learnable clinical skills. However, we need both. We need evidence-based practice to engage effectively with the science on which clinical interventions are based. We need values-based practice to link the science with the diverse values (including needs, wishes, concerns, beliefs and preferences) of individual patients and families.

In this chapter, we introduce values-based practice by way of two brief exercises that you may like to try for yourself. Being based on learnable clinical skills, values-based practice is better understood by 'doing than saying'. We then give a brief outline of values-based practice, illustrating, with two contrasting case histories, its importance in clinical care. We start with what may seem an obvious question, 'what are values?'.

EXERCISE 1: WHAT ARE VALUES?

This exercise comes in two parts:

1. Write down three words (or very short phrases) that mean 'values' to you.
2. Then ask someone else to try the same thing and compare what you have both written.

Note: It is important to actually write down your own three words – don't just think of them 'in your head'.

You are likely to find that everyone comes up with a different triplet of words. In values-based training, we usually do this as a group exercise. There are some overlaps but the range of words people come up with is remarkable. Figure 31.1 gives an illustrative list.

This exercise tells us two key things about values. Firstly, it highlights the diversity of meanings of the everyday term 'values'. This is important clinically. Values in clinical contexts are widely taken to mean 'ethics' or perhaps 'corporate' values (like the NHS core values on posters in clinical reception rooms).[1] But as Figure 31.1 shows, values are far wider than this.

A helpful way to sum up what values mean for clinical purposes is as anything *that matters*. In clinical decision-making, we have to find out what matters to our patients (we return to this below). Being aware of what matters to us (our own values) is a vital part of doing this effectively. What matters to managers and policymakers (resources) is also important in setting the context for clinical care. So, everyone's values matter in one way or another in clinical care. And of course, what matters varies from group to group and from individual to individual.

So the clinical context is one in which values are complex. Hence, it is not surprising that values in this context often come into conflict. This is why we need values-based as well as evidence-based practices. Values in healthcare are complex and conflicting. Values-based practice supports clinical decision-making where complex and conflicting values are in play.

The second thing we can learn from this exercise is that for all their diversity, values are not random. You can see this by asking yourself whether you disagree with the words other people come up with or with any of the words in Figure 31.1. What we usually find is that even though other people come up with quite different words, we readily agree one with another that all our words do indeed have something to do with values. If you came up with, say, 'principles', 'needs' and 'wishes', you might nonetheless agree that 'preferences', 'hopes' and other words in Figure 31.1 are also relevant.

As we get to grip with values, we realise that they are certainly more complex and conflicting than we generally recognise, and the need for systematic 'values-based practice' to support clinical decision-making becomes more apparent. There is another important rationale. As the following exercise demonstrates, we are all prone to making assumptions about values, which might be shorthanded as, 'Surely most people think like I do'. A 'surely' thought should act as a warning to us that an assumption is being made, and assumptions about values are the enemy of values-based practice.

•   Principles
•   Needs
•   Wishes
•   Preferences
•   Hopes
•   Ambitions
•   Concerns
•   Virtues, etc.

Figure 31.1 What values mean to me.

EXERCISE 2: IT'S YOUR DECISION

The idea of this second exercise is to imagine what you would do if given a forced choice between two competing treatments for an otherwise fatal disease. As you read the following scenario, try to avoid thinking about it in the abstract. Don't think about what people in general would choose or what the 'right' answer would be. Ask yourself, 'given me as I am now, at my age and in my life circumstances, what would I choose?'.

Here is the choice:

Imagine you have developed early symptoms of a potentially fatal disease. NICE[2] has approved two possible treatments:

- Treatment A – gives you a guaranteed period of remission but no cure.
- Treatment B – gives you a 50:50 chance of 'kill or cure'.

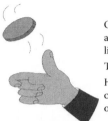

One option would have been to take my chance. A toss of a coin here and now offers me the chance of living well for the rest of my normal lifespan but if the coin comes down the wrong way I would die now.

The question for me is:

How long would my GUARANTEED survival have to be for me to choose this alternative option over the 50/50 life/death chance option?

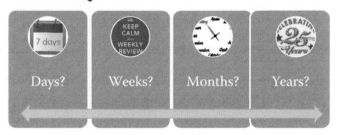

Figure 31.2 Choosing treatment A or B.

It's your decision – how long a period of remission would you want from Treatment A to choose that treatment rather than go for the 50:50 'kill or cure' from Treatment B?

As with our first exercise, it is important to write down your own period of remission – the period you would want to choose Treatment A over the 50:50 kill or cure Treatment B – rather than just thinking about it. You may not find this easy. Some people decide that whatever period A offered, they would 'want it over with' and go for Treatment B straight off. But look at Figure 31.2 and write down your own minimum period, whatever it is.

In a group exercise, people write down a great range of periods when faced with this scenario. Often, people sitting next to each other and who know each other really well come up with very different answers. They may be very surprised by this. You may be surprised that other people give very different answers from yours. However, when we think about why people come up with such different answers, we see that this is because different things *matter to them*: one person, say, may choose 20 years minimum because he or she has a young family and want enough time to see them safely grown up; another may choose only a year because the person is finishing a research project that he or she feels passionate about and that will take this time to complete. In other words, everyone brings different personal values to this difficult choice.

This second exercise reinforces the message about diversity of individual values – people choose different periods because there are different things that matter to them. However, the exercise also brings out the vital link between values and evidence. The evidence base in this imaginary scenario is the same for everyone. Yet, people make very different choices because their values are very different. This is why as we noted at the start of this chapter, we need values-based practice to link science, represented here by the evidence base of decision-making, with the unique values of individual patients and families.

AN OUTLINE OF VALUES-BASED PRACTICE

The overall process of values-based practice is shown diagrammatically in Figure 31.3. As this indicates, the core of values-based practice is 10 process elements covering clinical skills,

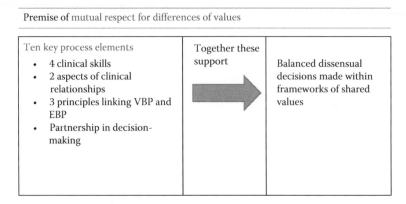

Premise of mutual respect for differences of values

Ten key process elements	Together these support	Balanced dissensual decisions made within frameworks of shared values
• 4 clinical skills • 2 aspects of clinical relationships • 3 principles linking VBP and EBP • Partnership in decision-making		

Figure 31.3 A diagram of value-based practice.

relationships, links with evidence-based practice and a particular take on partnership in decision-making. Building on a premise of mutual respect, these elements together support balanced decision-making within frameworks of shared values. Further details of these elements are summarised in Table 31.1.

The starting point for values-based practice is the first clinical skill listed in the table, raising awareness of values and of differences of values. The exercises above are aimed at developing this skill. Other awareness-raising exercises are given in the resources indicated in the Further Reading at the end of this chapter.

Besides awareness, reasoning about values, knowledge of values and communication skills are also important. Values-based practice indeed as we put it elsewhere is 'nothing without communication skills'.[3] As with so many clinical skills, the relationship here is two-way. Communication skills (especially for eliciting values and of conflict resolution) are important in values-based practice. However, values-based practice also brings in content to communication skills. It reminds us in particular to explore strengths as well as needs and difficulties. Values-based practice thus enriches the familiar ICE (ideas, concerns and expectations) to ICEStAR (adding strengths, aspirations and resources).

The clinical skills for values-based practice are most effectively deployed not by individuals working on their own but within clinical teams. The 'extended' multidisciplinary team of values-based practice brings in a range of diverse values as well as knowledge and skills to clinical care. This range of diverse values in turn is the basis of the values-based concept of person-*values*-centred care – care that starts from and builds on the actual rather than imagined values of the individual patient or family concerned. We return to the importance of person-values-centred care below.

All too often, values are thought to be somehow a counterbalance to the demands of evidence. They are not. They are fully complementary to evidence-based practice and equally essential to clinical decision-making. This is what the three linking principles shown in the table are about. They remind us in different ways always to keep both values and evidence in our clinical sights. David Sackett, writing in his role as the founder Director of Oxford's Centre for Evidence-based Medicine, defined evidence-based medicine originally as combining best research evidence with clinical experience and values.[4]

To understand how balanced decisions on individual cases can be made within frameworks of shared values, we need to consider the concept of dissensus. With *con*sensus, one or more perspectives are given up in favour of a shared view. Consensus is important in the processes

Table 31.1 The elements of values-based practice

Values-based practice	Brief definition
Premise of mutual respect	Mutual respect for differences of values
Skills – awareness	Awareness of values and of differences of values
Skills – knowledge	Knowledge retrieval and its limitations
Skills – reasoning	Used to explore the values in play rather than to 'solve' dilemmas
Skills – communication	Especially for eliciting values and for conflict resolution
Person-values-centred care	Care centred on the actual rather than assumed values of the patient
Extended MDT	MDT role extended to include a range and for value perspectives as well as of knowledge and skills
Two feet principle	All decisions are based on the two feet of values and evidence
Squeaky wheel principle	We notice values when they cause difficulties (like the squeaky wheel) but (like the wheel that doesn't squeak) they are always there and operative
Science-driven principle	Advances in medical science drive the need for VBP (as well as EBP) because they open up choices and with choices go values
Partnership	Decisions in VBP (although informed by clinical guidelines and other sources) are made by those directly concerned working together in partnership
Frameworks of shared values	Values shared by those in a given decision-making context (e.g. a GP practice) and within which balanced decisions can be made on individual cases
Balanced dissensual decisions	Decisions in which the values in question remain in play, to be balanced sometimes in one way and sometimes in other ways according to the circumstances of a given case

Note: EBP, evidence-based practice; MDT, multidisciplinary team; VBP, value-based practice.

of evidence-based medicine. We all try to reach agreement on the direction in which the best available evidence points. However, the balanced decisions that are the outputs of values-based practice are made by *diss*ensus. In dissensual decision-making, shared framework values instead of being given up one in favour of another, all remain in play to be balanced sometimes one way and sometimes in other ways, according to the circumstances of each individual case (see Figure 31.3).

WHY BOTHER?

Faced with remorselessly growing pressures on healthcare budgets and demands for 'through put', it is natural to ask 'why bother?' There is hardly time enough it seems to hear from our patients what's the matter *with* them. How can we go the extra mile to find out what matters *to* them?

Two stories illustrate how values-based practice can help us to work smarter not harder. Both stories are based on real events. The first is from clinical practice with biographical details changed. The second is from a recent Supreme Court case that as we describe has shifted the basis of consent in clinical decision-making decisively towards person-values-centred care.

KNEE-BENDS

A patient with a painful arthritic knee was referred to an orthopaedic surgeon for assessment for knee replacement. After the usual work-up, the surgeon made her sit down and told her he was pleased to say he could give her a prosthetic knee joint; the operation could be done in a month or two; she would need a period of physiotherapy but 18 months from now if all went well she would be pain-free.

As she got up to leave, she thanked the surgeon saying 'I'm so pleased, doctor, I'll be able to get back to my garden'. 'Well, tell me a bit more about that', the surgeon replied, inviting her to sit down again. The patient explained that it was not the pain in her knee that she was worried about. It was indeed painful but she could put up with that. What really mattered to her was that she had lost mobility to the point that she could no longer do her gardening.

The surgeon explained that while an artificial joint would in all probability give her a pain-free knee, the prostheses available offered only limited mobility. She would be no more mobile, and possibly less so, post-operation. The end result was that the patient opted for conservative management. Eighteen months later, she still had a painful knee but her mobility was restored to the point that she was happily back to gardening.

What matters to most people with painful arthritic knees is to get rid of the pain. It was natural therefore that those concerned in this patient's care had assumed that this was what mattered to her. However, this was *not* what mattered to her. And finding out what really mattered to her was a win-win for everyone. She got the treatment she needed. The surgeon had a satisfied patient. The health service budget was saved several tens of thousands of pounds in misdirected interventions.

Our second story carries the opposite message – neglecting what matters is a win for no one.

THE MONTGOMERY CASE

In 2013, a young woman with diabetes, Mrs. Nadine Montgomery, was delivered vaginally of a baby son. Sadly, the baby was born with severe disabilities arising from shoulder dystocia. This is a recognised risk for mothers with diabetes, but Mrs. Montgomery had not been offered the option of a caesarian section and decided to sue her health authority in damages.

The case ended up in the UK Supreme Court. The defence was that the gynaecologist had followed the practice of a body of her responsible peers in not warning Mrs. Montgomery of the risks of vaginal birth where she (the gynaecologist) considered these to be less than the risks of a caesarian section. This was in line with the 'prudent clinician' principle of consent on which until then clinicians had been able to rely on.[5] The court, however, drawing on a range of both legal precedents and evidence of contemporary standards of good practice, decided in favour of Mrs. Montgomery.[6]

The judgment is long but clinically nuanced. Its effect is to replace the 'prudent clinician' of the *Bolam* principle with an 'informed patient' principle of consent. The details though of how the patient becomes informed are all important. Informing the patient, the Montgomery judges spell out, does not mean 'bombarding the patient with technical information … (or) … demanding her signature on a consent form' (para 90). Nor does it mean just going along with whatever a patient wants: in Montgomery, as in values-based practice, clinicians' values matter too.[7] What the Montgomery standard of consent does mean is entering into 'dialogue' (para 90) with the patient to the point that the patient has sufficient understanding to make a choice that 'take(s) into account her own values' (para 115). Montgomery consent then is person-values-centred consent.

SUMMARY

In this chapter, we have described a clinical skills–based approach to working with values in healthcare called values-based practice. Our introductory exercises – the 'three words that mean values to you' and the forced choice between treatments – illustrate how values-based practice builds on raising awareness of values and other learnable clinical skills while working always in partnership with evidence-based practice. Our two case histories illustrate the importance of working more effectively with values as well as evidence. This is important if person-centred care is to be genuinely person-*values*-centred care. Person-values-centred care is in turn important if our interventions are to be targeted in a cost-effective way and according to contemporary (Montgomery) standards of consent.

Values-based practice for all that is no panacea. To the contrary, it is but one of a growing toolkit of ways of working with values in healthcare. Besides ethics and law, other important tools in the toolkit include health economics and decision analysis. Shared decision-making is the topic of a helpful on-line 'Advancing Quality Alliance' decision support resource. Values-based practice furthermore may be used as a whole or in parts. Each of the elements of our perhaps rather daunting diagram in Figure 31.3 may be used to good effect individually. The clinical stories in our *Essential Values-based Practice* (2012) illustrate the elements of values-based practice working separately as well as together. The tools in the values toolkit as a whole moreover must be used always in partnership with the evidence-base of decision-making.

Values-based practice, as just one of the tools in the values toolkit, and as a partner to evidence-based practice, has found a growing range of applications across mental health and primary care (see website below). The recently launched *Collaborating Centre for Values-based Practice* at St Catherine's College in Oxford is supporting the development of similar approaches in surgery and a number of areas of secondary care.[8]

CONCLUSIONS

We drew on examples from the specialist domains of orthopaedics and obstetrics, and yet the primary care message is no different.

In our model of values-based practice, we start by setting aside any assumption that we understand the way that others think. Then, if we reinforce our communication skills by asking specific 'values' questions like, 'what does your skin mean to you?', we are in a position to work with our patient in values-based reasoning. By drawing on the best available clinical evidence that aligns with the patient's values, we can achieve balanced dissensual decision-making within a shared framework of values.

Try it at home in your own practice and see for yourself how values-based practice supports your clinical care. Before long, you may find yourself using the same processes outside the consulting room and in the boardrooms where policy and community planning are discussed.

REFERENCES

1. http://www.nhs.uk/NHSEngland/thenhs/about/Pages/nhscoreprinciples.aspx [accessed 18 June 2016].
2. Strictly, National Institute for Health and Care Excellence; but invariably abbreviated to 'NICE'.

3. Fulford, K.W.M., Peile, E., and Carroll, H. (2012). *Essential Values-Based Practice: Clinical Stories Linking Science with People.* Cambridge: Cambridge University Press, p. 4.

4. Sackett, D.L. Straus, S.E., Scott Richardson, W., Rosenberg, W., and Haynes, R.B. (2000). *Evidence-Based Medicine: How to Practice and Teach EBM* (2nd ed.). Edinburgh: Churchill Livingstone.

5. *Bolam v Friern HMC* [1957] 2 All ER 118.

6. *Montgomery v Lanarkshire Health Board (Scotland)* [2015] UKSC 11. On appeal from: [2013] CSIH 3; [2010] CSIH 104. https://www.supremecourt.uk/cases/uksc-2013-0136.html [accessed 18 June 2016].

7. Fulford et al., 2012, *op.cit.*

8. E-Learning for Healthcare. (2012). *Introduction to Shared Decision Making.* http://cs1.e-learningforhealthcare.org.uk/public/SDM/SDM_01_01/d/ELFH_Session/7/session.html?lms=n#overview.html [accessed 18 June 2016].

FURTHER READING

The website for the *Collaborating Centre for Values-based Practice* includes a detailed reading guide covering the theory and practice of values-based practice. It also includes a number of downloadable learning resources. See valuesbasedpractice.org and follow the links to 'More about VBP'/'Reading Guide' and 'More about VBP'/'Full text Downloads'.

The authors' *Essential Values-based Practice: Clinical Stories Linking Science with People* describes the applications of values-based practice across a range of areas of both primary and secondary care through a series of extended case histories based on everyday clinical scenarios (managing low back pain, adolescent diabetes, mild hypertension, etc.). Chapter 14 of *Essentials* gives a worked example of how a GP practice worked together with their local patients' forum to develop their own framework of shared values.

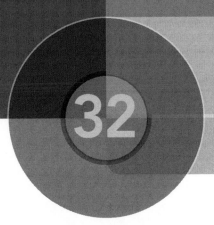

Adopting an alternative worldview: Perspectives from postmodernism

32

CHRIS CALDWELL AND SANJIV AHLUWALIA

IMAGINING A POSTMODERN WORLD

Imagine a person (and this will be me – CC) driving down a narrow, tree-lined lane. You are sitting next to me and there are other people, including my fellow author – SA – and maybe a dog, a child and a grandparent) in the back of the car. My eyes look at the road ahead and using the rear-view mirror, I can also see behind us. My ears listen to the sounds inside the car. I may be able to hear sounds outside the car, especially if the windows are open, or perhaps I imagine the sounds outside the car based on what I see.

My hands are on the steering wheel, my feet work the pedals and my body sits in the seat next to you. My head is there too. Every moment as the car progresses down the lane, I experience many different things. And inside my body, my inner self or selves may or may not be with you. Inward looking, I may be in many different places, using my body in multiple different ways, seeing, hearing, smelling, feeling, thinking, from moment to moment as we drive down the road.

And you – you are with me but you are experiencing the world from your own multiple perspectives, all slightly different from mine. Those in the back of the car and the dog – all have yet another set of experiences, all slightly different again. As we travel, others watch us: other people, animals, trees and birds in the sky, perhaps also spirits or angels. This is another host of different perspectives on the experience of us in the car, on the lane, driving, in our worlds. Every moment we move from the past through the present and into the future, looking back through the rear-view mirror to the past and ahead – many different pasts, presents and futures.

From the above text you will now have imagined a very complex, multilayered, interwoven 'picture' which is a representation of our everyday 'realities', a frame through which to view our practice as healthcare professionals working in primary care. Perhaps tangled and muddled, perhaps exciting, perhaps daunting, perhaps fun, perhaps frightening, depending on the perspective upon it we choose to take. Nevertheless, this is our unique individual living world – a world of multiple, simultaneous and ongoing experiences, some noticed, some captured, some lost and many learned from. In this chapter, we explore how adopting an approach, which instead of seeking to view everyday reality through one single dominant 'frame', seeks to hold open the multiplicity, and approach decision-making in practice through adopting such a worldview.

THE POSTMODERN PARADIGM

Thomas Kuhn[1] defined a 'paradigm' as a constellation of values, beliefs and methodological assumptions, tacit or explicit, which together make up a broader worldview. Kuhn observed that over the history of science, a number of paradigm shifts could be observed where a new perspective with greater explanatory power challenged the dominant view and eventually overcame it. In this way, science experienced a continual conceptual revolution. Whilst Kuhn limited his analysis to science, Foucault (1972),[2] through his concept of 'episteme', and, more recently, Best and Kellner (1997) have extended this analysis to contextualise a major transformational paradigm shift to the postmodern, which incorporates all intellectual and artistic disciplines and which impacts in all aspects of culture, society, values and practices of everyday life.

Dramatic technological, cultural, environmental and societal changes since the early 1920s have resulted in the emergence of multiple, often competing, so-called postmodern discourses in the aesthetic, scientific, philosophical, social and intellectual domains, and a theory war between these new theories and the received modern perspective. Best and Kellner[3] refer to this transformational shift as the 'postmodern turn,' a shifting into a space that is largely uncharted, not only offering new possibilities but also presenting challenges and danger. The roots of the postmodern turn can be traced back to some of the great social thinkers of the nineteenth century such as Nietzsche, Marx and Kierkegaard.

There is no consensus definition of postmodern. It is often seen in the popular press as synonymous with any novel contemporary social movement with global relevance across all aspects of societies. Academically, it is still hotly contested. Postmodern theorists such as Best and Kellner, argue, however, that it is precisely because postmodernism has multiple genealogies and disparate trajectories that somehow coalesce that this emergent, not-yet-dominant paradigm is significant and pertinent, as we attempt to develop and thrive in an increasingly complex, dynamic age. We concur with Best and Kellner and argue that postmodernism is therefore a very appropriate frame for approaching contemporary primary healthcare.

UNDERSTANDING POSTMODERNISM THROUGH ART

Engaging with ideas from postmodernism provides an opportunity to challenge previously held rules and even to confront for the first time some of one's deeply held (but perhaps untested) personal beliefs. Adopting a postmodern perspective, rather than the binary perspective of modernism, provides an opportunity to hold open more than one possible explanation for a situation as experienced, and in doing so offers the potential to contain anxiety – not simply accept and internalise or dismiss even or avoid. As a result, one can work with complex situations rather than seeking to understand, work through or control them or alternatively be consumed and worn out.

There is no better way to appreciate and explore this perspective than through engaging with postmodern art. In this section, we draw on the work of three artists: Paul Cezanne, Pablo Picasso and David Hockney. Through his work, Cezanne developed a postmodern theory of variability and stability which influenced many subsequent artists and which helps expand on the postmodern paradigm. Cezanne's theory focuses on the following:

- Multiple and simultaneous viewpoints – that moment to moment 'reality' is in fact experienced from an infinite number of 'angles' and is made up of many concurrent 'realities'.
- Interlocking moments – 'reality' as experienced is concurrent and continual, each event merging into and out the previous and the subsequent.
- A synthesis of space and figure – reality as experienced is a combination of the 'object' of the experience and the space in between.
- Rejecting the positivist notion of a single isolatable event – everything is related to what comes before and then subsequently as well as being subsumed within its own 'space'.
- The event containing the viewer – in opposition to the positivist modern perspective, postmodernism argues that we are all part of our own experiences and therefore can never be objective of that event.
- Presenting the human as non-exceptional – Cezanne asserts that human beings are no more important than any other element in the 'reality' of any single experience.

Picasso[4] powerfully adopts and further develops Cezanne's depiction of postmodern theory in his work. Turning to postmodern as a means to express his own feelings about the atrocities of war, most famously, he created 'Guernica', a 7.7 m mural depicting the bombing of a Basque country village.

Another postmodern artist whose work has had a profound influence on the practice of one of us is David Hockney, an artist famed for depicting the same, or very similar images, from incrementally differing perspectives. In the 1980s, Hockney[5] created a series of massive collages of the Grand Canyon made up of hundreds of photographs, each taken from a slightly different angle. Later, this image was included in his 2011 Royal Academy exhibition, 'A Bigger Picture', which also comprised massive and multiple representations of the countryside of the East Riding of Yorkshire over the four seasons, depicting at the same time incremental changes but with an overall radical effect, yet with the same patterns repeating on an annual basis.

Cezanne helps us to see that life as we experience it in relationship to another is complex and to attempt to simplify or reduce it is to fail to appreciate its rich and interconnected whole, which brings both beauty and ugliness, pleasure and pain, often at the same time. Hockney[6] is pre-occupied with what the world looks like and how human beings represent it, challenging us to look 'long and hard' in order to 'really see'. Through his art, Picasso helped himself and others to share feelings about how the events of their everyday reality (in this case the Spanish civil war) were impacting on them personally, and as a consequence to bear with the hideousness of the situation and remain resilient.

As healthcare professionals facing the ever increasing complexity of the day-to-day world of our practice, the postmodern perspective could provide a helpful frame through to reflect on our own everyday reality. Taking some time out to visit a gallery to convene with the representations of works of art might be a means for us to appreciate our own practice and in doing so to consider the many different perspectives and perceptions which are brought to bear on any single situation. Creating our own 'art' through painting, creative or reflective writing, photography or engaging with some other presentational form might help address some of the deep issues linked to differing perspectives in our health practice. This process might also sustain resilience to continue to practice, to work within complex, changing and conflicting situations, to hold the anxiety that this inevitably creates and use it constructively to move forwards working with it, rather than feel pressured by positivism to seek to understand, control and resolve.

USING A POSTMODERN FRAME IN CLINICAL PRACTICE

The following is a brief account of reflections of one of us (CC) on an everyday experience and the image created represents that experience. Through reflecting using writing (Box 32.1) and artistic expression (Figure 32.1), She found that she was able to better make sense of that experience. The process of inquiring into her practice through writing and painting led me to reflect on my own practice and the experiences she have working with leaders and practitioners within healthcare. How easy it is, when many people have worked together for many years, to assume we all share the same perspective, that we share values, ways of knowing and perceiving when this is so often not the case. Such assumptions can so often lead to failing of change initiatives.

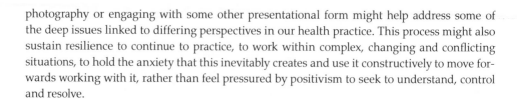

Box 32.1: Perspective and perception in action.
The appraisal: Three different observations over 2 days

On Thursday I arrived at work to find Bola and Eve deep in conversation. Bola soon came in to see me and told me that they had been talking about Eve's appraisal. Eve had her appraisal the day before with her line manager, Dana. Dana had mentioned an experience that Eve had been involved in. It had started positively but had ended on a less positive note. Bola told me that Dana had previously asked her to work with Eve on a number of issues and that she thought Eve was improving as a result. She was disappointed that Dana hadn't spoken to her before the appraisal. Bola was worried that the feedback Eve had received would now result in this progress being lost.

Later that day Dana came to see me. She told me that she had completed Eve's appraisal and that whilst it had started well, it had ended badly. She felt that she had praised Eve on the improved efficiency of her work and her professionalism. She felt that her suggestion for further improvement was received well but things had gone downhill once Dana had refused Eve's request for funding to undertake a course which Dana didn't think was relevant to Eve's work. Both parties left the appraisal feeling that it had not been a success.

When I then reported my conversation with Dana back to Bola she was very surprised. There had been no mention in Eve's account of the request to study and Eve's interpretation of the suggestion for improvement had been received in a very different way than Dana seemed to have meant it. She didn't know whom to believe.

Four people involved in this one situation. Four different perceptions of, and four different perspectives on, the same situation. Each perception made up of the inner and outer worlds of the individual concerned. Each seeking her own perception of success. No one intending a negative consequence but nevertheless it had a negative outcome. We worked over a period of many months to try to resolve things I tried to get us to step into each other's shoes, to enter each other's' worlds and come to resolution. It became clear that one person was not going to allow resolution to happen and it ended quite dramatically.

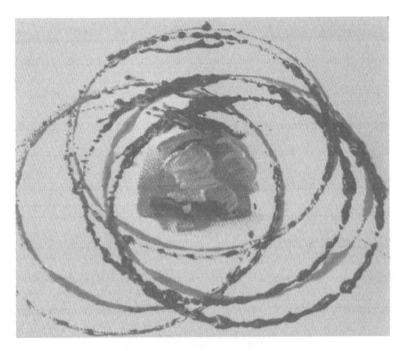

Figure 32.1 This image was created during the process of inquiry linked to the example in Box 32.1 and represents how it felt to be in that specific experience.

Adopting a postmodern frame offers the opportunity to appreciate the many different perspectives on this potentially baffling complex context in order to work through dilemmas and to consider new approaches to exploring possible options for taking action. Each person, whether clinician, patient, manager or policymaker, brings to any single situation their own unique perspective (as Cezanne suggests), presenting not one but many different 'truths' in their needs from healthcare and preferred solutions and therefore opportunities for moving forward. Holding open simultaneously, and appreciating (though not necessarily agreeing with) each other's situation through metaphorically stepping into their shoes and walking around in them as so famously recommended by the lawyer, Atticus Finch, in Laurie Lee's *To Kill a Mockingbird*,[7] can sometimes transform situations, dissolve conflicts and allow the humanity of person-to-person relationships to return.

This everyday experience was nevertheless a very stressful experience for everyone involved in the situation described in Box 32.1. In adopting a postmodern frame through reflective work, enabled an appreciation of the complexity and attempt a range of approaches to try to treat everyone with care but at the same time care for oneself.

APPLYING A POSTMODERNIST FRAME TO PRIMARY CARE

Working in primary care is recognised to be challenging. Uncertainty arises from conversations between healthcare professionals and their patients as well as amongst each other. Such conversations are often messy, complex and unpredictable. A postmodernist mindset has much to offer the clinician working in such an environment. As Cezanne and others suggest,[8] reality is emergent and evolving rather than fixed, change is a non-linear process, that we cannot be observers without at the same time being participants, and the whole is greater than the sum of the parts. Postmodernist thinking therefore encourages us to consider all human interactions to be uncertain, chaotic and open to multiple interpretations. Clinicians and patients are conversational partners whose views are 'partial, contested and situated rather than impartial, beyond argument and universal'.[9]

Such an approach to conversations in primary care has a number of implications:

- It invites clinicians to use their own experiences, ideas and reactions to help patients and colleagues make sense of 'their own world'.
- It invites clinicians to use ways of knowing[10] in their interactions with patients and colleagues that move beyond the simplistic biomedical model that has developed within the past 30 years.
- It encourages the development and use of professional judgement in helping patients deal with the inherent uncertainty they face in their lives.
- It generates potential solutions to intractable problems that might otherwise not be apparent.
- It reignites a sense of connectedness and authenticity with oneself and others that is often excluded in modernist and positivist influences on healthcare.

The challenges of healthcare provision partly relate to the way it is currently organised. We work in a system that is largely fragmented into silos and built around rational/technical and hierarchical solutions to many of the wicked problems we face. The postmodernist approach brings with it a need for a different kind of leadership – a postmodern leadership. Leaders with the ability and confidence to work collectively and collaboratively; leaders who are transparent, open and engaging; who can bring about and communicate clearly a shared vision and goal with the patient and what matters to them at its heart. This kind of leadership fosters trust to build individual and group confidence, facilitates and supports groups to work together through cycles of action and reflection, focusing on the relational and conversational as well as the technical, process and outcome-orientated approaches that have come to dominate modern healthcare.

Delivering effective primary care is viewed both in the UK and internationally as fundamental to bringing about the transformational revolution in healthcare, which achieves the 'triple aim' of good population health, experience of care and per capita cost.[11] Primary care providers and those commissioning it, under the pressure of ever growing demands on their services, also feel they bear the brunt of the challenge. They are where the buck stops and are faced with an increasingly large pile of documents, demands from the government and policymakers, all urging them to choose from what feels a myriad of potential options in order to bring about 'The' ultimate solution which can be 'Bottled, distributed widely and sprinkled 'liberally'. And yet, postmodernist thinking offers insights to such challenges by reminding us that solutions that are likely to succeed tend to be local, context-specific or situated, limited and difficult to transplant to other areas or situations.

CONCLUSIONS

The authors believe that the world is made of multiple perspectives that enrich our lives, provide challenges and create space for opportunities to emerge. An appreciation of the arts and use of reflective writing can genuinely help individuals to connect with themselves and with those around them. Postmodernist thinking has profound implications for primary healthcare in terms of conversations between individuals, the nature of leadership and the dangers of looking for universal solutions out with local contexts.

REFERENCES

1. Kuhn, T. (1970). *The structure of scientific revolutions.* Chicago, IL: Chicago University Press.
2. Foucault, M. (1972). *The archeology of knowledge.* London: Routledge Press.
3. Best, S. and Kellner, D. (1997). *The postmodern turn.* New York: Guildford Press.
4. Picasso, P. (1937) Guernica, Oil on canvas, 349 × 776 cm., Reina Sofía National Museum, Madrid, Spain.© 2012 Estate of Pablo Picasso/Artists Rights Society (ARS), New York, NY. http://www.tate.org.uk/art/artworks/picasso-weeping-woman-t05010. Accessed 9 March 2016.
5. Hockney, D. (1982) Grand Canyon Looking North, photocollage, 114.3 x 252.7 cm. Royal Academy, London 21 January — 9 April 2012. http://www.hockneypictures.com/exhibitions/pace09/pace09_11.php. Accessed 9 March 2016.
6. Gayford, M. (2011. *A bigger message: Conversations with David Hockney.* London: Thames & Hudson. p. 27.
7. Lee, H. (1960. *To kill a mockingbird.* Michigan: Popular Library, University of Michigan.
8. Ahluwalia, S. and Launer, J. (2012). Training for complexity and professional judgement: Beyond communication skills plus evidence. *Education for Primary Care* 23(5): 317–319.
9. Tavabie, A. and Ahluwalia, S. (2016). *General practice specialty training: Making it happen.* Chapter 9. pp. 93–102. London: RCGP.
10. Carper, B.A. (1978). Fundamental patterns of knowing in nursing. *Advances in Nursing Science* 1(1): 13–24.
11. Stiefel, M. and Nolan, K. (2012). *A guide to measuring the triple aim: Population health, experience of care, and per capita cost.* IHI Innovation Series white paper. Cambridge, MA: Institute for Healthcare Improvement, (Available on www.IHI.org).

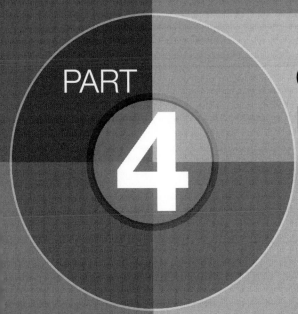

PART **4**

ON JUSTICE AND RESOURCES

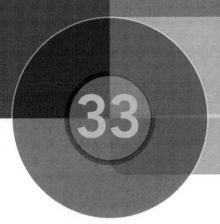

Beyond rationing: The ethics of commissioning in and by primary healthcare

33

DENNIS COX AND ANDREW PAPANIKITAS

INTRODUCTION

In any developed and integrated service healthcare service, and especially in state-funded healthcare services, there is a central process whereby services are planned, selected and funded: in a word – commissioned. In this chapter, we discuss the ethics of commissioning healthcare services. Commissioning for primary healthcare represents a particular interest in the English National Health Service (NHS). Since 2012, English general practitioners have been involved in commissioning healthcare – and we draw heavily on insights from ethical guidance developed for the British Royal College of General Practitioners by Oswald and Cox.[1] As with other chapters in this book, however, we hope that our discussion is of wider interest in jurisdictions beyond English primary healthcare, or even state-funded healthcare services. Any healthcare provider that purchases an array of services and is accountable in some way, whether to its users or its owners, 'commissions' those services. We will restrict ourselves to discussion of the ethics rather than law or national guidelines, though we acknowledge that the latter are often based on ethical principles.

Commissioning is often discussed as a form of resource allocation or rationing in a health-care system, catering to established need as well as possible using existing resources. It goes beyond a simple resource allocation process; it broadly involves four stages:

1. Identify the need (referred to as needs assessment)
2. Identify capacity to meet the need (referred to as tendering)
3. Delivery of service from that capacity (referred to as procurement)
4. Evaluation of the service (referred to as contract management). Evaluation should be linked to ways of improving or replacing a service that is inadequate.

The above definition matches that of the NHS in England: 'commissioning is the process of planning, agreeing and monitoring services'. Such a simple definition makes it difficult to disagree that health services funded from general taxation should be planned, agreed and monitored.

There is a major problem with the above definition, namely that in a realistic account of commissioning, resources are limited and therefore a rationing process is also required. There may be competing needs and corresponding capacities to meet the need. Therefore, however well resources are allocated, someone will be dissatisfied. The idea, that if healthcare services are commissioned very well and utilised in a scrupulous manner then rationing will not be necessary, is sometimes offered as a counterargument. Brody states that the two principal arguments for waste avoidance are: firstly, that we should not deprive any patient of useful medical services, even if they are expensive, as long as no money is being wasted on useless interventions, and secondly, that useless tests and treatments cause harm. Treatments that will not help patients cause complications. Similarly, diagnostic tests that will not help patients risk false positive results that may in turn lead to more tests and complications. Even if waste is eliminated, however, increased need (such as that caused by an ageing population) and increased capacity to meet the need (such as advances in healthcare technology) mean that this is a major but one-time saving.[2] We suggest that waste avoidance of this type is a duty for commissioners and healthcare professionals alike, but that, in the absence of unlimited resources, rationing is not quite so avoidable.

Rationing represents a major component of the ethical difficulties inherent in good commissioning. However, we suggest that rationing is only one albeit major aspect of the ethics of commissioning: Each stage of commissioning implies a set of ethical and philosophical issues that require attention. For the purpose of this chapter, we will discuss what a healthcare need is and what ought to count as healthcare, the tension between maximising good and respecting individuals and the ethical management of conflicts of interest. We will include duty to a defined patient or group of patients as a conflict. Finally, we will consider the role of patients in commissioning and resource allocation.

THE PHILOSOPHY AND ETHICS OF NEEDS ASSESSMENT AND TENDERING

Before comparing healthcare needs and services to meet those needs, commissioners must first have an understanding of what is a health need and what is properly considered a healthcare service. The philosophical questions that initially arise may not be ethical (to do with good and bad, right and wrong actions) but epistemological (questions about truth, knowledge and belief).

A surprising lack of thought is given to the idea that the question, 'What is good health?' depends upon the answer to the question, 'What is health?' In 1948, the World Health Organisation made the claim that health is a 'state of complete physical, mental and social wellbeing, and not merely the absence of disease or infirmity'.[3] By this definition, few if any might achieve 'health'. Philosophical accounts of health include those which relate to functional and statistical normality (implying that worse than normal is unhealthy and better than normal is enhanced), and those relating to human flourishing (whilst more holistic these can also be unhelpfully open-ended).[3,4] Regardless, a basic exploration of what we mean by health can be useful for commissioners and clinicians alike. An argument for this is that some healthcare interventions may restore physical function or correct a biochemical anomaly but do not contribute to meaningful health for a patient, whilst others might be arguably mutilating or physically harmful but enable better overall health.

There are a number of things that, arguably, contribute to good health, that are not within the remit of healthcare providers, and therefore are not paid out of money allocated for healthcare. These might include:

- Enforcement of legislation to reduce air pollution in cities and towns
- Traffic calming measures such as speed bumps to reduce road traffic accidents
- Long-term care to assist the elderly and chronically infirm with activities of daily living
- Health education in schools, advocating healthier lifestyles and the avoidance of risky behaviour.[5]

However, there are a few areas that are open to debate. This may be because of debate around whether they address a healthcare need (e.g. treatment of unexplained infertility), or where the theoretical rationale for the treatment or evidence regarding its efficacy is disputed (e.g. homeopathy and other alternative and complementary healthcare practices). A further area of debate concerns those areas of public spending that have an impact on the resources of others. For example, early discharge of frail patients from hospital may impact social welfare budgets, and inadequate social welfare provision may result in unnecessarily excessive or inappropriate episodes of healthcare.

SCENARIO: CONTINUING FUNDING FOR A CHARITABLE ORGANISATION WHICH OFFERS A REFUGE FOR BATTERED WOMEN (ADAPTED FROM OSWALD AND COX[1])

The commissioning organisation (CO) has been part-funding a local refuge for many years. The refuge is valued in the community and has been a spending commitment for successive health COs. Money is tight for the CO and they have to review all of their spending. Local government is providing 20% funding for the centre but cannot provide any additional funding.

All members of the CO recognise the importance of the centre, and the good done by the refuge, and that it ought to be funded for reasons of justice, given that it is vital to the interests of the vulnerable and disadvantaged group. Nevertheless, a majority of members on the board feel that such a service falls outside the scope of their healthcare commissioning responsibilities, and the CO's published aims (the most relevant of which is 'maximising health benefit through commissioned health services'). Some members voice their concern that without a refuge, the health of affected women and their children would suffer, and that lives would be put at risk. In order to give the centre the opportunity to find alternative sources of funding, the board agreed on an intention to maintain funding for the coming year, provide half of that funding for the following year and then to stop any further funding. However, given the potential impact of stopping funding, it was agreed that the chair would consult with the local health and well-being board before any decision was announced.

THE TENSION BETWEEN MAXIMISING GOOD AND RESPECTING THE FAIRNESS TO INDIVIDUALS

Oswald and Cox[1] suggest that there are two main approaches to resource allocation:

1. A utility-maximising rationale like quality-adjusted life years (QALYs), which can provide absolute but arguably unfair answers to the difficult questions arising in resource allocation
2. Fair processes such as 'Accountability for reasonableness', which propose no solutions other than processes by which policymakers can reach and justify their own conclusions.

In the 1980s and 1990s, economists elaborated the concept of quality-adjusted life years (QALYs) as a measure of the utility, expressed in healthy years of life, to be gained from healthcare.[6-8] A healthy year of life is worth 1.0 QALY, and a year of life at 70% of full health is worth 0.7 QALYs. At its simplest (and there are many variants, interpretations and applications), the QALY was proposed as a means to assess which healthcare treatments yield the greatest benefit, and thus how to allocate scarce resources. In the UK, QALYs have been, and still are, used by bodies such as the National Institute for Health and Clinical Excellence (NICE) to make resource allocation decisions on new medications and other technologies. NICE also deploys elements of the fair processes proposed by Daniels and Sabin.[9]

There have been many debates about QALYs.[10,11] One major criticism is that they systematically discriminate against the elderly and those with short life expectancy (who have less life and health to gain) and against disabled people (who have less health to gain). More generally, many philosophers reject approaches like QALYs that aim to maximise utility, and some have concluded that it is not possible to agree a fair and publicly acceptable rationale for allocating healthcare resources.[12] They argue that there is too much disagreement on the numerous ethical questions that arise when making such decisions. Indeed, the disagreement is not only on how to distribute resources fairly but also more fundamentally over what a healthcare system should aim to achieve.

Because of this lack of consensus, Daniels and Sabin propose that the only reliable guidance that can be given to policymakers is that they use fair, transparent and accountable processes to develop and justify their resource allocation decisions.[9] For Daniels and Sabin, legitimacy relies on fair processes for setting priorities in healthcare resource allocation. Their 'Accountability for reasonableness' framework provides four conditions that must be met by commissioners. These are as follows:

- *Publicity:* Rationing decisions made, and their rationale, must be made public.
- *Relevance:* The rationale on which decisions are made must be reasonable (i.e. based on evidence and relevant reasons), taking account of how the organisation provides value for money and meets varied healthcare needs.
- *Revision and appeals:* There must be a mechanism for individuals to challenge and dispute decisions, and for the organisation to learn and revise its policies.
- *Regulation:* There must be either external or self-imposed mechanisms for enforcing the first three conditions above.

A number of countries, including Norway, Denmark, New Zealand and Israel, have attempted to engage the public in explicit priority setting for healthcare. In general, these countries have favoured fair processes over utility-maximising approaches like QALYs.[1] The involvement of citizens in healthcare resource allocation is famously celebrated in the case of Oregon (USA).[13]

Fair processes are useful but commissioning bodies do require principles for morally consistent and hence 'fair' decision-making. Oswald and Cox suggest here two principles that commissioning bodies could consider of adopting.[1] The two principles are:

1. Every person's life has intrinsic value and is worthy of equal concern, and it matters how every life proceeds.
2. Each of us has a personal responsibility for the governance of our own life. This principle is not directly applicable to adults and children lacking the capacity to make autonomous decisions.

They choose these ethical principles for a number of reasons: Firstly, they can be used as a basis to address many of the fundamental ethical dilemmas that arise in commissioning. Secondly, they should be widely acceptable to, and consistent with the values of, the vast majority of citizens in Western democracies. They can unite people who might hold different belief systems, even though they have different reasons to accept it, and may disagree about when human life begins. Thirdly, the two principles are relatively simple, and easily understood. However, they dismiss the 'Four Principles' widely taught in medical education settings as being more relevant to clinical decision-making rather than rationing. A Four-Principles[14,15] approach, using a framework where beneficence (doing good), non-maleficence (not harming), respecting autonomy (in so far as one is able) and justice (treating equals equally and unequals unequally according to the morally relevant inequality) are treated as prima facie (ought to be followed unless they conflict with a more important expression of a principle), seems more nuanced. If one includes the concept of scope added by Gillon – the notion of to whom and to what extent the principles apply this arguably satisfies the same criteria for their use in decision-making.

CONFLICTS OF INTEREST

A conflict of interest can occur when an individual's ability to exercise judgement in one role is impaired by their obligation in another because of the existence of competing interest(s). Conflict may just as easily be generated by personal interest (e.g. if a commissioner has a vested financial interest in a provider of services) as by duty (e.g. if a commissioner perceives themselves to be under a strong study to someone – this could be to a particular patient population). Conflict of interest may be generated by conscientious objection to certain medical practices such as contraception and abortion services.

There is nothing inherently wrong in having conflicts of interest, and seeking to avoid or eliminate them entirely is unlikely to be possible or desirable for clinical commissioning groups. However, if they are not managed effectively, and commissioners are perceived to be misusing their powers, the consequences will be serious. It could undermine the confidence of providers and regulators in the probity and fairness of commissioning decisions, damage patients' confidence in the independence of healthcare professionals and ultimately destabilise public confidence in the system as a whole. In system where resources are inadequate to meet demands, it is even more important that the integrity of those decisions cannot be criticised.[13] According to Oswald and Cox, conflicts can be avoided and managed by:

- *Doing business properly*
  If clinical commissioning groups get their needs assessments, consultation mechanisms, commissioning strategies and procurement procedures right from the outset, then conflicts of interest become much easier to identify, avoid or deal with, and should withstand scrutiny.
- *Being proactive, not reactive*
  Substantial conflicts of interest can be avoided by being clear and transparent on what is acceptable before individuals are even elected or selected to be a commissioner; by inducting commissioners properly and ensuring they understand their obligations to declare conflicts of interest; and by agreeing in advance how a range of different situations and scenarios can be handled, rather than waiting until they arise. Conflicts of interest should be considered and declared not only on appointment but also before each decision-making meeting.
- *Assuming that individuals may not always be sensitive to conflicts of interest*
  Most individuals involved in commissioning will seek to do the right thing for the right reasons, but they may not always do it the right way due to lack of awareness of rules and procedures, insufficient information about a particular situation or lack of insight into the nature of the conflict. Rules should assume that people will volunteer information about

conflicts themselves and absent themselves from decision-making where they exist, but there should also be prompts and checks to reinforce this.

- *Being balanced and proportionate*

Rules should be clear and robust but not overly prescriptive and restrictive. Their intention should be to identify and manage conflicts of interest, not eliminate them, and their effect should be to protect and empower people by ensuring that decision-making is efficient as well as transparent and fair, but not constrain people by making it overly complex or slow.

SCENARIO: POTENTIAL CONFLICT OF INTEREST OVER NEW SERVICE TENDERING (ADAPTED FROM OSWALD AND COX[1])

Dr A is a member of a commissioning organisation (CO) and has a long-standing interest in and commitment to improving health and social care services for older people. She has worked closely with local geriatrician Dr B for many years, including working as her clinical assistant in the past. They have developed a number of service improvement initiatives together during this time and consider themselves to be good personal friends.

Recently, they have been working on a scheme to reduce unscheduled admissions to hospital from nursing homes. It involves Dr B visiting nursing homes and doing regular ward rounds together with community staff. It has been trialled and has had a measure of success which has been independently verified by a service evaluation. They would now like to extend the pilot, and the healthcare organisation that employs Dr B has suggested that a local tariff should be negotiated with the CO for this 'out-reach' service.

However, the CO has decided instead to run a tender for an integrated community support and admission avoidance scheme, with the specification to be informed by the outcomes of the pilot.

Due to her own involvement in the original pilot, association with the incumbent provider and allegiance to her friend and colleague, Dr A may be considered to have a conflict of interest when it comes to making decisions about the specification of this service and the award of the contract. She should probably not be involved in developing the tender, designing the criteria for selecting providers or in the final decision-making, even though she is a local expert. If the CO has clear prompts and guidelines for its members, this should be obvious to Dr A, who should decide to exempt herself, but may feel frustrated by this.

If the CO was clear at the outset about its commissioning priorities and strategy and its procurement framework (setting out what kind of services would be tendered under what circumstances), its decision to tender for the service should not have come as a surprise to the trust, or to the individuals involved.

COs will need to ensure that they do not discourage providers, or their own members, from being innovative and entrepreneurial by being inconsistent or opaque in their commissioning decisions and activities.

PUBLIC INVOLVEMENT IN HEALTHCARE COMMISSIONING

It has been suggested above that public involvement in priority setting for healthcare is a good thing. Those whose health is in question are, after all arguably, best placed to advise commissioners on their needs and whether healthcare provision is adequately matched to those needs. Moreover, there have been arguments that if people are rational and self-interested, they should create a society that looks after the neediest in it (provided that they do know what their own future holds – described as the 'Veil of ignorance' in a major work on political philosophy).[16] A 'patient-led' healthcare service implies giving the public a role in deciding where to put the resources in healthcare. This might involve seeking public opinion in the commissioning itself, or commissioning to allow the patient to choose from plurality of competing providers (e.g. through personal healthcare budgets). There are three problems with this approach that policymakers and practitioners should consider; patient choice does not solve the problem of rationing, how to advocate for (and protect from exploitation) those who cannot make effective choices and epistemological differences between commissioners and the general public about what constitutes healthcare.

Sheehan argues that, from the outset, patient choice and empowerment are irrelevant in decisions about scarce resources. He uses the following thought experiment: A baker has one loaf and three customers. Each customer has autonomously chosen to purchase a loaf of bread before they enter the bakery. In selling the loaf to any one of his customers, the baker would respect that customer's autonomy. His problem is precisely that he cannot respect all of their autonomous choices. He must decide which customer gets the loaf and which person's autonomy he should respect. He might sell the loaf to the first person into the shop, adopting a first come, first served principle of justice. He might divide the loaf into three so that everyone gets an equal but unsatisfying share. There are many more ways of approaching distributive justice here, each of which decides between autonomous choosers rather than respecting their choices. Resource allocation decisions in healthcare are necessarily decisions between patients, and so do not involve considerations of respect for patient choice.[17] Sheehan follows this argument to its logical conclusion and argues that clinicians are just as potentially conflicted, and therefore commissioners require a fair and clear rationale for decision-making (whoever is applying it). So, like the customers at Sheehan's bakery, someone will be unhappy. If local priorities mean that (for example) people in Oxford do not get a service that is provided in London, a dissatisfied person in Oxford might use a phrase like 'postcode lottery' to describe the unfairness of being denied something that he needs because of where he lives.

Commissioners need to consider how public that public involvement ought to take place, lest the commissioning agenda be dominated by one powerful lobby group, or more local decisions determined by the loudest and most articulate people rather than the neediest. There is a literature that argues that the poorest and neediest in the society are the least able to access healthcare, described by Tudor-Hart as the inverse care law.[18,19] When offering choice at the interface between healthcare and patient, Owens, Heath and others talk of patients abandoned to their autonomy by consumer model of patient autonomy.[4,20,21]

SCENARIO: WHEN TO LISTEN TO ACTIVE PRESSURE GROUP (ADAPTED FROM OSWALD AND COX[1])

The local Parkinson's disease group is very active and attends every board meeting asking questions about Parkinson's. They believe that the disease is inadequately managed in the area. It is not a priority mentioned in any of the commissioning organisation's policy documents. There is pressure to increase provision, with the local leader of the town council starting to ask questions via the local newspapers prompted by the local interest group. Furthermore, the Parkinson's group proposes to pump-prime investment by providing a nursing team free of charge for 2 years on the understanding that the funding will continue from the local healthcare organisation.

In drawing up the relevant policy document, the commissioners had spelt out their aims of maximising good subject to fairness, and their underlying ethical principles. They used these as explicit criteria when assessing and establishing the priorities for spending in the Joint Strategic Needs Assessment. As a result, the board feels that sufferers from Parkinson's disease were treated fairly in the needs assessment relative to other groups. For these reasons, they are reluctant to make any promises about increased funding when the pump priming expires in 2 years. Members were also concerned about whether a nursing team funded by the charity would blend in as part of the team and whether or not they would be prepared to follow guidelines developed by the commissioners. The board decides against any additional funding at this stage, but to investigate further the claims that local standards of provision are sub-standard. Given the level of local pressure and media attention, the chair of the commissioning group asks for a meeting to be set up with the town council leader and a representative from the Parkinson's disease charity in order to fully understand their concerns. It is agreed that after that meeting, the board will consider making a press release.

The third problem is a more fundamental one that has already been visited twice in this chapter, that policymakers, clinicians and the public may disagree over what is health and what is healthcare.[4,22] Disagreements are epistemic differences rather than ethical ones. Rogers illustrated this using a Scottish child health programme. The programme included a community participation initiative including a series of public meetings to inquire what extra services might be provided. One of the services requested was baby massage. However, at the time, there was no research evidence to support this as effective in improving health. Given resources were limited, officials decided not to provide the service based on their belief it would not work.[22,23]

CONCLUSION

The core argument for primary healthcare workers' involvement in healthcare commissioning relies on the healthcare worker having a holistic approach to patients, their families, communities and public health. However, the exploration of the inherent ethical issues in commissioning is relevant to all commissioners of healthcare. Commissioners of healthcare must consider not just the ethical sources of disagreement inherent in such decisions, but also the epistemic. Epistemic concerns such as what is health and who counts as a person are about 'what is?', and, 'how ought we to act?' may well follow from them.

Principles for ethical decision making are not unproblematic. Oswald and Cox acknowledge the problems and sources of disagreement implicit in their two principles of every person having intrinsic value, and the principle of everyone having responsibility for their own health. Similarly, the four principles plus scope approach do not provide immediate answers but a method of seeing the morally relevant concerns. It is not the principles that are balanced against one another but the issues that they uncover.

It is a well-rehearsed position that commissioning and resource allocation decisions ought to be ethically 'sound'.[14] They ought to withstand public scrutiny, and those without justification re-examined and possibly excluded – for worked examples, we recommend reading Oswald and Cox's guidance for British GP commissioners.[1] Commissioning is about resource allocation and therefore about justice, advocacy and waste avoidance. It is also about respecting the personhood of those whom it claims to serve – we have raised some of the issues inherent in public participation. However, when considering the stages of commissioning, we find that it is also about conflicts and confluences of interest, fostering the flourishing of practitioners as well as patients (the two are codependent). A consideration of all of the ethical and philosophical theories, and empirical evidence of patient and practitioner behaviours, is beyond the scope of this chapter. However, we hope that the reader takes away an introductory understanding of commissioning as more than rationing, and the complexity inherent in both. Moreover, that, though this may make decision-making harder, it also makes it better.

REFERENCES

1. Oswald M, Cox D. Making difficult choices: Ethical commissioning guidance to general practitioners. In: *RCGP*, editor. London: Royal College of General Practitioners; 2011.
2. Brody H. From an ethics of rationing to an ethics of waste avoidance. *The New England Journal of Medicine* 2012; **366**(21): 1949–51.
3. Misselbrook D. Aristotle, Hume and the goals of medicine. *Journal of Evaluation in Clinical Practice* 2016; **22**(4): 544–9.

4. Owens J. Creating a patient-led NHS: Some ethical and epistemological challenges. *London Journal of Primary Care (Abingdon)* 2012; **4**(2): 138–43.

5. Papanikitas A. *Medical ethics and sociology.* 2nd ed. Edinburgh: Elsevier/Mosby; 2013.

6. Williams A. The value of QALYs. *Health and Social Service Journal* 1985; **18**: 3–5.

7. Williams A. QALYS and ethics: A health economist's perspective. *Social Science & Medicine* 1996; **43**(12): 1795–804.

8. Brock DW. Quality of life measures in health care and medical ethics. *The Quality of Life* 1993; **1**: 95–133.

9. Daniels N, Sabin JE. Accountability for reasonableness: An update. *BMJ* 2008; **337**: a1850.

10. Mooney G. QALYs: Are they enough? A health economist's perspective. *Journal of Medical Ethics* 1989; **15**(3): 148–52.

11. Cubbon J. Unprincipled QALYs: A response to Harris. *Journal of Medical Ethics* 1992; **18**(2): 100.

12. Holm S. The second phase of priority setting. Goodbye to the simple solutions: The second phase of priority setting in health care. *BMJ* 1998; **317**(7164): 1000–2.

13. Spicer J. Oregon and the UK: Experiments in resource allocation. *London Journal of Primary Care (Abingdon)* 2010; **3**(2): 105–8.

14. Gillon R. Medical ethics: Four principles plus attention to scope. *BMJ* 1994; **309**(6948): 184–8.

15. Beauchamp TL, Childress JF. *Principles of biomedical ethics.* 6th ed. Oxford: Oxford University Press; 2009.

16. Rawls J. *A theory of justice.* Original ed. Cambridge, MA: Belknap Press of Harvard University Press; 1971.

17. Sheehan M. It's unethical for general practitioners to be commissioners. *BMJ* 2011; **342**: d1430.

18. Hart JT. The inverse care law. *Lancet* 1971; **1**(7696): 405–12.

19. Tudor Hart J. Commentary: Three decades of the inverse care law. *BMJ* 2000; **320**(7226): 18–9.

20. Heath I. A wolf in sheep's clothing: A critical look at the ethics of drug taking. *BMJ* 2003; **327**(7419): 856–8.

21. Emanuel EJ, Emanuel LL. Four models of the physician-patient relationship. *JAMA* 1992; **267**(16): 2221–6.

22. Braunack-Mayer A. The ethics of primary health care. In: Ashcroft R, Draper H, Dawson A, McMillan J, eds. *Principles of healthcare ethics.* 2nd ed. London: Wiley; 2007: 357–64.

23. Rogers WA. Feminism and public health ethics. *Journal of Medical Ethics* 2006; **32**(6): 351–4.

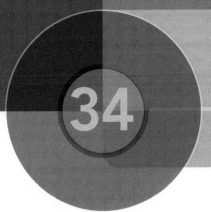

The moral atom: Mapping out the relational world of healthcare professionals

34

IOANNA PSALTI

INTRODUCTION

People might universally regard health as a personal core value necessary to fulfil other values such as independence. Healthcare services are expected to be ethically driven and healthcare professionals to maximise the health of the patients. Reformations of the National Health Service (NHS) in England have however forced awareness that at system level, health is only one value among others, while increasing healthcare marketisation has challenged ethical behaviour at personal level. In this chapter, multiple theoretical perspectives are brought together in a bricolage approach[1] to understand:

- The complexity of the relational world of the healthcare professional (social psychology concepts)
- How unethical behaviour and decision-making can appear (behavioural ethics)
- The emerging ethical challenges in healthcare, whether moral dilemmas or moral distress (organisational, relational and differential ethics).

The moral atom of a healthcare professional is the basic unit of the moral ecosystem of healthcare presented in the related chapter infra. The moral atom maps out the relational world of healthcare professionals and it aspires to inform change management, for example, at times of changing expectations from one's role as part of a greater ecosystem (e.g. gatekeepers to specialist care and resource allocation) or when managing dualities in personal development (clinician vs. entrepreneur businessman, whether in a private or a public healthcare system, partnership to a GP practice, network or hospital). The moral atom points to the benefits of the integrated care ethics framework which brings together learning from relational and differential thinking, and descriptive (behavioural ethics), prescriptive (health economics) and normative approaches (clinical and business ethics). This expanded framework does not separate clinical decisions and business management. Instead, it suggests that one may inform the other.

THE MORAL ATOM

The English NHS reforms of 2012 have changed the practice of medicine: the patient–physician relationship is now in interaction with the employer organisation, community, state and resources and placed in a competitive market (competitors, investors), with pressure from regulatory bodies to deliver quality and health outcomes. The moral atom for a healthcare professional is defined here as a network of relationships between the individual and other entities (people, social groups, organisations, institutions, etc.), which are morally significant for the individual to be in moral and emotional equilibrium. These relationships encompass those imposed by the professional environment of the individual working in a health service (as defined elsewhere in this book) with additional relationships prescribed by the social identity of the specific individual (cultural, spiritual, ethnic, etc.).

The moral atom is analogous to the social atom[2] of social psychology developed by J.L. Moreno who postulated that the smallest social structure in a community – 'the nucleus of relations' – cannot be less than two persons, and as a result we can only be understood within our personal/social context.[3] In parallel, the healing process can only exist within a personal or social context, as a relation between the patient and the healthcare professional bound by a moral contract 'to do no harm'. The moral atom is the 'nucleus of the healing relation' and despite it being influenced by the system surrounding it, it preserves one's agency as it allows for personal choices in some spheres. The moral atom demands attentiveness and responsiveness to multiple commitments at multiple levels, individual, institutional, organisational and collective, and it helps in visualising how changes in responsibilities may challenge core professional and personal values at the individual level.

Figure 34.1 shows the changes in size, complexity, structure and social goals of the moral atom for a healthcare professional in relation with time. Relationships arising from other aspects of the social identity of the individual such as ethnicity, gender, etc are neither discussed nor shown graphically for the sake of simplicity. Prior to 1948, the personal responsibilities of a healthcare professional were to the patient as payer, to the regulator and to one's self as owner of a private practice, that is, financial and other self-care (Figure 34.1a). The NHS formation installed the state as public payer for the health services (Figure 34.1b), with a tremendous expansion to the moral atom after 1990 (Figure 34.1c) as the health service gradually moved away from the GP's own home, a setting with a single moral position and low uncertainty and risk at business level. The practice of medicine was placed under new regulatory and audit bodies (QOF, Monitor, Competition and Markets Authority, etc.), with added obligations to community and environment (population health outcomes, resource allocation) and to larger provider organisations (organisational performance, sustainability of business). The risk has effectively been relocated from the state on to the individuals and the organisations they work for, with the need to assess and manage uncertainty at all levels – individual, organisational, institutional and collective (societal and environmental). Conflictual organisational and clinical obligations became inherent to one's multi-role in the healthcare ecosystem, particularly as advocate of patient and gatekeeper within a social context (resource allocation). Cases of burn-out linked to moral and emotional distress as a result of such conflictual obligations may benefit from a holistic approach to ethical behaviour that integrates awareness of the multilevel uncertainty, with improved capacity for self-care, moral resilience and moral courage at the individual level.

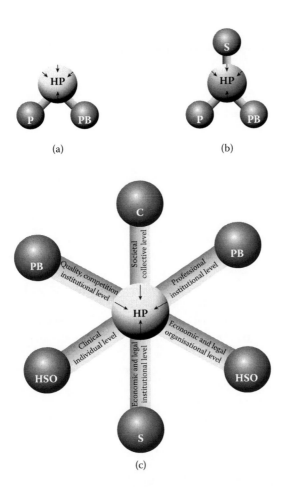

Figure 34.1 The moral atom for a healthcare professional (HP) in terms of personal responsibility towards Patients (P), professional training and accrediting bodies (PB), other regulatory bodies (RB), the Health Service Organisation (HSO) within which they work, the Community (C) and State (S) within which their HSO operate. → denotes responsibility to one's self: (a) pre-1948, (b) 1948–1990, and (c) 1990 to today.

RETHINKING THE ETHICAL FRAMEWORK

The moral atom model as depicted in Figure 34.1 highlights that any personal action in the healing process is explicitly situated in an array of professional responsibilities towards other stakeholders within the community (and the natural environment). Framing the provider–patient relationship as part of a greater and highly differentiated environment (patients, healthcare professionals, administrators, industry, etc.) highlights the art of healing as a relational activity made possible because of where it takes place and highlights the need to create a collective moral agreement from the perspectives of all stakeholders (clinical, managerial, patients, etc.) and the diversity of moral viewpoints arising from the diversity in socioeconomic status. Market mechanisms and healthcare reforms (integrated care, the new primary care models) increase the population of the moral atom as shown in Figure 34.1c and bring in obligations to the collective face-to-face with obligations to the individual.

The appeal to community as a norm is significant. It demands expansion of the traditional definition of ethics from the moral duty and obligation at individual level to the ethics of community centring the communal over the individual as the primary locus of moral agency analogous to that reported for education.[4] The moral responsibility of providers becomes the engagement in communal processes as they pursue the moral purposes of their work and address the ongoing challenges of daily life and work in their specific community settings (individual practice, hospitals, healthcare networks, etc.). The ethics of community supports the concept of distributive justice to inform decisions in priority setting and fair resource allocation, achieving equity and highlighting the need to reinterpret the ground principles that inform traditional clinical ethics in order to address the new locus of moral agency in: (1) market conditions where market success depends on whether providers can choose to compete (competitor autonomy and choice), all providers can compete (universality) at equal terms (fairness and justice) and with no adverse impact to population health (beneficence and maleficence) and (2) community settings where the delivering of services is expected to be in best interest of society to improve population health outcomes and prevent harm by tackling unnecessary interventions (overdiagnosis, overscreening and overtreatment). With the exception of autonomy, perhaps meaningful only at individual level, beneficence and non-maleficence apply with focal variations. More specifically, beneficence in trust, with locus the business, applies in the manager's obligation to see all parties in a commercial endeavour prosper on the basis of created value with the differential diagnosis criteria to balance the interests of business, patients and community. This is similar to the beneficence in trust, with the focus on community as the moral atom operates under an unwritten covenant between physician, patient, organisation and community based on the needs of patient, community and health service organisation, the physician's expertise and on mutual trust and communication.

Healthcare delivery has changed greatly since 1948, demanding an expansion in the role of ethical education beyond the ethics needed for the practice of medicine and into moral mentoring in an everlasting evolution of the greater ecosystem. Integrated care is shared care between clinical, organisational and institutional settings, each setting having a plurality of moral positions with high uncertainty both in technical and in moral terms. The new skill-mix at healthcare delivery (care team) and at commissioning level (CCGs) includes GPs, hospital doctors, nurses and pharmacists. Obligations and potential conflicts may be addressed differently by different healthcare professionals at emotional and practical level. Emerging new power differentials further increase uncertainty and risk in the system as the hierarchy of knowledge and roles in decision-making are challenged, whereas expectations and norms in professional attitudes and behaviour have to be redefined before the highly differentiated teams are able to deliver. For example, what is appropriate as health outcome or resource allocation? How can one inform and evaluate appropriateness (in behaviour, metrics, etc.) arising in multidisciplinary teams of the new primary care models? The degree of satisfaction with either resource allocation or outcome or performance depends on whose definition and expectation it fits,[5] clinicians, researchers, ethicists, politicians or patients themselves. Managing the dynamics of an enlarged and differentiated care team may demand additional exploration at personal level on how power is defined, amplified and misused (whether under- or overused) in all the relevant contexts (medical employee–patient, employee–manager or employee–community), what responsibilities are assigned to the power role and how one can carry out ethical monitoring of such new power differentials. It is the perspective of relational responsibility rather than autonomy that is important in a marketised healthcare as is the acceptance of shared risk and vulnerability, engagement in a highly differentiated system and emerging new risks such as business sustainability under competition.

Bridging the gulf between morals and the hard nature of business demands a framework that is pragmatic regarding the challenges to be addressed, relevant to the contemporary healthcare ecosystem and acceptable by the plurality in moral viewpoints and moral expectations. Normative or prescriptive frameworks are limited because:

- They concentrate on the individual instead of one's place in a system. Clinical ethics around autonomy or beneficence focus on the 'value-producing' stage of the care process and the responsibility for patient–physician relationship, ignoring the total system. Business ethics focuses on evaluating the moral acceptability of the actions of management and employees instead of the responsibility in designing processes ethically.
- Singular moral orders have legitimacy issues for decisions at organisational or collective level in morally pluralistic workplaces and marketplaces. An ethical behaviour informed by values defined by the experience and expectations of a particular professional group or sector may be perceived as the oppressive use of power of one professional group.
- Cognitive guidelines to manage ethical lapses assume that moral dilemmas are interpreted in a conscious manner and morality is a stable personality trait that can be developed. The principal–agent models[6] of business ethics assume individual self-interest, and possibly even greed, suggesting that individual employees may put their own interests before those of the organisation or its shareholders[7] despite the regular occurrences of unethical behaviour with no self-interest at its core such as cases of gaming the system to benefit individuals in need.[8] Yet, research on morality, intuition and effect suggests that moral judgements and interpretations are the consequences of automatic and intuitive affective reactions rather than conscious reasoning processes, with anchoring values operating in the cognitive models of moral decision.[9]

Understanding the relationships and the cross-interactions in the healthcare ecosystem is essential in learning how one should work in relation to the clinical workplace, the marketplace, the community and the greater environment. In other words, how to do what is morally right for the patient, being socially responsible and without ruining one's career or organisation. A relational ethics approach[10] acknowledges the ethical significance of the interdependencies in the moral atom, understands both patient and healthcare professionals as embodied selves situated within families and communities, and underscores the need to address issues of power and vulnerability at both patient and healthcare professional levels. The fundamental nature of relational ethics is that ethical commitment, agency and responsibility for self and to the other arise out of concrete situations which invariably involve relations between two or more people and affect two or more people.[11] The responsibility vector is however bidirectional – if healthcare professionals have a duty to patients, employees, community, state, regulators, etc., then these social actors also have duties to healthcare professionals. Viewing the patient–provider relationship as one of human beings within a social context may also provide insight in cases of gaming with no self-interest at its core. 'Dr Robin Hood' occurrences remain acceptable, innocuous practice, as a result of implicit social cognition processes that fade the 'ethics' from an ethical dilemma (ethical fading).[12] On the one hand, the provider is propelled into action having perceived patients as being treated unfairly by the system and on the other hand, others fail to notice such acts as fraudulent, considering them as 'compassionate' not because they are morally uneducated, but because of the social context. The question is whether Robin Hood would still be upheld as a hero if he redistributed wealth taken from a noble leader who himself undertook philanthropic deeds, instead of from an unfair tyrant.

The moral basis for decisions can further be strengthened by differential consideration of actions and knowledge to evaluate appropriateness and ethical perspectives in an increasingly differential healthcare and differential society. Such differential approach, although important in fairly balancing the inherent trade-offs between satisfying immediate user needs and maintaining other system functions, must be supported by explicitly formulated values. Quantitative knowledge may be necessary regarding ecosystem responses to service use and their impact (local, regional, short- or long-term) within their specific socioeconomic, political and cultural settings (health economics). For example, in Norway, cost-effectiveness has a central role only alongside the health-loss criterion – the priority of an intervention increases with the expected lifetime health loss of the beneficiary in the absence of such intervention.[13] Prescriptive approaches are encountered in medicine under conditions of increasing uncertainty as in cases of clinical trials and oncology treatments where conflictual obligations to the patient care and medical progress[14] are resolved via moral evaluation that integrates scientific and technical evaluation into the diagnosing of moral facts (differential ethics).

Descriptive approaches such as behavioural ethics may also assist in better understanding one's own behaviour and increase awareness about other factors affecting our moral judgement such as the existence of a variety of ethical blind spots – implicit bias, temporal lens, failure to notice others' unethical behaviour[15]; how empathy and sympathy can change with shifting circumstances and can be ends to themselves, felt without giving rise to action; and that moral values (personal, organisational and communal) can be subverted by changes in their position in a hierarchy of values depending on external (e.g. political system) and internal (e.g. the time of one's life) conditions.[16] The latter becomes important if the moral basis of decisions at personal level is prescribed by a specific hierarchy of values. Any change to such hierarchy, as for example, at times of distress, may have an impact on the prosocial orientation (a combination of beliefs, attitudes and values that is associated with helpful actions[17]) and precipitate different decisions (and hence actions) of questionable morality.

The nature of contemporary healthcare demands ethics research focusing on finding empirically testable strategies to mitigate unethical behaviour in healthcare settings. Above all, it asks for an integrated care ethics framework.[18] The framework, currently under development, integrates the basic principles of clinical ethics with more descriptive approaches such as behavioural ethics and health economics as shown in Figure 34.2.[18] Above all, such framework

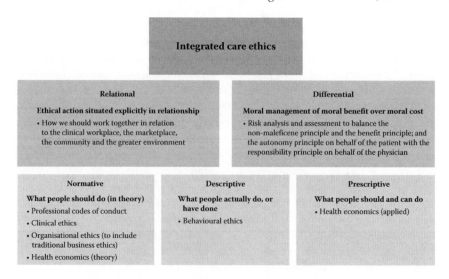

Figure 34.2 The integrated care ethics framework comprised relational and differential thinking integrated with normative, descriptive and prescriptive approaches.

addresses the demands of the marketisation of healthcare by bringing together relational thinking for the mutual acceptance of uncertainty and vulnerability and differential thinking for respect and responsibility for awareness of different value systems, for example, cultural perceptions about the patient–physician relationship, which may impact clinical decisions.

Only then can mutual trust be formed.

CONCLUSIONS

The complexity of the healthcare environment means that healthcare professionals need to learn how to live with uncertainty, not in it. Any healthcare reform will need 10–15 years before the changes it brings about can be managed effectively. Continuously in the media we hear about professional identity crisis of doctors, burn-out and career changes. If these are symptoms of unmanaged expectations from both career planning and working conditions, then responsibility falls on the training of healthcare professionals to support people during such a period, a type of bottom-up change management while turning out workers that are both resilient and responsible towards their patients and the community they serve.

REFERENCES

1. Kincheloe JL. Describing the Bricolage: Conceptualizing a New Rigor in Qualitative Research. *Qualitative Inquiry* 2001; 7(6): 679–692.

2. Remer R. Social Atom Theory Revisited. *International Journal of Action Methods* 2001; 54(2): 74.

3. Cukier R. *Words of Jacob Levi Moreno: A Glossary of the Terms Used by J. L. Moreno.* 2007, pp. 47–51.

4. Furman GC. The Ethic of Community. *Journal of Educational Administration* 2004; 42(2): 215–235.

5. Lolas F. Differential Ethics in Global Mental Health. *JAHR – European Journal of Bioethics* 2015; 6/2(12): 247–254.

6. Jensen MC, Meckling WH. Theory of the Firm: Managerial Behavior, Agency Costs and Ownership Structure. *Journal of Financial Economics* 1967; 3: 305–360.

7. De Cremer D, van Dick R, Tenbrunsel A, Pillutla M, Murnighan JK. Understanding Ethical Behavior and Decision Making in Management: A Behavioural Business Ethics Approach. *British Journal of Management* 2011; 22(1): 1–4.

8. Edge RS, Randall Groves J. (Eds.). *Ethics of Health Care: A Guide for Clinical Practice.* Florence, KY: Delmar Learning. 2005, pp. 125–126.

9. Brand CM, Oaksford M. The Effect of Probability Anchors on Moral Decision Making. Proceedings of the 37th Annual Meeting of the Cognitive Science Society, Cognitive Science Society; Pasadena, California, July 22–25, 2015, pp. 268–272.

10. Austin WJ. Relational ethics. *The Sage Encyclopedia of Qualitative Research Methods.* Given LM (Ed.). Thousand Oaks, CA: SAGE. 2008, pp. 748–749.

11. Bergum V, Dossetor J. *Relational Ethics. The Full Meaning of Respect.* Hagerstown, MD: University Publishing Group; 2005.

12. Tenbrunsel AE, Messick DM. Ethical Fading: The Role of Self-Deception in Unethical Behavior. *Social Justice Research* 2004; 17(2): 223–236.

13. Ottersen T, Førde R, Kakad M, Kjellevold A, Melberg HO, Moen A, Ringard Å, Norheim OF. A New Proposal for Priority Setting in Norway: Open and Fair. *Health Policy* 2016; 120(3): 246–251.

14. Sass HM. Ethical Considerations in Phase I Clinical Trials. *Onkologie* 1990; 13: 85–88.

15. Sezer O, Gino F, Bazerman MH. Ethical Blind Spots: Explaining Unintentional Unethical Behaviour. Special Issue on Morality and Ethics Gino F, Salvi S (eds). *Current Opinion in Psychology* 2015; 6: 77–81.

16. Gouveia VV, Vione KC, Milfont TL, Fischer R. Patterns of Value Change during the Life Span. Some Evidence from a Functional Approach to Values. *Personality and Social Psychology Bulletin* 2015; 41(9): 1276–1290.

17. Staub E. The Roots of Helping, Heroic Rescue and Resistance to and the Prevention of Mass Violence: Active by Standership in Extreme Times and in Building Peaceful Societies. In *The Oxford Handbook of Prosocial Behavior*. Schroeder DA, Graziano WG (Eds.). Oxford University Press; 2015, pp. 696–697.

18. Psalti I, Paschke M. *Integrated Care Ethics: Moral Action in a Changing Environment*. Manuscript in preparation. 2016.

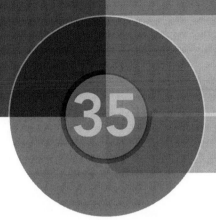

Moral ecosystems: Exploring the business dimension in healthcare reforms

35

IOANNA PSALTI AND MICHAEL PASCHKE

Healing is an art, medicine is a profession but healthcare is a business.[1]

INTRODUCTION

The serial transformation of the NHS in England since the 1990s has caused an ongoing debate around public service markets, with corporate business structures arising in the practice of medicine, and retail clinics appearing in large grocery stores next to fruits and vegetables. Whether such changes commodify or professionalise the commissioning and delivery of healthcare, the bottom line is that they remove the 'invisibility cloak' over the link between medicine and profit, long preserved largely by free access to health services. Old concerns around healing as a profitable activity re-emerge, particularly on the impact of executive boardrooms on clinical decisions at 'bedside' and on how to ensure ethical market stewardship.

The topic of healthcare as a profit sector has become particularly uncomfortable since the introduction of managed care – a controversial mix of 'medicine, workers' rights and business profits' – and the perpetual 'dying' and 'resurrection' of the purchaser–provider split (a mechanism that separates the formulation of policy from its delivery, aiming to create provider competition through contractual obligations and organisational separation from third-party payers). Such quasi-market arrangements in healthcare precipitate complex and often 'hidden' dynamics among a plethora of stakeholders, themselves not readily identifiable. In recognising the many types of scholarly endeavour that apply to healthcare business, we bring stakeholder theory from organisational management and business studies together with ecology concepts to explore the ethos of the health system. We propose the moral ecosystem as an exploratory tool for the intricacy of the healthcare system and the impact of health reforms, with particular reference to the delivery of health services. The model responds to policy and organisational contexts with the evolution of NHS England as case study.

THE MORAL ECOSYSTEM: RESPONSIBILITIES IN DESIGNING AND DELIVERING HEALTHCARE

Stakeholder theory has joined business, capitalism and ethics by placing business management into a fiduciary relationship with stakeholders and the business itself in terms of organisational sustainability. Business is viewed as a system creating value for all stakeholders – those entities (individuals and groups) who can 'affect or be affected by the realisation of a company's objectives',[2,3] with human beings being viewed as people rather than means to ends. Stakeholders are drawn from the socioeconomic and political environments within which the organisation is operating and they are differentiated into internal (elements within the organisation such as owners, employees, etc.) and external (parties which are not part of the organisation but can affect or be affected by its activities). Stakeholder theory is, therefore, distinctly different from shareholder theory, with emphasis on financial value and a focus of responsibility solely onto shareholders. Patients, doctors, professional associations, hospitals, government, industry, suppliers, etc. are all stakeholders in healthcare with a shared vision, health and well-being. They are bound to each other with a plethora of interactive relationships in a symbiotic and organic way, making up the healthcare ecosystem,[4–6,*] in an analogy to biological ecosystems. Such ecosystems are of different scales depending on the size of population coverage, for example, national healthcare systems, hospital chains and general practitioner (GP) networks, and of different types depending on the nature of the ecological relationships, that is, on what basis the stakeholders are connected. A moral ecosystem is defined by the set of moral links among the stakeholders, the sum of both accountability (regulatory or legal) and moral responsibility relationships as prescribed by the agreed goals of the specific system.

Figure 35.1 shows the simplest moral ecosystem of a health service provider and the dynamic web of dyadic moral links among its stakeholders. The provider can be an organisation (GP/dental practice, a polyclinic, hospital, clinic or pharmacy retailer) or a professional individual (GP, specialist, nurse, dentist or pharmacist) with single occupancy at the internal stakeholder level: a single individual holding the roles of owner, manager and employee and with no partners. The core external group comprises those stakeholders without whom healthcare activity would not be possible: patients, professional bodies that train/accredit/regulate professional conduct, payers and suppliers (products/services bought directly by the provider, e.g. consumables and diagnostic services). This system operates under public funding and in the absence of market mechanisms, for example, a GP practice in post-NHS formation era in the UK with services being free at the point of use, and physician–patient relationship being governed solely by the medical code of conduct of the General Medical Council. Prior to 1948, this moral ecosystem would be even simpler, with services being mainly funded by the patient.

The system design of the UK NHS created a peculiar, potentially vulnerable moral ecosystem with central planning of service delivery, public financing and ownership of production based on monopolies and dualities in roles:

- A state monopoly (and duality) in both the provision of hospital care (emergency and specialist care) and the training of doctors and nurses

---

* Since the 1960s, ecological concepts were introduced in healthcare to study the use of health services for future resource allocation and population-based healthcare research. The ecology model presented in this chapter arises as a result of healthcare reforms and should not be confused with the medical ecology model of 1960s healthcare developed for resource allocation and assessed use of primary, secondary and tertiary healthcare in public, private and mixed-finance systems on the basis of sociodemographic characteristics (population-based registers). The two models have different focus despite the commonalities between some of their concepts, for example, resource consideration.

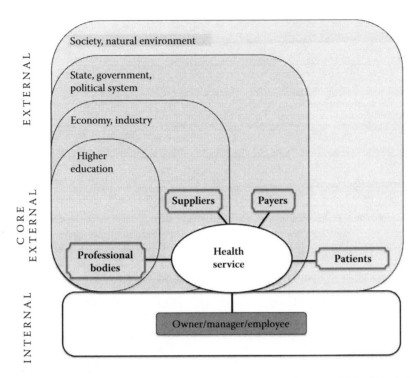

Figure 35.1 The moral ecosystem for a health service provider and the moral links (lines in bold) among stakeholders within a given socioeconomic and political operating environment and in the absence of market mechanisms.

- A monopoly employer (NHS)
- A general practice monopoly in primary care provision managing 99% of the UK population[7] under a public–private hybrid referral model and independent contractor status for GPs
- Duality in GP's role, as gatekeeper/coordinator to specialist care, and as owner of private enterprises organised around a profitable partnership model similar to law or accountancy firms.

Other aspects of the system design relied on public–private models such as the leasing of NHS buildings from the private sector under the Private Finance Initiative contracts, the importing of private patients to UK hospitals and exporting of health services to foreign markets under the National Health System Overseas Enterprise (NHSOE), supplementing income during funding decreases in 1988.[8]

Universal access to care has probably rendered any ethical concerns around the monopolies, and the business dimension at general practice or at hospital level, relatively unimportant. At least they have been largely taken for granted. The persistent aura of the Hippocratic oath ideals and historic restrictions at trade level, for example, on advertising[9] and the sale of goodwill[10]* in NHS practices (with professional ostracism or imprisonment for non-compliance), enhanced the 'self-image' of the medical occupation as a liberal profession, instead of paid agents of the state,[11] with absolute reliance on the professional codes of conduct for governance and immunity to 'greed' and 'self-interest'. The subtle 'occupational' and 'sector' stereotyping,

---

* Goodwill is the difference between the actual physical value of something and the price that somebody is prepared to pay for it. Its sale yields significant financial returns without selling the whole business.

typical among public as a result of psychosocial attribution process,[12–14] has been further fuelled by free access to services; healthcare became effortlessly the 'noble cause' sector, with doctors and nurses selflessly serving the community, in contrast to for-profit sectors being perceived as 'greedy' or 'immoral'.

Although not exactly a market, healthcare provision in the UK has therefore historically been linked to someone's profit. A series of health reforms, often referred to as marketisation or commoditisation of primary care, and facilitated by the increasing integration of digital solutions at clinical level, have recently begun to challenge perceptions as to whose profit it was and whose market it was becoming. Managed care, the NHS exercising its power as the dominant purchaser, and the growth in private providers including walk-in emergency treatment centres[15] are largely perceived as erosive of the traditional primary care system. Such changes have however been revolutionary in instilling responsibilities across all stakeholder groups: at patient level, such as self-managing chronic conditions, at clinical level, such as value consciousness in healthcare professionals for resource allocation and at government level, such as the provision of a fair competitive environment that does not harm patients.

POPULATION DIVERSITY IN THE MORAL ECOSYSTEM: THE IMPACT OF INTEGRATED CARE AND MARKET MECHANISMS

The moral ecosystem is a dynamic system, responsive and sensitive to changes such as the series of paradigm shifts in thinking about health across Europe in the early twenty-first century: from curing to wellness and prevention,[16] from treating single diseases to 'patient-' and 'population-oriented' care and coordinating services around people's needs.[17] Reforms of macroscale (national healthcare system) and microscale (individual healthcare settings, for example, GP practice and hospital) occurred at organisational, administrative and clinical level, focusing on primary care, chronic diseases and multimorbidity. Integrated care* rose as the strategy for improved health outcomes, quality of care and patient satisfaction.

In England, integrated care, a policy goal since the 1960s and a statutory duty since 2012,[18] introduced new primary care models with increasing reliance on market mechanisms (competition, decentralisation, patient choice) for their funding. The introduction of new system goals has changed the demographics in both the number of stakeholder groups and the 'spatial' distribution of a given group in terms of environments. This has precipitated a marked 'genetic' differentiation within and among stakeholder groups: that is to say, distinctly different groups within one environment. For example, there are now different public regulatory bodies for quality, price setting, etc., where payers span state and industry domains [being public, private (out-of-pocket), insurers or a mixture].

Figure 35.2 shows the unequivocal population diversity in the moral ecosystem of a health service as a result of the introduction of market mechanisms and the responsibility in resource allocation, as in the case of the NHS England with its overall policy and system goals being integrated care,[19] competition and patient choice. The obligations of a health service are defined by the system and the natural environment surrounding the patient–provider relation. Non-market approaches in Scotland, Wales and Northern Ireland will therefore prescribe ecosystems different to that shown here. A marked differentiation of the internal stakeholder group into owners, employees, managers and partners is precipitated by payment reforms such

---

* Integrated care is defined as the horizontal and vertical integration in healthcare delivery through dissolution of the historic institutional separation between primary, hospital and social care, whether commissioned or provided by local authorities.

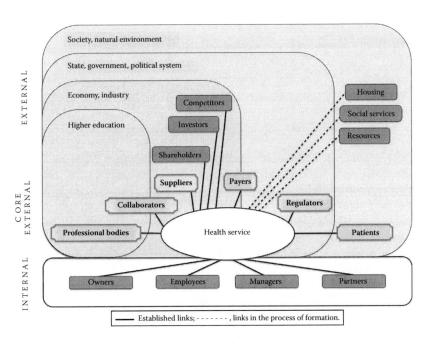

Figure 35.2 The moral ecosystem for a health service provider under market mechanisms.

as pay-for-performance and the increasing management of health by networks of care around the polyclinic concept[20,21] (co-location of a range of services in super-surgeries or federations). The core external group includes collaborators as a result of managed care and reorganisation of care around Vanguard schemes,[22] which integrated primary and acute care systems or multispecialty community providers. Public regulators of course have different mandates and they now include the Care Quality Commission, the Audit Commission (for financial governance), the Competition and Markets Authority (for anti-competitive behaviour of providers or commissioners) and NHS Improvement[23] to tighten the link between financial discipline and service quality.[24]

Investors, shareholders and competitors have been added to the external group by changes to the purchasing function[25] in the NHS, the formation of GP-led clinical commissioning groups (CCGs) and the removal of historic restrictions (on advertising ban, the sale of goodwill and boundaries of GP catchment areas). The latter in particular has allowed an increasing diversification in the production of health services, for example, the 'building of private health systems' by independent providers (private, non-profit, voluntary sectors). These may be in strategic locations near patients' homes like pharmacies or out-of-hours walk-in clinics in large grocery store chains of high visibility, traffic volumes and accessibility. Such provision of services includes social and primary care services of GP practices, urgent care centres and minor injury units, and although it is still funded by public contracts in England, it is similar to activities funded through the USA health insurance system such as the Henry Ford Health System[26] in southeast Michigan, with the Quick Care Clinic[27,*] as its most recent addition.

New moral links (Figure 35.2: dashed lines) are created, as financial and regulatory control of social services and housing sector devolves from the state to the primary care providers.

---

* This venture is modelled along the boutique retail blueprint, administered by a certified nurse practitioner targeting largely self-pay patients.

Consolidation of the reforms will 'rehouse' the new stakeholder groups into the core external group, with the state retaining partial control in the periphery of the system.

Being a service provider and a business precipitate an array of internal and external objectives for a provider: clinical (quality and health outcomes) and organisational (financial, profit and sustainability, service level, compliance performance). Given the social context of health provision, internal stakeholders need to think 'but is this right?'[28] for *all* stakeholders (internal and external) before undertaking actions individually or collectively for the realisation of *any* objective.

In reality, a provider's ecosystem is more complex than that shown in Figure 35.2. Stakeholders have their own subsystems with variations in scope and perceptions, for example, employees are differentiated into medical, nursing, technical, support and infrastructure. Changes in subsystems may affect ecosystem functions in countless scenarios, expanding the web of stakeholder interactions with cross-pair linkages appearing between the dyadic relations. Increased regulation and standards monitoring may result in withdrawal of some services by for-profit private providers, with detrimental impact on health equity. Rural areas are particularly vulnerable to this.

Private health insurance coverage through employment reaching a critical level may present the opportunity for withdrawal of state support, with consequent impact on patient choice. Single ownership of the entire supply chain through mergers and acquisitions, for example, a health insurance company owning the dominant provider in a geographic region, become crucial if the company has interests in the housing sector and owns *both* health and social services. Abuse of position can occur by restricting provider (preferred providers) or conditions covered for treatment or accepted for housing. Competition in attracting and retaining patients, staff, suppliers, etc. creates additional relationships and strain.

SUSTAINABILITY AND THE 'ETHOS' OF THE HEALTH SYSTEM

The corporate world has long recognised the importance of the link between sustainability and social/environmental responsibility in attracting and retaining customers.[29] Similarly, the sustainability of the greater ecosystem of healthcare (national or multistate health system) depends on the health system taking responsibility for the production of services and products which are effective, safe and accessible to all citizens. Social responsibility in improving equity and environmental responsibility in the use of resources will address over/under-diagnosis and over/under-treatment. These components of sustainability are in addition to compliance with governance measures and building capacity to balance turbulence, uncertainty, dependency and stability in stakeholder interactions (Figure 35.3).

The social and environmental responsibilities of healthcare, effectively the ethical dimensions of sustainability, constitute the ethos of healthcare. We interpret this as the guiding beliefs and goals of a health system in itself shaped as it is by agreed strategy and programmes in health. It also includes the behaviour of components in addition to the healthcare delivery system such as the healthcare industry (suppliers/manufacturers of healthcare products/technologies), Information and Communications Technology (ICT) services, research organisations, system planning bodies (whether market participants or government), trade unions and charities. The ethos of the health system demands proactivity and multi-directionality in stakeholder responsibility to one another: free access to care and citizen's responsibility in maintaining healthy lifestyles; community support of care settings and organisational responsibility for resources and health outcomes; responsibility in updating the training to equip healthcare

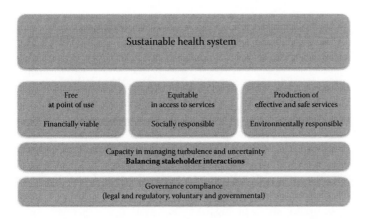

Figure 35.3 The components of sustainability in a health system.

professionals with changes in the marketplace. Perhaps above all lies providers' compliance with regulations, and provision of policies ethical in their mandate and scope.

The quasi-market character in the government-funded and new incarnation of NHS England is largely defined by patient choice and provider competition. Quasi-markets are planned with a third party (purchaser), allowing market entry to providers/products/services so that the purchaser and provider are distinct entities (in effect, a purchaser–provider split). Market success depends on moral design and moral monitoring of such technical aspects of market mechanisms (structures, incentives and their measures), with differentiation in the decision-making process that includes patients and healthcare professionals as stakeholders even for uncomfortable decisions. Currently, there is little reference to how the CCGs will ensure a fair competition among providers or the avoidance of perverse incentives that trigger gaming or distort clinical priorities.[30] Or, what happens with quality of care and competition in the absence of a market such as when there are dominant providers in rural areas.[31] Above all, how patient choice is framed and offered by the system, given that such key policy objective for the success of market competition is not influenced by service costs. Is payment by results really translated as 'money follows patients'[32] or do patients follow money because of how patient choice is framed? It should be recalled that removal of GP catchment areas brought 'consumer autonomy' as a remedy to earlier system failures to improve efficiency as with the independent sector treatment centres in 1990 in the UK.[33] Monitoring how patient choice is implemented instils morality in market design. Patient choice may be compromised when in-network alliances operate at referral level to support colleagues, or when collaborators or partners of the service (whether affiliated or independent) 'cream skim' undetected. Choosing patients for reasons other than their need for care can occur under fixed payment schemes (e.g. choosing less ill patients[34]) or when one's income and reputation are enhanced through research in a particular disease by imposing access restrictions to the general population.

Limitations in existing delivery infrastructure, for example, in case of a sole provider in rural area, automatically restrict patient choice, unless patients are willing to travel elsewhere. The emergence of new providers, although enhancing competition, runs opposite to the quasi-market goal of maximising efficiency. There is a lack of clarity in incentives for purchasers to compare available services, particularly as it is difficult to assess providers both in terms of value for money and the effectiveness of interventions in everyday clinical settings, in the absence of evidence. Not only political will and commitment are essential if low performing providers are either to improve or disappear under competition, but also emerging evidence has shown that improved outcomes are more likely associated with adopting organisational innovations rather than the introduction of market arrangements.[35] As a result, the rhetoric of quasi-markets launched as the means to improve quality and equity in health services in the 1990s may not match reality; quasi-markets appear to have brought a shift from improving equity and social justice to a maximisation of value for money and consumer choice instead.

Linking choice to competition and markets also ignores the complexity surrounding choice at patient level and the relational aspects between patient and provider. Figure 35.2 shows how such relation is not only around the patient's clinical needs but also socially embedded in a community with social, cultural and context-specific factors shaping patient views differently to the views of policymakers; after all, people are typically less concerned about provider choice and more about provider's proximity to home or retaining the public and universal aspects of their health system.[36] Drawing the patient into a pivotal role to merely increase competition within primary care for services also remains questionable, given the nature of healthcare as 'expert' or 'credence' service, similar to legal/financial advice or repair goods activities; the power differential governing the patient–physician relationship; and the information asymmetry at patient level.

External constraints such as policies at macro-level must be clear to prevent moral distress or confusion as a result of misinterpretations. Recent public procurement and competition rules[37] authorise anti-competitive behaviour in the commissioning of services by the NHS, if a qualitative cost-benefit analysis shows that it is in the (best) interest of healthcare users.[38] Such distortion of competition is open to abuse unintentionally, or intentionally, in the absence of clarification regarding what constitutes user's interests and how this will be agreed upon. The *Health and Social Care Act 2012* demands that almost all services must be competitively sourced and that commissioning groups treat providers in a non-discriminatory way, without favouring one over another on the basis of ownership. A 'sole provider' clause* is at odds with the commissioners' freedom to decide which services to tender[39] and becomes meaningless if transaction costs for tendering outweigh savings in service costs. Moreover, it can be used as a justification to avoid tendering, particularly in rural and remote areas with one provider as the only 'apparent' source of supply.

Other technical aspects cause further concern. Outsourced non-medical primary care services are business-to-business dealings (e.g. managing patient registration data or call/recall lists for screening). It is unclear whether service users are aware of such arrangements and whether such data are under the security required by the Information Governance Assurance Framework (IGAF) accreditation, as strictly speaking, these are not medical records. Such concerns become more important, given court rulings on company conduct in case of deviant behaviour: companies cannot commit a crime under the *Companies Act 2006* as they are not 'persons'.

Integrating the social care of vulnerable and underserved populations (older people, racial and ethnic minorities, low-income people, other marginalised groups) brings intergroup and intergenerational solidarity into the ethics discussion regarding resource allocation.[40] Can market mechanisms with an implicit pursuit for profit in healthcare be accepted as a means to an end? Such utilitarian moral basis for the marketisation of healthcare has to be examined regarding the type of solidarity (rational or constitutive) and the morality of the motivation argument ('authenticity' in motives).[41] We should ask: Is the extensive restructuring of NHS powered solely

---

* The clause states that there is no requirement to put contracts out to competitive tender 'where only a single provider is capable of providing the services'.

by the £20 billion target in efficiency savings or by an aspiration to evolve into an efficient, self-regulated organisation devoted to quality and value of patient care? Is patient empowerment a cost-saving means or true to commitment to put the citizen in the heart of the services? Such debates at the core of healthcare reformations are beyond the scope of this chapter but they influence what governance measures are needed and how healthcare professionals perceive their role in the marketisation of healthcare, in terms of both professional identity and personal integrity.

CONCLUSIONS

The introduction of quasi-markets in highly professional services becomes questionable due to imperfect competition and lack of markets. Responsibility for failure lies with the regulatory bodies in designing a genuinely achievable market structure and fair competition. Low demand for some services such as rare diseases, or low supply such as inadequate numbers of health professionals, can have an impact upon markets, as do incentives that influence how patient choice is applied in practice.

The moral ecosystem of healthcare system may throw light onto what system design and support can enable the 'Noble Cause' sector to become a 'Noble Business' and assist healthcare professionals to become objective advocates of their patients, contribute to an economical system and exercise self-care at the same time.

REFERENCES

1. Prescott JE. Chief academic officer at the Association of American Medical Colleges, as quoted in Adjusting, More M.D.'s Add M.B.A. *NY Times*. September 5, 2011.
2. Freeman RE. *Strategic Management: A Stakeholder Approach.* Boston, MA: Pitman; 1984.
3. Freeman RE, Wicks AC, Parmar B. Stakeholder theory and "the corporate objective revisited". *Organization Science* 2004; 15(3): 364–369.
4. White KL, Williams TF, Greenberg BG. The ecology of medical care. *New England Journal of Medicine* 1961; 265: 885–892.
5. White KL. The ecology of medical care: Origins and implications for population-based healthcare research. *Health Services Research* 1997; 32(1): 11–21.
6. Ferro A, Kristiansson PMD. Ecology of medical care in a publicly funded health care system: A registry study in Sweden. *Scandinavian Journal of Primary Health Care* 2011; 29(3): 187–192.
7. Royal College of General Practitioners. *The 2022 GP Compendium of Evidence*. RCGP; London, UK, 2013.
8. Rivett G. A guide to the NHS. Available from: www.nhshistory.net [Accessed 26 July 2016].
9. Irvine DH. The advertising of doctors' services. *Journal of Medical Ethics* 1991; 17: 35–40. doi: 10.1136/jme.17.1.35.
10. The New GMS Contract 2003: Investing in General Practice. Paragraph 7.21. p. 55. Available from: http://webarchive.nationalarchives.gov.uk/20130107105354/http:/www.dh.gov.uk/prod_consum_dh/groups/dh_digitalassets/@dh/@en/documents/digitalasset/dh_4071967.pdf [Accessed: 26 July 2016].
11. Barry J, Jones C (eds.). *Medicine and Charity before the Welfare State*. Taylor & Francis; London, 2003. p. 9.

12. Litvak PM, Lerner JS, Tiedens LZ, Shonk K. Fuel in the fire: How anger impacts judgment and decision-making. In: Potegal M, Stemmler G, Spielberger C (eds.), *International Handbook of Anger, Constituent and Concomitant Biological, Psychological, and Social Processes*. Springer; New York, 2010. pp. 287–310.

13. Weiner B. *Achievement Motivation and Attribution Theory*. Morristown, NJ: General Learning Press; 1974.

14. Chiarella M, McInnes E. Legality, morality and reality—The role of the nurse in maintaining standards of care. *Australian Journal of Advanced Nursing* 2008; 26(1): 77–83.

15. Midlands and Lancashire Commissioning Support Unit, NHS. *Urgent Care Models*. Available from: http://midlandsandlancashirecsu.nhs.uk/the-strategy-unit/publications/30-urgent-care-models-march-2015?path= [Accessed 26 July 2016].

16. Singh AR. Modern medicine: Towards prevention, cure, well-being and longevity. *Mens Sana Monographs* 2010; 8(1): 17–29.

17. Shortell S, Addicott R, Walsh N, Ham C. Accountable care organisations in the United States and England. Testing, evaluating and learning what works. Kings Fund; 2014. Available from: http://www.kingsfund.org.uk/sites/files/kf/field/field_publication_file/accountable-care-organisations-united-states-england-shortell-mar14.pdf [Accessed 26 July 2016].

18. Lewis RQ, Rosen R, Goodwin N, Dixon J. *Where next for integrated care organisations in the English NHS?* London: The Nuffield Trust; 2010.

19. Shaw S, Rosen R, Rumbold B. Perspectives shaping integrated care. In *An Overview of Integrated Care in the NHS What is Integrated Care*. Report. Nuffield Trust; London, 2011. p. 13.

20. Imison C, Naylor C, Maybin J. Under one roof: Will polyclinics deliver integrated care? King's Fund; 2008. Available from: https://www.kingsfund.org.uk/sites/files/kf/Under-One-Roof-polyclinics-deliver-integrated-care-Imison-Naylor-Maybin-Kings-Fund-June-2008.pdf [Accessed 26 July 2016].

21. NHS London. Healthcare for London: A framework for action. 2007. Available from: http://www.londonhp.nhs.uk/publications/a-framework-for-action/ [Accessed 26 July 2016].

22. *New Care Models: Vanguards—Developing a Blueprint for the Future of NHS and Care Services*. NHS; 2016. Available from: https://www.england.nhs.uk/wp-content/uploads/2015/11/new_care_models.pdf [Accessed 19 June 2016].

23. *What Do Leaders Want from NHS Improvement?* Nuffield Trust; 2015. Available from: http://www.nuffieldtrust.org.uk/node/4346 [Accessed 26 July 2016].

24. *Announcement on The Merger of Monitor and the Trust Development Authority*. Available from: http://www.ntda.nhs.uk [Accessed 26 July 2016].

25. Lewis R, Smith J, Harrison A. From quasi-market to market in the National Health Service in England: What does this mean for the purchasing of health services? *Journal of Health Services Research and Policy* 2009; 14(1): 44–51.

26. Henry Ford Health System, 2017. Available from: https://www.henryford.com/

27. QuickCare Clinic, 2017. Available from: http://www.henryford.com/body.cfm?id=61591

28. Pellegrino E. The medical profession as a moral community. *Bulletin of the New York Academy of Medicine* 1990; 66(3): 221–232.

29. Spiller R. Ethical business and investment: A model for business and society. *Journal of Business Ethics* 2000; 27(1–2): 149–160.

30. Mears A. Gaming and targets in the English NHS. *Universal Journal of Management* 2014; 2(7): 293–301.

31. Kähkönen L. Quasi-markets, competition and market failures in local government services. *Kommunal ekonomi och politik*. 2004; 8(3): 31–47.

32. Department of Health. A simple guide to payment by results. Gateway Ref: 18135. 2012. Available from: https://www.gov.uk/government/uploads/system/uploads/attachment_data/file/213150/PbR-Simple-Guide-FINAL.pdf [Accessed 27 July 2016].

33. Naylor C, Gregory S. Independent sector treatment centres. King's Fund; 2009. Available from http://www.kingsfund.org.uk/sites/files/kf/Briefing-Independent-sector-treatment-centres-ISTC-Chris-Naylor-Sarah-Gregory-Kings-Fund-October-2009.pdf [Accessed 26 July 2016].

34. Friesner DL, Rosenman R. Do hospitals practice cream skimming? *Health Services Management Research* 2009; 22(1): 39–49. doi: 10.1258/hsmr.2008.008003.

35. Tuulonen A, Kataja M, Syvänen U, Miettunen S, Uusitalo H. Right services to right patients at right time in right setting in Tays Eye Centre. *Acta Ophthalmologica* 2016; 94(7): 720–735. doi: 10.1111/aos.13168.

36. Fotaki M. What market-based patient choice can't do for the NHS: the theory and evidence of how choice works in health care. Centre for Health and the Public Interest; 2014. Available from: https://chpi.org.uk/wp-content/uploads/2014/03/What-market-based-patient-choice-cant-do-for-the-NHS-CHPI.pdf [Accessed 26 July 2016].

37. Explanatory Memorandum to the National Health Service (Procurement, Patient Choice and Competition) (No.2) Regulations 2013 No. 500. Available from: http://www.legislation.gov.uk/uksi/2013/500/contents/made [Accessed 26 July 2016].

38. Graells AS. New rules for health care procurement in the UK: A critical assessment from the perspective of EU economic law. *Public Procurement Law Review* 2015; 24: 16–30.

39. Hudson B. *Competition and Collaboration in the New NHS*. London: Centre for Health and the Public Interest; 2013.

40. Pavlokova K. Intergenerational solidarity of the public health care systems in Europe. *Acta VSFS* 2010; 4(1): 12–46.

41. Psalti I. Morality in the marketisation of healthcare and the authenticity dimension, London Journal of Primary Care, *In Press* (2017), Year, Volume, Pages to be assigned. To be accessible from http://www.tandfonline.com/loi/tlpc20

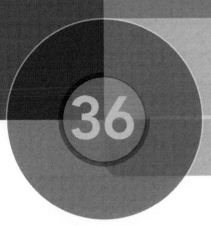

The duty of candour in primary care

36

SUZANNE SHALE

'Tis impossible to separate the chance of good from the risk of ill.'

David Hume
A Treatise of Human Nature

INTRODUCTION

This chapter is about voluntarily disclosing information to patients when something goes wrong in primary care. The professionals providing primary care [general practitioners (family physicians), district nurses, specialist nurses, podiatrists, physiotherapists, audiologists, paramedics and many others] encounter widely varying types of adverse events in very different contexts. I have selected examples that I hope will illustrate ethical dimensions of candour common to all.

Towards the end of the twentieth century, an ethical consensus began to emerge that clinicians owe a duty of candour to their patients. This means that patients should be told, without having to ask, when things go wrong in their care.

Why did it take so long for this consensus to emerge? The answer is probably that it was only in the latter part of the century that the health professionals began to discuss openly and study in depth what goes wrong in the course of healthcare. Even then, the focus has been on the dangers of hospital care. It has taken much longer to appreciate the risks to which patients are exposed in primary care.

It is commonly said that around 1 in 10 patients will experience unintended harm in hospital;[1-3] prevalence studies indicate that between 3% and 16% of hospitalised patients experience adverse events.[4] What about primary care? There is a paucity of studies, and so far the focus has been on patient safety in general practice (family physicians). It is now well recognised that understanding patient safety in primary care requires a different conceptual apparatus than that used for hospital medicine.[5] However, averaging across studies that use the most robust methods, it is estimated that some 1–2% of all family practice consultations in the United States and the UK may include some form of adverse event. For out-of-hours care, estimated error rates range from 2% to 6%. One Scottish study found that 11% of prescriptions written in primary care contained an error, whilst a record review of care home residents in England found one or more errors in 70% of residents' prescriptions. Missed or delayed diagnoses are known to constitute a source of significant harm and are probably under-represented in prevalence studies.[6,7]

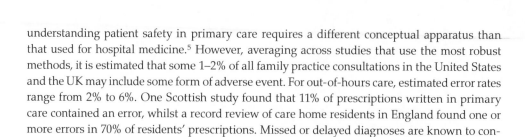

EXAMPLE 1

A patient who is a heavy smoker with a persistent cough is noted to have a suspicious lesion on a chest X-ray. The doctor asks administrative staff to arrange an urgent appointment with the patient. There is no answer on the patient's home telephone as he is on a holiday. The message to follow up is missed. Nine months later, the patient presents with shortness of breath and haemoptysis. He is admitted to hospital and diagnosed with lung cancer.

(Source: Care Quality Commission)[8]

Comment It is readily apparent in this case that mishaps have led to a delay in diagnosis, shortening the patients' likely lifespan. In England, this incident would trigger the statutory duty of candour.

Although severe harm may constitute a lower proportion of injuries in primary care than hospital care, cases of death and serious injury are of serious concern. In recent years, the Medical Defence Union has, for example, highlighted the high human and financial costs of failure to diagnose child brain tumours, meningitis and ovarian cancer.

WHY SHOULD PATIENTS OR FAMILIES BE TOLD WHEN THINGS GO WRONG DURING CARE?

The ethical consensus that now surrounds candour is relatively recent. A seminal paper on medical mistakes by Wu in 1991 mentions disclosure to patients almost as an afterthought.[9] At the beginning of the twenty-first century, authors still thought it necessary to outline the ethical arguments both for *and* against disclosure of harm to patients.[10,11] What has changed since these early articles are not the ethical arguments in favour of disclosure, but the institutional arrangements emerging in several countries that make it obligatory.[12]

Whenever an ethical practice is institutionalised, however, we run the risk of losing sight of why we do it. Disclosure can be an extremely demanding ethical practice, particularly when the harm is severe and emotions are running high. For this reason, it is important to be clear about the nature and scope of the ethical obligation that is being fulfilled.

GENERAL ETHICAL ARGUMENTS

Firstly, patients have a deep moral interest in what happens to their body. Candid disclosure of information, both before treatment and after it, respects this interest.

When patients are able to make autonomous choices, their moral interest in bodily integrity is promoted by respecting their decisions about what is done to them. This principle of respect for autonomy governs disclosure of information for the purposes of consent; when treatment and the risks that accompany, it must be properly explained. The same principle applies to disclosure of information about what has happened during any course of treatment. Patients and their families hold strong normative expectations that treatment effects, errors and untoward outcomes will be explained.[13–17]

Secondly, disclosing information about harm reflects the need for truthfulness in relationships with patients.

A duty-based or deontological ethical perspective views truth-telling as important for its own sake. The notion of candour, though, goes beyond simple truth-telling. Candour means volunteering information when a patient does not know enough to venture an inquiry. A narrow Kantian view would be that giving an untruthful answer to a direct question from a patient ('Have I been harmed?') would be absolutely wrong, but failing to volunteer information about harm might be morally acceptable. On the contrary, adopting the deontological reasoning of W.D. Ross[18], I would argue that prima facie duties of non-maleficence (doing no harm), fidelity (acting according to explicit and implied promises) and reparation (the duty to make up for wrongful acts done to others) taken together lead ineluctably to a duty of candid disclosure.

Looked at from a teleological perspective, honesty in medicine is important because it sustains trust between patients, professionals and organisations. One argument can be made from a broadly rule-utilitarian standpoint. People who need healthcare rely on the people who provide it. They have to be able to trust individual professionals, and trust the institutions that deliver care. Honesty is central to trust. Consistent openness and honesty directly benefits individual patients, and, through upholding trust in the institutions of medicine, indirectly benefits all current and future patients.

A critical importance of honesty can also be argued from a virtue ethical position. Practicing the virtue of truthfulness well, in appropriate circumstances, is a manifestation of the personal integrity of the clinician as well as a means of sustaining lasting relationships of trust with patients.[11]

Fourthly, a narrative ethical approach[19–22] points compellingly towards disclosing harm with care and compassion.

Patients and their families recount vividly the feelings of disorientation and destabilisation that follow in the wake of care going seriously wrong.[14,23–25] Following unexpected injury, they need to make sense of the unanticipated twist in their story. Ascribing some sort of meaning to events appears to be an important part of the process of recovery. This need to find meaning in misfortune is one reason patients and families insist on being reassured that the same kind of injury cannot happen again to someone else. The story of the past cannot be changed, but it can help shape the story of the future.

Finally, patient safety is a first priority for both deontological and teleological reasons.

'Being honest with patients and carers, providers of care are far more likely to be honest with themselves; and that is the foundation of a culture of improvement'.[26] Whether improvement is done to comply with the duty of non-maleficence, or whether it is done to maximise well-being, the only good thing that comes from healthcare harm is the lessons learnt from it.

PROFESSIONAL ETHICS, LEGAL AND INSTRUMENTAL REASONS FOR DISCLOSURE

Around the world, the ethical codes of many of the healthcare professions are now converging on a professional duty of candour. These professional ethical codes are accompanied by legal arrangements that vary widely between jurisdictions.[12] Although in common law jurisdictions, it may be possible to pursue a clinical negligence claim if a failure to disclose harm causes subsequent harm,[27] laws mandating candour in the wake of harm remain rare. However, several legal systems now provide some form of protection for apologies so that facts may be disclosed, and apologies offered, without automatically incurring liability for malpractice.[28]

England currently has some of the most stringent provisions of all for mandating disclosure. All care professionals in the UK are bound by an individual professional duty of candour. Their professional ethical codes were recently revised in order to reflect the statutory duty of disclosure that binds organisations in England. This statutory duty requires organisations to have systems in place to ensure harm is disclosed, and apologies offered.[29] The duty is enforced by regulators, and persistent breach may incur potential criminal liability by the organisation. There is also a contractual duty of candour, drawn in terms similar to the statutory duty, which binds any organisation that provides publicly funded care. The chief flaw in these apparently extensive and overlapping arrangements is that none of them can be legally enforced directly by patients. This leaves patients reliant upon others to hold professionals and organisations to account.

We have already identified ample reason to be candid. If any further argument is needed, there is some evidence that patients may be less likely to pursue malpractice claims against honest and empathetic clinicians who disclose and apologise when things go wrong.[30–32]

WHAT IS THERE A DUTY TO BE CANDID ABOUT?

Health professionals have a duty to be candid about both harm and error that leads to harm. Sometimes, things go wrong without error on the part of a practitioner: unavoidable falls, treatment side effects, unfortunate complications, and so on. In other times, things go wrong through error: misdiagnoses, prescribing errors, administrative failures and the like. The starting point for understanding obligations of candour is understanding that what is important for patients is receiving an explanation of what has happened, irrespective of whether the harm was caused by error or misfortune.

EXAMPLE 2

A patient had been taking warfarin for several years for stroke prevention from atrial fibrillation. His INR (coagulation rate) was stable and he attended a warfarin clinic monthly, at his GP's practice, for monitoring. He went to see his GP, complaining of a cough and shortness of breath, and was given antibiotics for chest infection. Ten days passed, during which his chest symptoms recovered. He then slipped at home and hit his leg, and developed an uncomfortable haematoma. When he attended the warfarin clinic for his regular check, his INR was found to be significantly outside of the desired range. It was likely that the antibiotic treatment had increased the anticoagulant effect of the patient's usual warfarin dose. The patient required vitamin K, and had to reattend the surgery every day for several days to recheck his INR value and modify his warfarin dose, until the INR value stabilised.

(Source: Care Quality Commission)[8]

Comment In this case, there was no obvious fault, but the patient experienced harm from a side effect of treatment. This incident would trigger the statutory duty of candour in England.

Fulfilling a duty of candour turns on health practitioners knowing that something has triggered the duty. The trigger may be a mistake (Example 3) or an untoward outcome (Example 4). In the case of a mistake, it is in the nature of mistakes that when we form the intention to act, we think we are doing the right thing. We do not think we are mistaken at that moment. Only after the action has been initiated do we find that it was mistaken,[33] possibly because we did not do the right thing, perhaps because we did the right thing in the wrong way. Medical care is a team activity, so that in some cases, it is only after care has been handed over to other professionals, and outcomes are known, that a mistake or harm is identified.

EXAMPLE 3

An ambulance crew attended a call for a patient who fell from scaffolding. On arrival, the patient was conscious but lying awkwardly, with a leg that was clearly fractured and twisted. Before carrying out a full assessment or immobilising the cervical spine, the crew repositioned the patient to straighten the leg. After repositioning, the patient was unable to move any of their limbs. At this stage, the spinal cord was immobilised. Later investigations identified that the patient had a cervical fracture and spinal cord damage. The patient was left with long-term paralysis from the neck down.

(Source: London Ambulance Service)[34]

Comment This was a tragic mistake thought to have been a right action at the time. Ambulance services face very different challenges from other primary care practitioners enacting their duty of disclosure. Crews often hand over responsibility to others soon after initiating treatment, and in many cases will only be able to comply with duties of disclosure if the subsequent provider advises them of the need to do so. Even if an error or harm is realised immediately, the midst of a medical emergency is not a propitious moment for open disclosure. Arrangements will have to be in place to ensure disclosure can take place at a later time. Moreover, ambulance crews rarely have any prior relationship with their patients unlike, say, district nurses. How the nature of the relationship affects disclosure has not yet been the subject of research.

Epistemic uncertainty, a constant in medical practice, makes complying with obligations of candour more complex.[35] It may not be apparent until sometime after events have occurred that harm has arisen. Even then, it may be difficult to discern that the initial error is the cause of the poor outcome.

EXAMPLE 4

A mother called her family practitioner, requesting a visit for her two-and-a-half-year-old son, who had a temperature of 41° with diarrhoea and vomiting. Later in the day, the mother called the practice again, telling the receptionist her child was 'floppy and lethargic'. A doctor visited the child at home. She noted that the child had been unwell for 24 hours and had a temperature of 39°. On examination, she found no abnormality, aside from a rash on the child's limbs, which she thought was not haemorrhagic. Some 5 hours after the doctor's visit, the parents took the boy to hospital where he was diagnosed with meningococcal septicaemia. He recovered, but unfortunately, both his feet and the tips of several fingers were amputated.

(Source: Medical Defence Union)[36]

Comment The issues in this case came to light 5 years after, when the parents sued on behalf of the child. Experts judged that delayed diagnosis had caused additional suffering; the family practice expert commented that where a child was described as unwell with a temperature of 39°, he would normally admit them to hospital. Because the child suffered an avoidable harm, such incidents ought to be disclosed. However, to comply with a duty of candour, the professionals involved in the case have to perceive that the duty applies. With hindsight, and knowing the outcome, others may judge that care was inappropriate when this is not apparent at the time.

IS THERE A DUTY TO BE CANDID ABOUT HARM IN THE PAST, AND ERROR BY OTHERS?

When it is a question of disclosure to the patients themselves, time having passed does not make any moral difference. All of the ethical arguments set out in the preceding section apply with equal weight when professionals discover harm that has occurred in the past (through clinical audit or record review for instance), or when they encounter mistakes made by other professionals. If disclosure would be made, on the facts known, to a patient injured in the

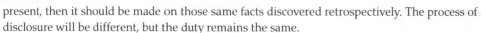
present, then it should be made on those same facts discovered retrospectively. The process of disclosure will be different, but the duty remains the same.

When a patient has died, is their survivors' moral interest in knowing about what has happened to their body analogous to the patient's own? Respondents in a UK study were uneasy about being open with bereaved relatives in cases where a patient had died some time before, when there may have been avoidable contributing factors, but the facts were unclear and likely to remain so.[35] Subject to the usual considerations of medical confidentiality, it could be argued that survivors with a very close emotional bond have a similar moral interest to the deceased in knowing what happened, which cannot be ignored even if time has passed and the facts are unclear. Those with significant financial dependency on the deceased may have their own legal interests to defend. This places them in a somewhat different position from survivors bound by purely formal ties of kinship, who had no emotional or social ties to the deceased.

It might thus be argued that disclosure should be made to those with a strong interest, but would be irrelevant to those with a weak interest. However, basing disclosure decisions on professionals' judgements about the nature of the bonds to survivors would be hard to justify; there is simply too much that professionals do not and cannot know about such bonds. (See also the discussion of therapeutic privilege, and of disclosure to bereaved parents, below.)

SHOULD PATIENTS ALWAYS BE TOLD WHEN THINGS GO WRONG?

There has been extensive debate about when it may be acceptable not to tell the whole truth in the realm of consent to treatment. In the context of consent, justifications have been offered *inter alia* for deceiving patients for research purposes, withholding information when patients decline it and for withholding information on the grounds of therapeutic privilege. There has as yet been little equivalent discussion of ethical justifications for withholding information about errors or harm where a presumption of openness otherwise prevails.

It is hard to envisage circumstances in which information about harm could legitimately be withheld for research purposes, but I do not underestimate the ingenuity of researchers. If there were thought to be good reason, it would have to be argued in the process of ethical review.

By analogy with reasoning on disclosure for consent purposes, there may be rare situations when a patient is offered, but reasonably declines, information about healthcare harm.

There may also be rare situations where a form of 'therapeutic privilege' could be invoked, on grounds that an emotionally fragile patient would suffer greater harm from candour than they would from concealment.[11] However, any claim of therapeutic privilege should be assessed with extreme caution. Firstly, there is an important difference between invoking therapeutic privilege in order to withhold information about diagnosis, prognosis and treatment, and invoking therapeutic privilege to withhold information about iatrogenic harm. The latter is arguably far more questionable, being susceptible both to self-serving justification on the part of the clinician and to patient and family suspicions of a cover-up. Secondly, the concept of therapeutic privilege has itself being called into question: a statement on therapeutic privilege issued by the American Medical Association, for example, averred that 'withholding medical information from patients without their knowledge or consent is ethically unacceptable'.[37]

Withholding information about iatrogenic harm would require an exceptionally strong justification. In principle, it would seem only to be acceptable in the short term (e.g. pending recovery) and only if other parties within the scope of confidentiality (family or other personal representatives for instance) were promptly informed.[16]

EXAMPLE 5

A 6-month-old baby has a treatable infection, but dies at home from septic shock following administrative errors by a telephone triage service and further delays in diagnosis. Her mother, a single parent, voices suicidal thoughts to several care professionals following the child's death. Shortly after the initial post-mortem, and in accordance with local procedures, a multi-agency case discussion is convened that includes all those involved in caring for the child. One of the aims of the meeting is to agree how information about the cause of death will be shared with her parents. Concerned about the mother's fragile emotional state and the well-being of her other children, the health visitor questions whether it will benefit her to explain the course of events and that the child's infection could successfully have been treated.

Comment Any parent whose child dies will experience unimaginable distress. But, does an elevated level of distress justify withholding information that the death was avoidable? In the United Kingdom, bereaved parents have been some of the most indomitable campaigners for openness following the death of children. In the UK, Will Powell, Josephine Ocloo, Clare Bowen, James Titcombe, Scott Morrish and Sara Ryan all fought tenacious battles to get the unvarnished truth about their child's death. It would appear that for bereaved parents, the psychological burden inflicted on them by concealing information about their child's death is significantly greater than the psychological burden suffered from knowing the truth at its worst. What is needed in these circumstances is not secrecy but thoughtful support.

WHAT SHOULD BE TOLD TO PEOPLE WITH IMPAIRED CAPACITY?

Turning to adult patients whose decisional capacity is impaired, fluctuating or non-existent, there has been scant discussion of their needs in the ethical literature. There are two questions to answer. Should other parties be told when an incapacitated patient has come to harm? Should patients who have partially impaired or fluctuating capacity be told about harm?

Whether other parties should be told is easily answered with reference to ethical principle (and varying legal provisions) for decision-making for incapacitated patients. Surrogate decision-makers (whether these are healthcare professionals, family members or other personal representatives) are standing in the shoes of the patient and must be informed. Those who are not surrogate decision-makers as such, but who hold legal rights to be consulted or informed about treatment decisions, must also be told. Thus, the view in England is that, consistent with the *Mental Capacity Act 2005*, the statutory duty of candour mandates disclosure to identify others if the patient lacks capacity.

In relation to patients with partially impaired capacity (e.g. people with learning disabilities), the issue is straightforward in principle, if not in practise: patients should be told what has happened to them, in ways that they are capable of understanding it, and given the support they need to come to terms with it. Notice that they must be told the truth *and also* supported, one of these alone will not do.

Where capacity fluctuates, disclosure would seem appropriate when capacity is present. However, the causes underlying patients' fluctuating capacity may generate difficult situations. For example, if the course of disease combined with opioid treatment is impairing capacity in a patient at end of life, the benefits of openness may appear to weigh less than the burdens of openness. The discussion of therapeutic privilege (above) suggests that in such a situation, information should be withheld only *in extremis*, and then, only withheld from the patient if other parties such as next of kin or personal representatives are informed.

WHAT AND HOW SHOULD CHILDREN BE TOLD?

This is a particularly pertinent question in the primary care context where children and young people may constitute a larger proportion of the overall patient population.

There is consensus among paediatricians that harm should be disclosed to the *parents* of immature minors.[38] This correlates with parents' own normative expectations of disclosure; one US survey of parents found near unanimity that all errors ought to be disclosed, regardless of severity.[39]

Disclosure to children, in particular older children, requires further consideration. National and local jurisdictions stipulate different ages at which young people are presumed to be competent to make their own treatment decisions. If the law presumes the young person is competent to decide (as it does in England at the age of 16), then they are competent for the purposes of disclosure too. However, many jurisdictions also provide for a developmental assessment of capacity so that children under the age of presumed capacity, who are capable of understanding the issues involved, are permitted to make their own treatment decisions. Where a child has been judged to have the maturity to make a treatment decision, does it follow that he or she has the maturity to cope with disclosure of harm? Most of the time the answer will be yes, particularly if parents have been involved in the treatment decision and the disclosure discussion.

However, assessment of capacity is generally decision-specific, so the degree of maturity required depends upon the treatment decision being made. Difficulties may arise if a child judged capable of consenting to minor treatment subsequently suffers major harm, difficulties compounded if they have been receiving treatment without the knowledge of their parents. These difficulties do not mandate against disclosure, but they are likely to make it a particularly complex task.

One interesting study of paediatricians' views on disclosure to children themselves supplied food for thought (but not normative guidance).[40] Virtually all thought it important to disclose to a child's parents, but fewer thought disclosure should be made to the child. Generally, they thought physicians and parents should decide together whether to disclose to the child, with many inclined to disclose to developmentally appropriate children over the age of about twelve. Unless the child asked them directly about what happened, most would defer to the parents' wishes if they were asked not to disclose.

WHAT SHOULD PATIENTS OR FAMILIES BE TOLD WHEN THINGS GO WRONG DURING CARE?

It would seem to be obvious that a duty of candour entails telling patients or their survivors everything that is relevant. This includes telling them, if an error was made, that an error was made. However, acknowledging error is the most challenging aspect of the duty of candour. Research reveals a 'disclosure gap': marked differences between what patients say they want from clinicians and what clinicians say they would provide. Patients and bereaved families consistently report wanting a full account of what happened that includes a statement of error if warranted, and wanting to hear what will be done to prevent a similar event in future. When clinicians' disclosure views have been studied, in the absence of mandatory disclosure laws, many would refer to harm without identifying error, provide details only if patients ask specific questions, infrequently volunteer an apology and rarely discuss the prevention of future errors.[15,16,41–43] This is why the statutory duty of candour in England has required not only candour but also an apology, and for the outcome of any investigation to be shared with the patient or their loved ones.

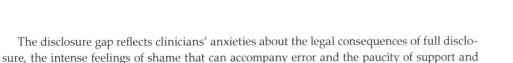

The disclosure gap reflects clinicians' anxieties about the legal consequences of full disclosure, the intense feelings of shame that can accompany error and the paucity of support and training for this difficult task.

CANDOUR AND APOLOGIES IN LAW

It has been widely recognised that the threat of legal proceedings inhibits open disclosure of error. For this reason, many jurisdictions have passed laws that protect apologies. Such laws generally stipulate that an apology cannot be treated as an admission of liability or be admitted to court as evidence of malpractice.[28,44]

Whilst protection of apologies is welcomed, it is not without difficulties. A 'partial' apology ('I'm truly sorry that this has happened') is a statement of sorrow or regret that does not include acceptance of responsibility. A 'full' apology, however, adds an explanation and acceptance of responsibility ('I'm truly sorry this happened. This is why it happened. This was our responsibility, and we let you down'.) What patients or their supporters want is full apologies.[45–47] The problem with apology protection laws is that whilst they invariably protect statements of regret, they do not always protect statements of responsibility. Health professionals therefore continue to feel exposed, and will do so until they receive unambiguous guidance on what they can say without exposing themselves to legal jeopardy.

The position in England is that apologies are protected by s.2 of the *Compensation Act 2006*. The offer of an apology as part of the duty of candour has been strongly supported by the NHS Litigation Authority (which in effect underwrites NHS organisations) and all of the medical insurance societies. The scope of the apology protected by the Compensation Act has not, however, been tested in court.

> ### EXAMPLE 6
>
> *An 86-year-old woman with a chesty cough and signs of a red and swollen leg was diagnosed with a chest infection, and discharged home from hospital. The community nurse agreed to visit, but due to high workload did not visit for 3 days. When she arrived, she found the woman had died. An autopsy confirmed the cause was pulmonary embolism. Clinical staff and managers from the hospital, together with managers from the community service, met the woman's daughters to explain the cause of death. The hospital doctor apologised specifically for the misdiagnosis, and the community service apologised for the delays in attendance by the district nurse.*
>
> *(Source: Nursing Times)[48]*

PSYCHOLOGICAL IMPEDIMENTS TO FULL DISCLOSURE

There is growing recognition of the psychological and social impact on clinical professionals involved in adverse events. (Wu introduced the term 'second victim' to describe this phenomenon.[49] It is catchy, but unfortunate. Patients and families view kin and other associates as the real 'second victims'; and it may not be helpful to label capable professionals, who often have strong coping skills, as 'victims'. I have therefore used clumsier but less contentious language such as 'involved professionals'.)

Whether adverse events were precipitated by misadventure or mistake, involved professionals experience intense emotions of guilt and shame, anxiety, anger and sadness. Feelings of guilt and shame are common whatever level of harm has occurred, whatever the healthcare profession and whatever the setting, whether primary or secondary care.[50–54]

Without appropriate education and support, guilt, shame, embarrassment and fear act as powerful impediments to compassionate disclosure of error.[55] Given how much is at stake for

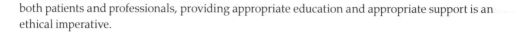

both patients and professionals, providing appropriate education and appropriate support is an ethical imperative.

WHAT'S THE BEST WAY OF TEACHING CANDOUR?

There has been very little research into educating clinicians in disclosure practice. However, study findings and practice wisdom suggest that communicating the presence of an *error* and *enacting* an appropriate apology are key challenges.[56] To be effective, educational programmes will have to confront the shame that accompanies an error, and foster the acceptance of responsibility that is the precondition for authentic enactment of an apology.

WHAT SUPPORT FOR CLINICIANS WORKS?

In a systematic review,[57] Seys found no consensus on what mechanisms are most effective. Many advocate some form of peer support which may include on-the-spot discussion ('disclosure coaching') with an experienced peer to prepare for the disclosure conversation. To support involved professionals in coming to terms with the impact of adverse events upon themselves, programmes commonly feature provision of confidential space for talking and listening, inquiring about colleague coping and facilitating open discussion of the error.

Among the most developed organisational systems is Scott's 'three-tier' approach to support[58] which moves through varying levels of severity. Tier one provides immediate reassurance, with support for open disclosure; tier two provides ongoing practical support; and tier three offers specialised emotional and therapeutic support. Each of these tiers draws upon the resources already available to large institutions.

CONCLUDING COMMENT

We often think of ethics as an attempt to answer the question: 'What ought I to do?' But as philosopher Margaret Walker points out 'One of our recurrent ethical tasks is better suggested by the question "What ought I – or better *we* – to do now?" after someone has blotted or torn the page by doing something wrong[59] [p. 6]'.

Disclosure is a critical part of the process that Walker and other philosophers describe as moral repair. Moral repair starts with acknowledgement that some wrong has been done, demands acknowledgement of the moral scope of the wrong and calls for acknowledgement of personal responsibility.[60] Compassionate disclosure is one of the first steps that must be taken after harm. It enables both professionals and patients to start the long process of reconstructing confidence in the system, rebuilding trust in professionals and professional competence and regaining hope for the future. Historically, medicine has been slow to rise to the challenge of repairing moral relationships after harm. It is difficult work but, for the good of all involved, it is a challenge that must now be met head on.

REFERENCES

1. Schimmel E. The hazards of hospitalisation. *Ann Intern Med.* 1964;60:100–10.
2. Steel K, Gertman P, Crescenzi C, Anderson J. Iatrogenic illness on a general medical service at a university hospital. *N Engl J Med.* 1981;304(11):638–42.

3. Brennan T, Leape L, Laird N, Hebert L, Localio A, Lawthers A, et al. Incidence of adverse events and negligence in hospitalized patients: Results of the Harvard Medical Practice Study. *N Engl J Med.* 1991;324(6):370–6.

4. Jha A, Prasopa-Plaizier N, Larizgoitia I, Bates D. Patient safety research: An overview of the global evidence. *Qual Saf Health Care.* 2010;19:42–4.

5. Daker-White G, Hays R, McSharry J, Giles S, Cheraghi-Sohi S, Rhodes P, et al. Blame the patient, blame the doctor or blame the system? A meta-synthesis of qualitative studies of patient safety in primary care. *PLoS One.* 2015;10(8):e0128329.

6. Houston N, Bowie P. The Scottish patient safety programme in primary care: Context, interventions and early outcomes. *Scott Med J.* 2015;60(4):192–5.

7. Anon. *Evidence Scan: Levels of Harm in Primary Care.* London: The Health Foundation; 2011.

8. Sparrow N. *Nigel's Surgery 32: Duty of Candour and General Practice: Care Quality Commission.* [updated 01 January 2016]. Available from: http://www.cqc.org.uk/guidance-providers/gp-services/nigels-surgery-32-duty-candour-general-practice-regulation-20 (accessed June 26, 2017).

9. Wu AW. Do house officers learn from their mistakes? *Qual Saf Health Care.* 2003;12(>3):221–6.

10. Wu A, Cavanaugh T, McPhee S, Lo B, Micco G. To tell the truth: Ethical and practical issues in disclosing medical mistakes to patients. *J Gen Intern Med.* 1997;12:770–5.

11. Smith ML, Forster HP. Morally managing medical mistakes. *Camb Q Healthc Ethics.* 2000;9(1):38–53.

12. Wu AW, McCay L, Levinson W, Iedema R, Wallace G, Boyle DJ, et al. Disclosing adverse events to patients: International norms and trends. *J Patient Saf.* 2017;13(1):43–49.

13. Iedema R, Sorensen R, Manias E, Tuckett A, Piper D, Mallock N, et al. Patients' and family members' experiences of open disclosure following adverse events. *Int J Qual Health Care.* 2008;20(6):421–32.

14. Iedema R, Allen S, Britton K, Piper D, Baker A, Grbich C, et al. Patients' and family members' views on how clinicians enact and how they should enact incident disclosure: The "100 patient stories" qualitative study. *BMJ.* 2011;343:d4423.

15. Levinson W. Disclosing medical errors to patients: A challenge for health care professionals and institutions. *Patient Educ Couns.* 2009;76(3):296–9.

16. Gallagher TH, Waterman AD, Ebers AG, Fraser VJ, Levinson W. Patients' and physicians' attitudes regarding the disclosure of medical errors. *JAMA.* 2003;289(8):1001–7.

17. Piper D, Iedema R, Bower K. Rural patients' experiences of the open disclosure of adverse events. *Aust J Rural Health.* 2014;22(4):197–203.

18. Ross WD, Stratton-Lake P. *The Right and the Good.* Oxford: Oxford University Press; 2002.

19. Charon R. Narrative contributions to medical ethics; Recognition, formulation, interpretation and validation in the practice of the ethicist. In: DuBose ER, Hamel RP, O'Connell LJ, editors. *A Matter of Principles? Ferment in US Bioethics.* Valley Forge, PA: Trinity Press International; 1994. pp. 260–83.

20. Murray TH. What do we mean by 'narrative ethics?' In: Lindemann Nelson H, editor. *Stories and their Limits: Narrative Approaches to Bioethics.* New York: Routledge; 1997. p. 3–17.

21. Lindemann Nelson H, editor. *Stories and their Limits: Narrative Approaches to Bioethics.* New York: Routledge; 1997.

22. Charon R, Montello M, editors. *Stories Matter: The Role of Narrative in Medical Ethics.* New York: Routledge; 2002.

23. Titcombe J. *Joshua's Story: Uncovering the Morecambe Bay NHS Scandal.* Leeds: Anderson Wallace Publishing; 2015.

24. Anderson-Wallace M, Shale S. Restoring trust: What is "quality" in the aftermath of healthcare harm? *Clinical Risk.* 2014;20(1–2):16–18.

25. Ocloo JE. Harmed patients gaining voice: Challenging dominant perspectives in the construction of medical harm and patient safety reforms. *Soc Sci Med.* 2010;71(3):510–16.

26. Dalton D, Williams N. *Building a Culture of Candour: A Review of the Threshold for the Duty of Candour and of the Incentives for Care Organisations to be Candid.* Surgeons RCo, editor. London; Royal College of Surgeons (England) https://www.rcseng.ac.uk/-/media/files/rcs/library-and-publications/non-journal-publications/duty-of-candour-review-final-report-2014.pdf (accessed June 26, 2017), 2014.

27. Wheeler R. Candour for surgeons: The absence of spin. *Ann Roy Coll Surg Engl.* 2014;96(6):420–2.

28. Vines P. Apologies and civil liability in the UK: A view from elsewhere. *Edinburgh Law Rev.* 2008;12:200.

29. Regulation 20 The Health and Social Care Act 2008 (Regulated Activities) Regulations 2014.

30. Kachalia A, Kaufman SR, Boothman R, Anderson S, Welch K, Saint S, et al. Liability claims and costs before and after implementation of a medical error disclosure program. *Ann Intern Med.* 2010;153(4):213–21.

31. Ho B, Liu E. Does sorry work? The impact of apology laws on medical malpractice. *J Risk Uncertainty.* 2011;43(2):141–67.

32. Boothman RC, Imhoff SJ, Campbell DA Jr. Nurturing a culture of patient safety and achieving lower malpractice risk through disclosure: Lessons learned and future directions. *Front Health Serv Manag.* 2012;28(3):13.

33. Paget MA. *The Unity of Mistakes; A Phenomenological Interpretation of Medical Work.* Philadelphia, PA: Temple University Press; 1988.

34. Anon. *Being Open and Duty of Candour Policy and Procedure.* Being Open and Duty of Candour Policy and Procedure London; London Ambulance Service. http://www.londonambulance.nhs.uk/talking_with_us/freedom_of_information/classes_of_information/idoc.ashx?docid=56087b0a-fcba-42b1-ba20-a6cd0f01bb2c&version=-1 (accessed June 26, 2017), 2015.

35. Birks Y, Entwistle V, Harrison R, Bosanquet K, Watt I, Iedema R. Being open about unanticipated problems in health care: The challenges of uncertainties. *J Health Serv Res Policy.* 2015;20(1 Suppl):54–60.

36. Moodley S. Meningitis case histories. *Good Practice.* 2013. Available from: http://www.themdu.com/guidance-and-advice/journals/good-practice-october-2013/meningitis-case-histories#sthash.uxnPGBv2.dpuf [Accessed 01 January 2016].

37. Bostick NA, Sade R, McMahon JW, Benjamin R. Report of the American Medical Association Council on Ethical and Judicial Affairs: Withholding information from patients: Rethinking the propriety of 'therapeutic privilege.' *J Clin Ethics.* 2006;17(4):302.

38. Garbutt J, Brownstein DR, Klein EJ, Waterman A, Krauss MJ, Marcuse EK, et al. Reporting and disclosing medical errors: Pediatricians' attitudes and behaviors. *Arch Pediatr Adolesc Med.* 2007;161(2):179–85.

39. Hobgood C, Tamayo-Sarver JH, Elms A, Weiner B. Parental preferences for error disclosure, reporting, and legal action after medical error in the care of their children. *Pediatrics.* 2005;116(6):1276–86.

40. Kolaitis IN, Schinasi DA, Ross LF. Should medical errors be disclosed to pediatric patients? Pediatricians' attitudes toward error disclosure. *Acad Pediatr.* 2015;16(5):482–8.

41. Birks Y, Harrison R, Bosanquet K, Hall J, Harden M, Entwistle V, et al. An exploration of the implementation of open disclosure of adverse events in the UK: A scoping review and qualitative exploration. *Health Serv Deliv Res.* 2014;2(20):1–195.

42. Gallagher TH, Garbutt JM, Waterman AD, Flum DR, Larson EB, Waterman BM, et al. Choosing your words carefully: How physicians would disclose harmful medical errors to patients. *Arch Intern Med.* 2006;166(15):1585–93.

43. Cox W. The five A's: What do patients want after an adverse event? *J Healthc Risk Manag.* 2007;27(3):25–9.

44. Vines P. Apologising for personal injury in law: Failing to take account of lessons from psychology in blameworthiness and propensity to sue. *Psychiatry Psychol Law.* 2015;22(4):624–34.

45. Allan A, McKillop D, Dooley J, Allan MM, Preece DA. Apologies following an adverse medical event: The importance of focusing on the consumer's needs. *Patient Educ Couns.* 2015;98(9):1058–62.

46. Mazor KM, Greene SM, Roblin D, Lemay CA, Firneno CL, Calvi J, et al. More than words: Patients' views on apology and disclosure when things go wrong in cancer care. *Patient Educ Couns.* 2013;90(3):341–6.

47. Peto RR, Tenerowicz LM, Benjamin EM, Morsi DS, Burger PK. One system's journey in creating a disclosure and apology program. *Jt Comm J Qual Patient Saf.* 2009;35(10):487–96.

48. Dix A. Adhering to new duty of candour guidance. *Nurs Times.* 2015;111(32–33):17–19.

49. Wu AW. Medical error: The second victim: The doctor who makes the mistake needs help too. *BMJ: Br Med J.* 2000;320(7237):726.

50. Harrison R, Lawton R, Perlo J, Gardner P, Armitage G, Shapiro J. Emotion and coping in the aftermath of medical error: A cross-country exploration. *J Patient Saf.* 2015;11(1):28–35.

51. Newman M. The emotional impact of mistakes on family physicians. *Arch Fam Med.* 1996;5:71–5.

52. Scott SD, Hirschinger LE, Cox KR, McCoig M, Brandt J, Hall LW. The natural history of recovery for the healthcare provider 'second victim' after adverse patient events. *Qual Saf Health Care.* 2009;18(5):325–30.

53. Mants T. Health care professionals' experiences after making errors in practice: An integrative review of the literature. Unpublished Masters Thesis, School of Nursing, University of Victoria, BC, 2015.

54. O'Beirne M, Sterling P, Palacios-Derflingher L, Hohman S, Zwicker K. Emotional impact of patient safety incidents on family physicians and their office staff. *J Am Board Fam Med.* 2012;25(2):177–83.

55. Ofri D. Ashamed to admit it: Owning up to medical error. *Health Aff (Millwood).* 2010;29(8):1549–51.

56. White AA, Bell SK, Krauss MJ, Garbutt J, Dunagan WC, Fraser VJ, et al. How trainees would disclose medical errors: Educational implications for training programmes. *Med Educ.* 2011;45(4):372–80.

57. Seys D, Scott S, Wu A, Van Gerven E, Vleugels A, Euwema M, et al. Supporting involved health care professionals (second victims) following an adverse health event: A literature review. *Int J Nurs Stud.* 2013;50(5):678–87.

58. Scott SD, Hirschinger LE, Cox KR, McCoig M, Hahn-Cover K, Epperly KM, et al. Caring for our own: Deploying a systemwide second victim rapid response team. *Jt Comm J Qual Patient Saf.* 2010;36(5):233–40.

59. Walker MU. *Moral Repair: Reconstructing Moral Relations after Wrongdoing.* Cambridge: Cambridge University Press; 2006.

60. Shale S. *Moral Leadership in Medicine: Building Ethical Healthcare Organizations.* Cambridge University Press; Cambridge, 2011.

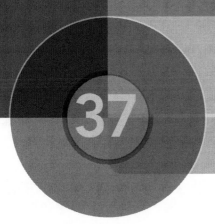

The inescapability of conscience in primary healthcare

ANDREW PAPANIKITAS

INTRODUCTION

Conscience in healthcare has by turns been seen as a moral and legal right, and as a source of harm and injustice.[1] It has also been discussed in terms of its potential in detecting and preventing unethical practice,[2] and debated as an essential feature of professional autonomy.[3] Conscience is variously described: it may accommodate a gut feeling that something is morally wrong as well as a more reflective insight into the impact of our actions.[2] Conscience is also inextricably linked to the notion of integrity – the virtue of acting in accordance with correct values, even when this is made difficult by circumstances.[4] In this chapter, I use two examples of conscientious objection – conscientious objection to involvement in abortion and conscientious objection to providing or facilitating complementary and alternative medicine (CAM). These emerged from a small qualitative study for a doctorate in medical education. They are presented as foci for a theoretical discussion with practical implications, rather than as a generalisable theory of conscience-manifest in primary healthcare. There is much discussion about what may legitimately be classified as conscientious objection. I will proceed on the basis that conscientious objection in healthcare is where someone refuses to do something based on a sincerely held belief, and that conscience is a feeling about the moral rightness or wrongness of a decision or a process of reflecting in action. This process is ultimately triggered by a belief with moral ramifications or a belief about the moral rightness and wrongness of a decision. The belief may be seen as a premise in an argument, upon which that argument depends. I will further argue that better understanding of conscience and conscientious objection is essential in the primary healthcare setting. Primary healthcare offers plentiful opportunity for difference of both beliefs and values that in turn generates the potential for conscientious objection. I invite the reader to consider the contexts discussed in this chapter in terms of what role conscience might have in healthcare. Because both abortion and complementary medicine elicit strong opinion, there is a danger that the chapter is read as an inadequate discussion of the rightness and wrongness of either. That is not the intention, but rather by juxtaposing them to offer ways of better understanding conscience in healthcare.

A NOTE ON METHOD AND DRAMATIS PERSONAE

Some of the verbatim quotations below are from a small qualitative study for a doctorate in medical education. The data presented here and the ensuing discussion are derived from 19 semi-structured interviews and one focus group. In both the interviews and the focus group, I started with general questions, such as 'Describe the setting in which you practice', and 'What kind of situations do you think of when you hear the phrase, "Ethical issues in general practice"?'. More specific questions revolved around sources of ethical guidance and support, including the question, 'If there was such a thing as a centre for primary health-care ethics, what do you imagine it might do?'. For example:

AP: If there were such a thing as a sort of fictional centre of primary care ethics, what do you imagine it might do?

Dr F (GP-Trainee): It would do research.

AP: What kind of research?

Dr F: It would do research on primary care ethics, it would do studies looking into, you know, how doctors are and . [pauses]

AP: So you're talking about empirical research?

Dr F: Yes. I think that's what would be one of the things. I think that it would offer, you know, if it was good, it would offer advice, it would be somewhere that doctors could turn to and – for help with ethical dilemmas. And I think that, I just imagine it would, you know, the doctors or the researchers within this fictional centre would write books on ethics and . . .

AP: Do people read books on ethics?

Dr F: No, not people I know.

Although this study contains no formal element of observation, I became immersed in my field: practising as a general practitioner (GP), facilitating ethics and communication skills at a medical school and co-leading a module in primary healthcare ethics for a Master's degree qualification. I attended further medical ethics training, participated in ethics education for GPs and attended general practice conferences. Whilst some participants were very happy to talk to me, whether they perceived a kinship with me, saw some benefit in taking part or had an opinion they wished to voice, others were more wary of someone who they perceived as knowing both general practice and ethics and therefore in a position to criticise at best and report them to the professional body at worst (though in no case was this actually necessary); metaphorically, some potential participants saw me as an ambassador and others saw me as a spy.[5] I also had an internal ethical tension, the desire not to interview anyone over whom I might be seen to have undue influence, for example, as a clinical supervisor or a tutor, which reduced participant availability. The study had approval from the Royal Free Hospital NHS research ethics committee, reference: 09/H0720/126. Longer discussions of my method are accessible elsewhere.[6,7]

Pseudonym (in alphabetical order according to randomly assigned letter)	Roles in academia, education, policy and practice	Gender	Location of practice
Prof A	Full-time academic/educator, international medical graduate (IMG)	Female	N/A (former GP overseas)
Dr B	GP partner, academic/educator/ leader, UK graduate	Male	Urban
Dr C	GP partner /educator/philosopher, UK graduate	Male	Rural
Dr D	GP Partner in first 5 years since qualification, IMG	Female	Urban
Dr E	GP partner, academic/ethicist/ educator, UK graduate	Male	Suburban
Dr F	GP trainee in final year of training, leader (medical politics), UK graduate	Female	Suburban
Dr G	Retired GP partner /educator/ leader, UK graduate	Male	Semi-Rural
Dr L	Non-GP clinician with PhD/ Full-time academic/educator, UK graduate	Female	N/A
Dr M	Sessional/Locum GP educator/ ethicist, UK graduate	Female	Urban
Dr N	Locum GP, No academic, education or leadership roles, IMG	Female	Urban/ Suburban
Dr O	Salaried GP/leader, UK graduate	Male	Rural
Prof P	Salaried GP/leader/academic, UK graduate	Male	Urban
Dr Q	Salaried GP, UK graduate	Male	Urban
Dr R	Salaried GP, academic/ philosopher/educator, UK graduate	Male	Suburban
Dr S	GP partner/educator/ethicist/ leader UK graduate	Male	Urban
Dr U	Sessional/locum GP and retired educator/leader, UK graduate	Male	Urban and rural
Dr W	Locum GP/leader/GP commissioner, UK Graduate	Male	Urban
Prof Y	GP Partner/academic/ethicist, UK Graduate	Female	Urban
Prof Z	Retired GP partner/academic/ ethicist, UK graduate	Male	Urban
Focus Group: Drs H.I.J.K. X.	GP trainees (none with any teaching or academic role), all UK graduates	1 male, 4 female	Urban

CONSCIENCE AND BELIEFS ABOUT THE MORAL STATUS OF THE FOETUS

There is a vast academic and educational literature on the ethics of abortion and much of it concerns whether healthcare workers ought to refrain from participating, or have the right to so refrain. Indeed, the literature on conscientious objection in medicine is principally focused on abortion.[1,2,8,9]

Conscientious objection to abortion stems from beliefs about the moral status of the human embryo. Some people may not regard the yet unborn as having full human status and therefore may view a termination of pregnancy as an extension of contraception or as a gynaecological treatment. The woman's right to choose whether to continue to be pregnant until delivery may be viewed as a value that trumps any notional rights of the foetus. Others may consider that the foetus has full human status from the moment of conception (a view often but not necessarily associated with sincerely held religious beliefs) or that the foetus increasingly acquires moral status from conception to birth.

Gillon suggests that these views are not ethical at all but epistemological. According to Gillon, two people may agree that killing people is wrong (the ethical question) but disagree over what counts as a person (the epistemological question).[10,11] This makes any kind of ethical discussion very difficult. It also makes conscientious positions either essential or misguided (depending on the observer's belief). Whilst UK law does not consider an embryo at any stage to be a person, someone who believes the embryo to be a person from the point of conception may consider abortion to be the same as murder.

CONSCIENTIOUS OBJECTION AS SOCIETAL DISCONTINUITY

In the UK mainland, there has been a historical prohibition on providing or facilitating treatment with the intention to cause an abortion.

> … the GMC … has tended to concentrate on the five 'A's of alcoholism, advertising, addiction, adultery and abortion (though since the legalization of abortion, the latter less so).[12]

The prohibition on abortion is also ascribed to a set of values derived from the Hippocratic Oath and subsequent declarations of the World Medical Association.[13] As such, the very term 'ethics' meant avoiding involvement in certain practices such as abortions, which came pre-labelled as unethical. Prior to 1967, in the UK, the law and professional guidelines offered a simple solution to most dilemmas concerning abortion – it was not allowed unless to save the life of the mother. This 'common law' justification[14] was broadly interpreted by courts but still represented a significant risk of criminal and career-ending prosecution for the doctor. This may well have reduced the requests for abortions as well as made it much easier to practise with a conscientious objection to the procedure. This did however mean that clinicians who believed that an abortion was necessary either refrained with a guilty conscience, or risked professional and legal ramifications in order to act in accordance with their beliefs and values.

Following the *Abortion Act 1967*, in the UK, the decision to refer for and carry out terminations of pregnancy was placed at the discretion of doctors, with the caveat that there was some scope for doctors to opt out. This opt-out was provided on the basis of sincere conscientious objection and the absence of risk to the life or severe risk to the health of the woman requesting the procedure.

The first question to ask therefore is, what is a sincere belief? Must it be a religious belief? It may after all be based on criteria other than religious. For example, if a clinician objects to performing an abortion for reasons of foetal viability or a particular stage of foetal sentience conferring moral worth, this would seem sufficient grounds for conscientious objection but does not depend on a religious belief.

Referral for an abortion has in effect generally become seen as legally permissible, and therefore, a refusal to participate or to refer is seen as refusal to provide a service to which the patient is entitled.[1]

Dr E: I would say it's reprehensible for somebody like Julian Savulescu to take the line that they did in the BMJ famously, about six years ago, to say that, you know, doctors with conscience should not be allowed to practice. It seems to me his argument that you do what the state says or otherwise you're not an ethical doctor, is an extremely flawed one. So you've got to face that brutalising pressure. You've got to face the pressure of having to deal with the very real emotional strains and conflicts that are going to arise in consultation with patients that, you know, you wouldn't otherwise have if you towed the party line.

Savulescu argues that doctors' consciences (and by implication those of any clinician) have little place in the delivery of modern medical care. He proposes that people who are not prepared to offer legally permitted, efficient and beneficial care to a patient because it conflicts with their values should not be doctors. He argues that a service which depends on the values of the treating doctor results in patients shopping around doctors to receive services to which they are entitled. This introduces inefficiency and wastes resources. The less-informed patients may fail to receive a service to which they are entitled – this inequity is unjustifiable.[1] The argument has rapidly found its way into educational materials as a view which GP trainees are encouraged to heed.[15]

CONSCIENCE, POWER AND SHARED DECISION-MAKING

Conscientious refusals to provide or indeed accept a medical treatment represent a clinician-centred and patient-centred use of power in the consultation. Discussions around areas such as abortion, where disagreements are shaped by epistemological differences of opinion as well as moral ones, serve as stark examples of the potential push and pull of values in the consultation. Dr G reflects on whether a GP has a right or duty to determine the outcome of the consultation.

Dr G: … the ethical issue for abortion for a doctor is not, is not just 'is abortion right or wrong?' but the ethical decision is given that I hold a view either way, have I the right to insist upon it? […]

Roger Neighbour comments on the morality of influencing patients' decisions in *The Inner Consultation*, a manual of consultation skills that is widely taught to and often referenced by British GPs.

What do you do if you have sound reasons for thinking one option is far better than the others, but the patient chooses the 'wrong' one? I never promised you an end to moral dilemmas. You could accept the patient's choice for the moment, and let time be the teacher; or you could use some of the more covert influencing techniques we shall be discussing shortly. Or you could ask your medical protection society. Or your priest.[16]

Neighbour answers his own question. If a GP can influence a patient in that same patient's best interests, then there are times when it is right to do so.

The doctor is credited with expertise, charisma and respect amounting to what Michael Balint called 'his apostolic function'. This lends 'doctor's orders' and authority which, while we may secretly consider it undeserved, we should be foolish not to use in the patient's interests.[16]

For Neighbour, medical 'authority' is one of many skills or attributes which can be used to the patient's good. His reference to the medical protection society and the priest illustrates the idea that whether, and the degree to which, a doctor 'influences' the patient may rightly or wrongly be affected by both professional and personal ethics.

The moral authority of a clinician becomes somewhat challenged if clinician and patient become aware that they have different values. This especially so if a clinician conscientiously refuses to provide or a patient conscientiously refuses to accept any particular treatment.

Dr R: It's actually a bit more complicated … Well, because you have to decide how much of that you're going to let, you're going to reveal to the patient, and how much you're going to get involved.

Clinicians such as Dr R might be aware that their reasons for refusing to provide something may not be accepted by the patient, especially if others clinicians might not refuse. This is a dilemma, because it more fully respects the autonomy of the patient whilst potentially undermining the therapeutic relationship by calling into question the clinician's motivations now and in the future.

ABSOLUTE AND NUANCED POSITIONS ON ABORTION-AVOIDANCE AND ENGAGEMENT

Abortion can be seen as issue that is sometimes invisible, and subject to both ethical avoidance and ethical deferral. A possible reason for abortion representing less of an issue is that in recent decades, patients have usually been able to self-refer to abortion services without ever seeing someone who might object. In areas in the UK that are well served by family planning clinics, this is perhaps an issue that might avoid the GP consultation entirely and become invisible as far as the ethics of practice is concerned. Importantly, it may mean that education about abortion and its attendant ethical issues needs to be provided in order to prepare the new GP for practice in areas that are less well served, or to counsel patients who are unable or unwilling to directly access an abortion service.

Dr R: I mean the structure is such that you don't actually have to make, decide whether or not they're going to have an abortion, because if you're not happy about it, there are easy ways round it, and, in fact, all you need to do now where I'm in, is give them a piece of paper with a phone number on basically, a little referral slip and they do the rest.

GPs with an ethical aversion to involvement in abortion may choose to use such redirection to avoid an ethically challenging encounter. Passing the patient a referral slip, however, is also a way of avoiding an uncomfortable and time-consuming discussion regardless of whether a GP strongly objects to abortion. A key problem with this approach is that the GP may be in a better position to counsel the patient, may have access to their full healthcare record and have established a relationship of trust. The patient may be unwilling or unable to access family planning series directly, and the GP may be able to deal with related issues, such as whether the patient is at risk of sexually transmitted illness or in an abusive relationship.

Dr R also expressed the opinion that if a GP holds a fixed ethical view regarding abortion, then dealing with requests is comparatively easier.

Dr R: I think it's fairly easy, perhaps comparatively easy for those people who consider that abortion is wrong in all circumstances. And it's probably fairly … It's pretty easy for those people who consider that a woman has a right to choose in all circumstances. … But I mean it's this thing about, which I have a continuing discomfort, because I don't have a black and white view … If you have a Hursthousian[17] view, which is what I have, that, you know, there are times when, with regret, one will decide that abortion is the least bad course.

It is perhaps surprising that despite a belief in foetal personhood or sanctity, and the discretion afforded to them by various jurisdictions, clinicians may still choose to have involvement in the decision to terminate a pregnancy. Here, a conscientious clinician might consider that a necessary evil ought not to be stripped of its difficulty. Conversely, a clinician who does not regard the foetus as a person, or believes that only the pregnant woman has the right to decide whether to continue with her pregnancy, might find such requests much easier. However, there is still such things as an outrageous request.

Prof Y: … on the whole I [am] always for abortion, unless it really is an outrageous request, but I always discuss it. So that would not be a problem for me.

The limit to Prof Y's favourable view is the outrageous request, and the condition of referral is discussion of whether this is the best course of action for the woman concerned. Even where there is consensus about the permissibility of abortion based on women's rights, there may be moral outrage for reasons other than the rightness or wrongness of abortion itself. For example, selective abortions for cultural reasons such as the preference for male heirs may provoke ethical disapproval from people who would otherwise regard themselves as pro-choice.

A conscientious objection also does not necessarily render the issue easy to avoid. Some Roman Catholic writers state that deferring to colleagues or to counselling services (who will facilitate abortions) does not absolve a GP of complicity. From the position of Watt and others, providing information or referring to a colleague (active avoidance of the issue) will often be morally wrong. To adhere to this more stringent form of conscientious objection, a GP ought to only refer to services and charities that will encourage and support a woman to go through with her pregnancy, and only to suggest colleagues who are opposed to abortion. Furthermore, they suggest that the discussion is an opportunity to find those requests that do not comply with the abortion act, and to give advice about the risks of the procedure in the hope that they will dissuade the patient from seeking an abortion.[18,19] Awareness of such advice makes conscientious objection much harder for GPs who hold a sincere belief in the sanctity of human life from the point of conception.

BELIEFS ABOUT THE EFFECTIVENESS OF TREATMENT AND ABOUT THE MORALITY OF ALTERNATIVE THERAPISTS

Conscience and conscientious objection reemerged in my study of ethics education in UK general practice in the context of refusal to facilitate CAM. Western medicine by definition excludes alternative systems – if science is truth, then alternatives to science and its conclusions are perceived by practitioners of Western medicine as delusions and lies. Ernst argues that complementary and alternative practitioners can be unethical in three key ways: their methods cannot be explained by Western science, their results cannot be substantiated and they have no robust professional oversight to regulate their behaviour.[20,21] By endorsing CAM therapies in any way, practitioners are accordingly acting outside of an officially recognised role and therefore, by definition, unprofessional according to Ernst's papers. Beliefs about the rightness and wrongness of facilitating CAM referrals based on beliefs about whether CAM works arose in my data.

Dr E: So if I can return to my sort of hobby horse about waste of money and so on, I practice in a very fashionable area, where I get lots of requests for... I'm asked to get a referral to the Royal Homoeopathic Hospital, my heart absolutely sinks because I personally think that homoeopathy is bunk and has no proven value at all and a total waste of money.

Beliefs about the morality of restricting treatment in the presence of waste raised further epistemological questions about what constitutes a beneficial treatment and what constitutes a waste. General practice (and healthcare more generally) in the UK claims to be scientific and evidence-based. This does not allow room for alternatives, especially with respect to the allocation of state funds. Practice '...in a very fashionable [geographical] area' implies articulate patients who are more involved in decision-making and less deferential to clinical authority. In the case of Dr E, this meant patients' requests that they felt they could not conscientiously accede to. When personal beliefs align with professional consensus and public consensus about what a healthcare service may provide – conscientiously adhering to the moral duties that follow seems more straightforward.

Dr W, a GP and healthcare commissioner, compared the UK with his experience of healthcare in China. In the latter context, maintaining a conscientious objection to CAM would be less straightforward.

Dr W: ... I was in China, and in China their medical model is definitely not a biomedical model the way we think of it. And they have a very inclusive approach. ... they have a very justifiable argument to say, well Chinese medicine existed long before Western medicine did. And there's something cultural around how in the West the doctors have approach, which has meant we've excluded many other things. And whereas their approach in China at the moment is, if you go to a, a Chinese hospital, actually they're dual trained or they're open to complementary – I wouldn't use the word 'complementary' there, open to what I describe as their mainstream medicine ... And things like acupuncture are about as standard as writing a prescription. And they do, if you speak to anybody about Chinese medicine, actually their formulations are not too different to how we formulate a diagnosis. So it's, it's an interesting one from that perspective. It's made me rethink actually my very rigid hard-nosed Western view.

The personal views of both DR W and Dr E on alternatives to Western medicine had softened with experience. However, both conscientiously would only use public funding for treatments that were endorsed by evidence-based medicine. Qualifying as a doctor in the UK implies that certain beliefs, for example, about science and evidence-based medicine, have been adopted.

PRIVATE HEALTHCARE AND CONSCIENCE

In my study, Dr W and Dr E both suggested that their attitudes were nuanced by the opportunity costs of alternative medicine. Clearly, there may be a spectrum of belief regarding the effectiveness of both Western medicine and its alternatives. In a context of unrestricted resources, the main limiting factor at a consultation and a commissioning level might be avoiding harm whilst maximising choice. Beliefs about the benefits of treatments might not weigh so heavily.

Dr W: [It has not] … changed what I have to do because I have to justify public finance, when it comes to making decisions here, but there is something around acknowledging that we have a very restrictive practice rather than an inclusive practice. … as a commissioner, I wouldn't go with the commissioning of a non-numerical, unquantifiable service with very little evidence base, because I just wouldn't be able to stand up and justify that as we cut other services where is there a lot more evidence to it.

In his paper on conscientious objection, Savulescu suggests that private elective medicine is an area where doctors might have more liberty to practice according to their values.[1] However, elective medicine implies a lack of urgent significant implications for patients' lives and health. Savulescu also argues that this does not absolve doctors of informing patients of relevant alternative risks and benefits in a reasonable, complete and unbiased way. However, if one has a conscientious belief that CAM works or does not work in a particular instance, it seems disingenuous to only offer it to those who are self-funded (if one believes it works) or only restrict it from those who are state-funded (if one believes that it does not). The key explanation is that private practice affords clinicians the freedom to offer a certain type of medicine, and patients to choose a certain type of medicine. By contrast, state-funded healthcare comes with a set menu of treatment options, shaped by the beliefs and values vested in the state and modified by professional bodies and patient organisations.

CONCLUSIONS

If this chapter does something coherent, it is to raise the possibility that, based on what healthcare workers (GPs in the case of my study) believe, they may conscientiously endorse or object to certain kinds of practice. Conscience and conscientious objection are perhaps over-attributed to religious perspectives, perhaps because the most discussed contexts are those where the major world faiths have something action-guiding to say. The unfairness of endorsing religious rather than secular values is raised as an argument against conscience.[1] I find it more interesting to extend conscience to secular as well as religious values, an approach that is evident in recent literature.[2,4]

Clinicians in the cultural West (e.g. doctors in the UK) are usually under a professional obligation not to allow their own values and beliefs to prejudice their work. However, given that they may be expected to influence patient's decisions, it is doubtful that they operate in a state of moral neutrality. The ability and duty of the UK GP to influence patients are remarked upon by GP educators[16] and the healer's power is commented upon in ethics more generally.[22] The ethically sensitive clinicians must decide how far they will allow their values to influence the patient, and how far they will allow their patients' values and choices to influence their actions. Intuitively, clinicians should attempt to influence and persuade patients to accept healthcare goods and avoid harms. However, they also ought to decide to what degree they should display their espoused values and beliefs, and acknowledge any particular source of moral values that the patient would consider to represent a conflict of interests. A declaration of beliefs may undermine the ability to persuade.

Others have suggested that conscientious objection in reproductive medicine is taken for granted in a manner that does not permit discussion of (and reflection on) clinician values, whilst at the same time, there is a profound and unjust intolerance of conscience in other areas of medical practice.[2] This general hostility towards conscience and conscientious objection has the potential to push conscientious objectors towards avoidance of an issue – whether this is by deferring decisions to others, or conspiring to avoid situations where one's conscience will be activated. I have written elsewhere about forms of ethics avoidance.[23] However, Birchley's argument that the hostility towards conscience as a concept makes reflection and discussion more difficult and therefore has an adverse effect on probity is a useful one. If healthcare professionals could reflect on times that they were swayed or not swayed by conscience, then perhaps we might see less prejudice and more reflective ethical decision-making.[2]

I have suggested that conscientious objection may in practice represent avoidance of ethical problems that were caused by differences in belief. There is an argument that this may at times represent an abandonment of patients in need. In cases involving a request for an abortion, there is a legal requirement for the clinician to make a judgement as to whether the circumstances meet the referral criteria. This judgement can be avoided by passing the request to a colleague or to a self-referral service. However, neither may be available, and complete avoidance may sometimes be neglectful of other duties such as child safeguarding.[24–26] Deferral may still place some doctors with sincere conscientious objections in difficulty as they may see this as a form of facilitation or complicity.

Healthcare workers need to be aware of their own religious and scientific beliefs and to reflect on how these influence the advice that they give to patients.[27] Beliefs in this instance may include beliefs about the moral status of the embryo or about the potential harm to the mother of continuing with or terminating a pregnancy. The idea that an abortion is a tragic necessity is one which some clinicians with a belief in the moral worth of the embryo may use to justify facilitating a termination of pregnancy. By contrast, someone with no such beliefs may still consider an abortion request to be outrageous. Similarly, there is evidence to suggest that clinicians may be placed in a position where they believe that particular treatments were useless, and a drain on resources, but the healthcare authorities have decided that patients are entitled to be referred for them. In this situation, ethical discussion may take on a tone of conscientious objection, on the basis of a belief that CAMs are harmful or ineffective. However, there is evidence that (for example) some GP may abandon their espoused values in day-to-day resource-allocation decisions.[28] A conscientious position based on ethics is more tractable than one based on belief. This may offer an alternative account to one that sees values and facts as similar kinds of belief.[9]

The source of conflict based on conscience lies in the values and beliefs that are held by the clinician, the profession, the state and the patient or patient's representative. This represents somewhat more complex power struggle than the one between medical profession, civil society and the state.[29] Arguments have been made that doctors (but by extension, any clinicians) with a conscientious objection to something the state has agreed to provide should be made to submit to behavioural therapy[30] or removed from practice.[1] This is problematic, because conscience represents a way in which unethical practices, some of which are based on unsound beliefs, may be identified and resisted. Better understanding is needed however of conscience, what it is, and the benefits and burdens that it carries. The features of conscience that are epistemological (related to belief itself) rather than moral require greater public understanding. That understanding should not be focused on one type of case such as abortion, if the case is not to eclipse the broader understanding that is possible. There is much scope for conscience to be a part of reflection in education, and there is no reason why conscience should be inextricably linked with a theistic religion. Indeed, unless the beliefs and values (whatever their source) of clinician, patient, profession and state are somehow always in perfect alignment, conscience and conscientious objection are inescapable features of clinical practice.

REFERENCES

1. Savulescu J. Conscientious objection in medicine. *BMJ* 2006; **332**(7536): 294–7.
2. Birchley G. A clear case for conscience in healthcare practice. *Journal of Medical Ethics* 2012; **38**(1): 13–17.
3. Papanikitas A. Doctors should do as they're told—Myth or reality? *Journal of the Royal Society of Medicine* 2009; **102**(1): 40–2.
4. Colaianni A. A long shadow: Nazi doctors, moral vulnerability and contemporary medical culture. *Journal of Medical Ethics* 2012; **38**(7): 435–8.
5. Ives J, Owens J, Cribb A. IEEN workshop report: Teaching and learning in interdisciplinary and empirical ethics. *Clinical Ethics* 2013; **8**: 70–4.
6. Papanikitas A. Ethicality and confidentiality: Is there an inverse-care issue in general practice ethics? *Clinical Ethics* 2011; **6**: 186–90.
7. Papanikitas A. Methods. From the classroom to the clinic: Ethics education and general practice. PhD Thesis. King's College London, London, 2014, pp. 40–75.
8. Benn P. Conscience and healthcare ethics. In: Ashcroft RE, Dawson A, Draper H, McMillan JR, eds. *Principles of healthcare ethics*. 2nd ed. London: Wiley; 2007, pp. 345–63.
9. Jackson J. Personal beliefs and patient care. In: Ashcroft RE, Dawson A, Draper H, McMillan JR, eds. *Principles of healthcare ethics*. 2nd ed. London: Wiley; 2007, pp. 339–44.
10. Gillon R. Medical ethics: Four principles plus attention to scope. *BMJ* 1994; **309**(6948): 184–8.
11. Gillon R. Is there a 'new ethics of abortion?' *Journal of Medical Ethics* 2001; **27**(Suppl 2): ii5–9.
12. Armstrong D. Professional discipline. In: *An outline of sociology as applied to medicine*. 4th ed. Oxford: Butterworth Heinemann; 1994, p. 107.
13. Campbell AV, Higgs R. Choices. In: *In that case: Medical ethics in everyday practice*. London: Darton, Longman and Todd; 1982, pp. 1–19.
14. Herring J. Common law defences [contraception, abortion and pregancy]. In: *Ethics and medical law*. 6th ed. Oxford: Oxford University Press; 2016, p. 306.
15. Naidoo P. Ethical frameworks. In: *Cases and concpts for the new MRCGP*. Bloxham, Oxon: Scion; 2008, pp. 304–8.
16. Neighbour R. Checkpoint 3 (Handover): Communication skills. In: *The inner consultation*. 2nd ed. Oxford: Radcliffe Publishing; 2007, pp. 176–201.

17. Hursthouse R. Virtue theory and abortion. *Philosophy and Public Affairs* 1991; **20**(3): 223–46.

18. Delaney M. General medical practice: The problem of cooperation in evil. *Catholic Medical Quartery* 2006; **58**(2): 6–13.

19. Watt H. Co-operation problems in general practice. *Catholic Medical Quartery* 2008; **58**(3): 26–33.

20. Ernst E. The ethics of complementary medicine. *Journal of Medical Ethics* 1996; **22**(4): 197–8.

21. Ernst E. Ethics of complementary medicine: Practical issues. *The British Journal of General Practice* 2009; **59**(564): 517–19.

22. Brody H. The essence of primary care. In: *The Healer's power.* New Haven, CT: Yale University Press; 1992, pp. 56–61.

23. Papanikitas A, Lewis G, McKenzie-Edwards E. Should GPs avoid making ethical judgements? *The British Journal of General Practice* 2016; **66**(649): 441–2.

24. Papanikitas A. General practice, clinical intention and the Sexual Offences Act 2003. *London Journal of Primary Care* 2009; **2**: 146–50.

25. Bow S. Singling out the double effect—Sexual health advice and contraception are hically distinct. *London Journal of Primary Care (Abingdon)* 2015; **7**(5): 92–5.

26. Papanikitas A, Spicer J. Singling out the double effect—Some further comment. *London Journal of Primary Care (Abingdon)* 2015; **7**(5): 96.

27. Papanikitas A, Self-awareness and professionalism, InnovAIT, 2017; 0: 1–6 (online advance publication), DOI: 10.1177/1755738017710962

28. Berney L, Kelly M, Doyal L, Feder G, Griffiths C, Jones IR. Ethical principles and the rationing of health care: A qualitative study in general practice. *The British Journal of General Practice* 2005; **55**(517): 620–5.

29. Salter B. Who rules? The new politics of medical regulation. *Social Science and Medicine* 2001; **52**(6): 871–83.

30. Whiting D. Should doctors ever be professionally required to cahnge their attitudes? *Clinical Ethics* 2009; **4**: 67–73.

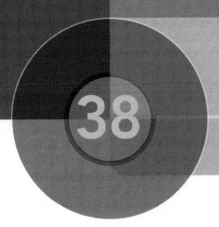

Professional self-care in primary care practice – An ethical puzzle

EMMA McKENZIE-EDWARDS

38

For the ancients, as Foucault claims, the care of the self was the foundational principle of all moral rationality. The care of the self is the ethical transformation of the self in the light of the truth, or, transformation of the self into a truthful existence.[1]

Is this an idealised philosophical concept or an ethical imperative? In this chapter, I attempt to consider the ethical challenges faced by the healthcare worker who is trying to consider themselves in the workplace and the limits to this self-consideration.

In his discussion in *Primary Care Ethics* about whether doctors should observe a moral duty to care for themselves, Andrew Dicker outlines a reasonable (and often repeated) argument that the public have a right 'not to consult a doctor who is not fit to fulfil the ordinary duties of a doctor'.[2] If healthcare professionals accept the premise that there is a need for clinician self-care in any sustainable model of healthcare practice, then clinicians need the skills with which to identify the challenges and the skills with which to balance self-care against patient care and other duties. In this chapter, I will examine some of the 'puzzle pieces' of professional self-care – some recently described and some ancient – before seeing if they can fit together into a coherent approach. Primary healthcare (particularly UK general practice) may offer a context in which to examine the phenomenon, and where good may result from doing so. Arguably, UK general practitioners are the only people who need to learn about ethical self-care, I intend that the reflections in this chapter should be transferable. Indeed, some concepts, such as surface and deep acting, have been transferred from other professions' experiences.

GOING BEYOND THE CALL OF DUTY

Medicine has a special place in the overwork and efficiency culture of the day. This cultural debate is about success, achievement, the limits of efficiency and what it is to be human.[3]

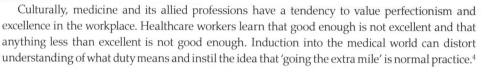

Culturally, medicine and its allied professions have a tendency to value perfectionism and excellence in the workplace. Healthcare workers learn that good enough is not excellent and that anything less than excellent is not good enough. Induction into the medical world can distort understanding of what duty means and instil the idea that 'going the extra mile' is normal practice.[4]

In a perfectionist framework, there is no distinction between what is required and what is beyond requirement and optional.[5] The National Health Service (NHS) in the UK has allowed some room for the values-based and vocationally-driven culture to flourish, but discussion about the enlarging 'credibility gap' between rhetoric and reality in clinical care provision[6] leads us to acknowledge the potentially limitless need and demand for healthcare provision in the primary care setting.

In her discussion about moral failure, Tessman holds that autonomous individuals maintain the safe position of always being able to choose not to be exceptional. The moral agent may struggle to meet the moral requirements from which they are not released.[7]

This combined medical culture of perfectionism, excellence and fear of failure and harming patients makes healthcare workers a particularly vulnerable professional group who may struggle to make the decision not to be exceptional. The unsustainable option of going beyond the call of duty cannot be the ethical norm in the long term.

PUTTING THE PATIENT FIRST

It has not always been the priority of the primary healthcare worker to 'put the patient first'. Less than 100 years ago, before the formation of the NHS, doctors prized efficient working for financial gain above prioritising patient need. The General Medical Council (GMC) now demands that doctors 'put patients first'.[8] Clinicians in first world countries are influenced by at least three other potentially competing factors of additional GMC-enforced directive and regulation, marketplace and target-driven care and the needs of their own families and loved ones. In low and middle-income countries, the additional pressures of extremely limited resource and overwhelming clinical need complicate the picture.

Healthcare workers are prone to stress, work long hours with complex physical and emotional issues and in addition have multiple social demands: career and work related, household responsibilities, relationships and personal goals. While it could be argued that these issues are not unique to healthcare work, healthcare workers do differ in that they have the unique professional concern of the fear of causing harm to a patient through inadequate or inappropriate care provision. They learn to distinguish what is normal and what is not healthy for those they care for but can often be short-sighted when it comes to recognising and dealing with these elements in themselves.[9]

In primary care, work is done in close physical and emotional proximity to the patient. The community setting places the healthcare worker in the heart of the patient's life and often involves visiting their home and interacting with members of their family. It can become difficult to see clear boundaries to duty in this situation.

What is it that prevents the healthcare worker from following the advice they are likely to offer their patient to self-care? Those who prize attainment, achievement and ambition or those who are dedicated vocationally will all be at risk of overwork and neglecting their own self-care. The professional codes demanding that patients are put first also limit the ability of the healthcare worker to step away. If the primary issues separating self-care of the clinician from self-care of the patient are the individual and collective notions of duty and obligation as a medical professional and the difficulties demarcating the boundaries, perhaps one of the barriers to self-care lies with the individual clinician and their personal values and beliefs. These may be closely related to the individual's sense of self and threatening them uncomfortable or even damaging to the individual.

SELF-CARE OR CARING SOCIETY?

Doctors are trained to respect patients as persons but there is no explicit demand or expectation of reciprocity from the patient. This lack of mutual respect and disassociation from social context places undue pressure on the clinician. With no society-endorsed boundaries, patients increasingly accept encouragement from the political arena to view medical services as a 'convenience store'. Contractual changes are afoot to make that a reality.

Tessman considers the relationship between the person whose needs are without limit and the person who is morally required to respond to these needs as complicated by the inevitability of moral failure. That this is a 'specific form of wrongdoing' that can only potentially be mitigated by forgiving the person for not fulfilling such a requirement.[10]

Are we obliged to consider forgiving ourselves in advance for this failure? Do we not also have a right to consider our own individual needs as valid? I suggest that the answer to both questions is yes.

It becomes a conflict then between duty and self-interest. As healthcare workers are generally trained to prioritise the patient above themselves, they are likely to feel like they are failing in or even violating their duty of care if they ever prioritise their own needs. In heavily regulated professions where decisions can mean the difference between life and death, fear of failure or implied incompetence is palpable.

Fear of perceived failure can plunge the clinician into anxiety that their livelihood or identity is threatened, which makes for a very powerful ethical barrier to admit to the need for self-care or assistance from others.

Is the inevitable end of this road culpable inability to provide best care? Healthcare workers fearful of this outcome and having limited options to effect change in their working patterns may be provoked to strike. How may this be ethically justifiable? Heyd suggests that the autonomy of the individual gives him special reason to 'fulfil his own needs before getting involved with the fulfilment of other people's needs. In this sense, rights precede duties'.[11]

Averting this would involve much greater community engagement and agreed, shared goals and responsibilities between professional and patient. There is an argument that society more broadly ought to better look after those who are its guardians: healthcare, police, fire-service and the military.

WHO CARES FOR THE CARERS?

As Chuck the intern put it in Shem's novel *The House of God*:

How can we care for our patients, man, if nobody cares for us?[12]

It can be difficult to find evidence of self-care training in healthcare curricula. When it does arise, it often focuses on alcohol and drug misuse or perceived 'unhealthy behaviour'. Postgraduate medical education has begun to acknowledge the issue, but often focuses on one specific area (such as burnout or moral distress) or technique (such as the Balint movement), rather than considering the global issues and broad principles.

Striving for high quality care is an aim lauded by NHS England:

And when we strive for high quality care, we must do so for everyone, including those who are vulnerable.[13]

They are speaking about patients of course. However, if healthcare workers are a vulnerable group, they need particular care and support to enable them to adequately perform their role.

Recommendations about clinical or professional supervision and its role in this area have been made by a number of bodies in the UK including the Care Quality Commission.[14] Clinical supervision can provide opportunity to reflect on, review and modify practice and identify training and continuing development needs. Importantly, supervision can help healthcare workers to manage the personal and professional demands created by the nature of their work. There has been limited implementation of structured supervision in the primary care environment. Where it is used regularly and meaningfully, supervision has the potential to help staff feel valued and address developmental needs in a challenging environment.[15]

DO DOCTORS HAVE AN ETHICAL OBLIGATION TO ENGAGE WITH THEIR OWN EMOTIONS?

A physician who allows his patients to move him emotionally will enrich his own experience of doctoring.[16]

Halpern attempted to persuade clinicians to move away from detached concern towards emotionally engaged empathy. She argued the validity of emotions in clinical practice for positive and therapeutic intervention, the need to learn to recognise them and use them constructively in the service of empathy.

Studies about emotional labour, a term first coined by Hochschild in 1983 when she described the dramaturgical perspective of air hostess and customer interactions, have considered the psychological trauma that can result from needing to assume an identity 'surface and deep acting' in a job.[17] Grandey[18] reviews the theories underlying emotional labour, and defines it as the process of managing both experience and expression of feelings to support or achieve organisational goals. Risks of this management include withdrawal, reduced job satisfaction and changes in performance.

Psychologists have found that the management of emotions can be associated with health problems such as cancer and heart disease.[19–21]

Not engaging with emotions, as Kerasidou and Horn argue, has a negative effect on doctors, increasing stress and anxiety and predisposing them to emotional burnout and mental suffering. It also prevents doctors from caring for their patients effectively and appropriately. Assuming '– that these two aspects of the doctor are integrally connected, then paying much more attention to the doctor as a person, and attending to their emotional and physical wellbeing should be a priority too'.[22]

Lack of emotional self-care therefore can have serious consequences, affecting performance, job satisfaction and even physical health. Ethically, avoiding emotional engagement or routine surface or deep acting in the professional role without adequate 'decompression' could be regarded as irresponsible behaviour.

CONCLUSION: ARE THERE ANY ANSWERS TO THIS ETHICAL PUZZLE?

I have suggested that ethical self-care is needed for good medical practice to take place. The limitations to this self-care include medical and societal cultural demands and restraints and the personal fear of the healthcare professional of potentially causing harm.

If a person's values originate more in the community and society that they happened to be born into than more innate aspects of self, then perhaps they can also be shaped by the culture that they live and work in.[23] Defining the need for self-care in the early stages of healthcare education and equipping students with the tools needed to self-care may help validate the issue in medical culture.

The notions of self-care and colleague care could be linked. An undertaking to work as a group 'looking out' for each other in the workplace reduces the pressure to self-care but of course only works if all workers buy-in to the idea. A move from personal private solutions to our problems towards working with others to achieve reform.[24] Acknowledging that new and emerging pressures on each generation of clinicians creates their own challenges and needs could aid this endeavour. Ballatt and Campling talk about reforming the culture of health-care through kindness or kinship. If we re-evaluate self-care as a part of kinship shared and expressed, we may have found a path forward.[25]

A range of methods have been suggested to enable critical reflection of emotional work and how it affects the healthcare workers' own emotional health, to both develop the empathic 'muscles' and as a shield to prevent burnout.[26–28] Narrative writing can be particularly effective at promoting reflective writing.[29] Bibliotherapy can offer insight and emotional context. The *House of God* is one of several novels that highlight the dehumanising effect of healthcare and offers the reader the insight that they are not alone and not failing by comparison with their peers.

Sir Theodore Fox, editor of the Lancet 1944–1965, supported the identification of general practice with a form of ethical self-cultivation.

> Never, I believe was there more need that the doctor should be a cultivated person, respected for his own sake and his knowledge of men and things, whose way of life gives him leisure and balance and a chance to reflect. Even if little can be done about it today, let us note that professional freedom should include freedom from overwork and financial anxiety on the one hand – and from too many household duties on the other.[30,31]

Fox's interpretation of continuing formative development of the primary care physician as fundamental encapsulates the idea of professional freedom in a balanced environment. The tensions of external workload pressure and lack of time to think, with no room for creativity and growth in primary care, are ever more palpable and this professional freedom is threatened. Safeguarding this freedom and space to reflect may seem, at first glance, to be a luxury. When considered in the context of ethical self-care, it can be reinterpreted as a necessity. It is every healthcare professional's responsibility to recognise the importance of self-care and strive to maintain equilibrium between their professional role and their personal care and development. The regulatory bodies of the profession and the government ought to also realise that this equi-librium is essential to running a sustainable health service, supporting it both financially and in regulatory edict. Society has a responsibility to acknowledge that healthcare workers are a valuable asset to a country's function and prosperity and ought to use such a precious resource responsibly and thoughtfully.

Healthcare professionals are people, just as those they care for. Healthcare professionals should care for themselves and their colleagues because they are people. The Kantian respect for person, 'never treat a person merely as a means, but always as an end', comes full circle.

REFERENCES

1. Foucault, M. 1994. The ethics of the concern for self as a practice of freedom. In P. Rainbow (Ed.), *Ethics: Subjectivity and Truth. Essential Works of Foucault 1954–1984.* Transl. R. Hurley et al., The New York Press, New York, p. 284.
2. Bowman, D., Spicer, J. 2007. *Primary Care Ethics.* Radcliffe Publishing, Oxford, pp. 137–147.
3. Bunting, M. 2004. *Willing Slaves: How the Overwork Culture Is Ruining Our Lives.* HarperCollins, London, p. xxvi.
4. Oxford University Hospitals NHS website. http://www.ouh.nhs.uk/about/vision-and-values/default.aspx [accessed 01 March 2016].
5. Tessman, L. 2015. *Moral Failure: On the Impossible Demands of Morality.* Oxford University Press, Oxford, p. 221.
6. Heath, I. 2008. *Matters of Life and Death: Key Writings.* Radcliffe Publishing, Oxford, p. 94.
7. Tessman, 2015, *op. cit.,* 228.
8. General Medical Council. 2013. *Good Medical Practice. Duties of a Doctor.* General Medical Council, London.
9. Gautam, M. 2011. *Irondoc: Practical Stress Management Tools for Physicians.* 2nd edition. Partner Publishing, Ottowa, Canada.
10. Tessman, 2015, *op. cit.,* 252.
11. Heyd, D. 1982. *Supererogation.* Cambridge University Press, Cambridge.
12. Shem, S. 1978. *The House of God.* Putman Publishing Group, New York.
13. NHS England website. https://www.england.nhs.uk/about/our-vision-and-purpose/imp-our-mission/high-quality-care/ [accessed 01 March 2016].
14. The Care Quality Commission. 2013. *Supporting Information and Guidance: Supporting Effective Clinical Supervision.* Care Quality Commission, Newcastle.
15. Barriball, L., While, A. and Munch, U. 2004. An audit of clinical supervision in primary care. *British Journal of Community Nursing, 9,* 389–397.
16. Halpern, J. 2003. What is clinical empathy? *Journal of General Internal Medicine, 18*(8), 670–674.
17. Hochschild, A.R. 1983. *The Managed Heart: Commercialization of Human Feeling.* University of California, London.
18. Grandey, A.A. 2000. Emotional regulation in the workplace: A new way to conceptualize emotional labor. *Journal of Occupational Health Psychology, 5*(1), 95.
19. Gross, J. 1989. Emotion expression in cancer onset and progression. *Social Science and Medicine, 28,* 1239–1248.
20. Pennebaker, J. 1990. *Opening Up: The Healing Power of Confiding in Others.* Morrow, New York.
21. Steptoe, A. 1993. Stress and the cardiovascular system: A psychosocial perspective. In S.C. Stanford and P. Salmon (Eds.), *Stress: From Synapse to Syndrome* (pp. 119–141). Academic Press, London.

22. Kerasidou, A. and Horn, R. 2016. Making space for empathy: Supporting doctors in the emotional labour of clinical care. *BMC Medical Ethics*. Volume 17:8, p. 10.

23. Burton, N. 2010. *The Art of Failure: The Anti Self-Help Guide*. Acheron Press, Oxford, pp. 77–78.

24. Bunting, 2004, *op. cit.*, xxv.

25. Ballatt, J. and Campling, P. 2011. *Intelligent Kindness: Reforming the Culture of Healthcare*. RCPsych Publications, London.

26. Halpern, J. 2001. *From Detached Concern to Empathy: Humanizing Medical Practice*. Oxford University Press, Oxford.

27. Wald, H.S. and Reis, S.P. 2010. Beyond the margins: Reflective writing and development of reflective capacity in medical education. *Journal of General Internal Medicine, 25*(7), 746–749.

28. Schön, D.A. 1983. *The Reflective Practitioner: How Professionals Think in Action* (Vol. 5126). Basic Books, New York.

29. Charon, R. 2001. Narrative medicine: A model for empathy, reflection, profession, and trust. *JAMA, 286*(15), 1897–1902.

30. Hayward, R. 2014. *The Transformation of the Psyche in British Primary Care, 1880–1970*. A&C Black, London, p. 111.

31. Fox, T.F. 1965. *Purposes of Medicine [The Harveian Oration for 1965]*. RCP, London.

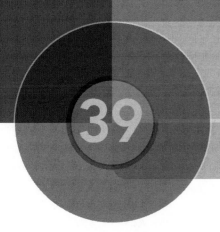

Global primary care ethics

39

BRIDGET KIELY AND CARWYN RHYS HOOPER

INTRODUCTION

Since the beginning of the Industrial Revolution, the world has witnessed a remarkable transformation in human health. For most of human history, average life expectancy is believed to have hovered around 35 years and many people lived lives that conformed to Hobbes' infamous description: 'nasty, brutish and short'. However, rapid improvements in hygiene and healthcare during the modern era had a revolutionary effect on human well-being and by the end of the twentieth century, well over half the people of the world lived in countries where life expectancy was over three score and 10 years.[1]

This has been an extraordinary achievement, but improvements in global life expectancy have been deeply uneven and a significant disparity continues to exist between high- and low-income countries. Life expectancy in Malawi remains almost half that of Japan, and people born in sub-Saharan Africa live, on average, for 20 years less than their European counterparts.[2] Much of these differences can be attributed to childhood (especially under five) mortality. In Chile, for example, the under 5 mortality rate is about 10 per 1000 live births, but in Cote d'Ivoire it is closer to 100 per 1000 live births.[2] Inequalities in maternal mortality are equally stark and also contribute significantly to global inequalities in life expectancy. The difference between maternal mortality in Slovenia (~10 per 100,000 live births) and Sierra Leone (~1400 per 100,000 live births) neatly illustrates this point.[3] The reasons for these gross inequalities in maternal and childhood mortality are many and complex. However, part of the explanation is that healthcare, especially basic primary care, is not easily available, accessible or affordable in the poorest parts of the world. Indeed, the majority of women in sub-Saharan Africa still give birth without a skilled birth attendant.[2]

In this chapter, we argue that there is a growing and overlapping consensus that the most egregious examples of global health inequalities must be rectified. We will also defend the empirical claim that affordable and accessible primary care service is a necessary, if not sufficient, condition for improving the health of the globally worst-off. Finally, we will discuss how primary care professionals in high-income countries can help ensure that basic primary care is available to all.

THE ETHICAL IMPERATIVE TO IMPROVE GLOBAL HEALTH

Few would deny that the world would be a better place if everyone had the opportunity to live a long and healthy life.[4] Most would also agree that there is something morally warped about a world where a million children die on the day they are born.[5] However, although there is widespread agreement that there is something seriously awry about a world where so many poverty-stricken people die very prematurely, there has traditionally been less agreement about the moral necessity to do something about this appalling state of affairs. The main reason for this is because significant changes to the global order, including a significant redistribution of global resources, are needed to create and maintain a physical and social environment that would enable most people to live reasonably long and healthy lives.

It is true that some people have long held the view that there is an ethical imperative to ensure that the worst-off are helped irrespective of the scale of the changes that this would necessitate at the global level. The best-known advocate of this idea is Peter Singer. In brief, Singer argues that we should prevent morally bad things from happening if we are capable of doing so and if we do not sacrifice anything of comparable moral importance in the process. This is a demanding philosophy, but it is difficult to argue that there are many material goods whose moral value outweigh the value of a child's life. In other words, if we take Singer's central claim seriously, we will be hard-pressed to avoid the conclusion that a significant redistribution of global resources is morally necessary. And even if we adopt Singer's less radical version of his central claim, it still seems highly likely that there was a strict obligation to ameliorate the very worst examples of global health inequalities.[6]

Singer's uncompromisingly utilitarian outlook is probably unrivalled in its contemporary radicalism. However, a number of deontologists have also defended the claim that there is a moral imperative to help the worse-off even if this requires significant global changes. Thomas Pogge, in particular, has put forward a powerful argument that some developed nations historically caused significant harm to less developed nations (e.g. via the slave trade) and that many of them continue to cause harm by creating and imposing a world order that disadvantages the worst-off. He goes on to argue that those who inflict harm must stop doing so and must provide some kind of restitution for the harm that they have already perpetrated.[7] This argument is less radical than the utilitarian argument discussed above because it is an implication of this deontological worldview that no one is obliged to rectify gross inequalities in global health unless they have been caused by injustices. Nevertheless, in a world where historical and contemporary rights violations are pervasive, the scale of the redistribution of global resources that Pogge's arguments demand is still very significant – and certainly sufficiently significant to necessitate remedying the situation of the worst-off.

Many people find either Peter Singer's or Thomas Pogge's arguments very compelling. However, not everyone accepts the premises of their arguments or the far-reaching conclusions they draw. Risse, for example, takes aim at the empirical claim that the global poor are harmed by the global order and tries to argue that the global order actually benefits the global poor.[8] Other philosophers object to Singer and Pogge's cosmopolitanism – that is, the idea that all human beings are, or should be, citizens of one community. Non-cosmopolitans offer different reasons why cosmopolitanism, especially in its strict form, is untenable, but the claim that tends to unite this group is that the duties that we owe to compatriots are often superior to the duties we owe to non-compatriots.[9]

Nevertheless, although there remains much philosophical resistance to the stronger claims of cosmopolitanism, there is a growing and overlapping consensus in the bioethical community that there is an ethical imperative to tackle the very worst examples of global health inequalities. This was evidenced, to an extent, during the recent Ebola epidemic when bioethicists of many different normative stripes argued that it was morally incumbent on the world as a whole to spend the resources that were needed to tackle the problem.[10,11]

There are a number of reasons for this normative shift towards accepting some core duties to the very worst off. Firstly, there is recognition that the costs of changing the global order to significantly improve the lives of the very worst-off are not as substantial as was once thought. This is not to say that the investments needed to solve the worse problems are negligible, but the relative success of the United Nations (UN) Millennium Development Goals neatly demonstrates what can be done with relatively little resource redistribution.[12]

Secondly, there is a better understanding that seemingly local problems that are often associated with regional poverty can cause global harm. Severe Acute Respiratory Syndrome (SARS), the H1N1 virus, Ebola and Zika have all recently demonstrated that a failure to monitor and control outbreaks of novel infectious disease in poorer regions of the world can wreak considerable human and economic damage all over the world.[13–16] This means that more developed nations that wish to protect their own interests and the human rights of their own citizens need to assist less-developed countries to develop their healthcare and disease surveillance systems. If they do not, global security will be under threat and even wealthy nation states will be unable to fulfil the normative duties they owe to their own citizens.

Thirdly, those who are committed to the idea that beneficent duties to help others, or the demands of distributive justice, primarily apply to groups or communities of people that interact and trade with each other have started to wake up to the nature and scale of globalisation. Almost every country on earth is now deeply embedded in the global economy, and this means that most people are now directly or indirectly affected by the rules of global trade and global institutions like the World Trade Organization. Even more importantly, the very poor are often significantly affected by these global governance and trade rules without having much, if any, say about them. Globalisation, in other words, has brought almost everyone into a closer social, and, thus, normative, relationship. Indeed, it is partly for this kind of reason that Beitz[17] believes that Rawls' famous principles of distributive justice, including the difference principle, should apply across the global community, not just within the borders of different sovereign states.

We do not wish to overstate the case. There are still some people who reject the claim that there is a strict moral obligation to help even the worst-off. There also remains much debate as to where the duty to provide the opportunity for health falls – that is, whether the duty bearer should be individual agents, national governments or the international community as a whole. However, many people now accept that we must help the worst-off, especially if we have harmed them. And, as the forces of globalisation advance – and as the social, cultural and economic ties between nation states grow – it seems highly likely that ever more people will come to accept that the worst examples of global health inequalities are not simply morally repugnant, but that there are strict ethical requirements to rectify them. This, incidentally, will be a great boon to policymakers, activists and healthcare professionals because a broad and overlapping agreement that there is an imperative to act will allow more people to focus on the best methods to eradicate the worst instances of global health inequalities instead of being distracted by the more fundamental question of whether there is a moral requirement to do anything in the first place.

EMPIRICAL EVIDENCE FOR GLOBAL PRIMARY CARE

It would be foolish to claim that the only way to reduce global health inequalities is through the provision of healthcare. Equitable access to healthcare is one of the wider determinants of health and is required along with a range of other measures to address current health inequalities.[18] This is also recognised by the World Health Organisation (WHO), which states that health 'is a fundamental human right and that the attainment of the highest possible level of health is a most important world-wide social goal whose realization requires the action of many other social and economic sectors in addition to the health sector'.[19]

Four decades ago, the WHO Alma Ata Declaration identified universal access to primary care, as part of a comprehensive national health system, as an important factor in ensuring equal opportunity to reach a level of health that would allow people to live economically and socially productive lives.[19] Having a primary care–based system also allows more equitable access, through geographical accessibility and by providing a health service that can meet the individual needs of the local population, and not only disease-specific or age-specific services. While access to HIV treatment is vital, if systems are just built around a single disease, this leaves people with other diseases, such as diabetes, with little access to treatment. There has been a great focus on reducing child mortality, but going forward, this should not be at the expense of the healthcare needs of older people. Primary care offers a holistic person-based approach, providing care from the cradle to the grave. There is increasing empirical evidence that these attributes of primary care contribute to its effectiveness in reducing mortality, reducing hospital admissions, improved user satisfaction and overall more effective use of resources.[20] Recent evidence also supports the idea that healthcare systems with primary care at their core are the most effective and equitable means of achieving global health.[21]

Despite the WHO declaration and the evidence supporting the generalist approach of primary care, 400 million people still lack access to primary care, and many attempts to develop primary care systems instead focus on a package of basic care, concentrating on priority diseases and age groups, rather than a generalist approach.[22] Often 'primary care' posts in low- and middle-income countries are staffed by healthcare workers with limited training, isolated from the rest of the systems, and are only equipped to deal with a limited range of acute ailments, rather than provide preventative services or ongoing care for long-term conditions.[20]

Resource constraints have been the main drivers of this approach, with the argument that it is better to treat some rather than none, but one of the advantages of primary care is that it provides a trusted source of first contact with the health system. To trust a system, people have to believe that it will address their needs, whatever they may be. There is increasing concern that this approach can reduce trust in the overall health system, perhaps violating one of the founding principles of health ethics.[23] Without this trust, people turn to alternative unregulated private providers or traditional healers, possibly delaying access to appropriate care, fragmenting the system and weakening the surveillance capacity of the national health system. This problem was all too apparent during the recent Ebola outbreak in West Africa, with people staying at home or visiting traditional healers, delaying diagnosis and allowing more members of their community to be exposed to the virus.[24] People also need to trust a system in order to present for preventative care. The consequences of untreated hypertension are all too apparent in lower middle-income countries with rising incidence of heart attack and stroke, now counting for an increasing number of years of life lost.[2]

While good primary care is not cheap, it is certainly more cost-effective than a system relying on hospital-based specialists alone and provides more equitable access, particularly for rural populations, who may otherwise lack access to healthcare professionals. Primary care is the hub from which patients are guided through the health system.

The National Health Service (NHS) system is one of the strongest primary care–based systems in the world, and despite having fewer doctors per head of population and spending less than the Organization for Economic Cooperation and Development (OECD) average, provides an, equitable and effective service,[21] providing at least one of the conditions necessary for the equal opportunity to live a reasonably healthy life. All the evidence supports that a person centred holistic approach and continuity of care are key in building the trust needed for an effective system, in turn an important step in reducing global health inequalities.[20,25] Knowing this, we do not think it is acceptable that primary care in low- and middle-income countries can be interpreted differently and delivered in a more limited way.

GLOBAL PRIMARY CARE ACTIVISM

We have argued in the previous section that there is an ethical imperative to help the globally worst-off and that the provision of adequate primary care may well be the most effective 'healthcare delivery' means of tackling the worst examples of health inequalities. As mentioned previously, the NHS has a strong primary care system at its core and has been hailed as one of the most equitable and effective systems in the world.[21] Primary care professionals working in such a system are uniquely placed to assist in the development of a truly global provision of primary care and, thus, to have an impact on global health inequalities. However, although primary care professionals who have a very cosmopolitan outlook will likely believe that they have strong duties to the globally worse-off, others will reasonably argue that due to their obligations to patients in their own country, they can only play a limited role abroad. We accept that the demands of caring for one's own patients mean that the amount of time available to care for others is often severely limited. However, we believe that it is incumbent on all primary care professionals to advocate for importance of primary care at home and on the global stage. This is crucial in order to ensure that primary care receives adequate recognition and funding and that the drive to achieve access for all is maintained.

While making the argument for the ethical imperative to reduce global health inequalities, we have mainly focused on changes and improvements in low-income countries, but neither the issues nor the benefits are solely in lower-income countries. While seen as a key enabler for further reductions in health inequalities globally, universal access to healthcare is a current political debate in the United Kingdom, with increasingly restricted access to primary healthcare for certain migrant groups.[26] Fees for access are being suggested, but this runs the risk of reducing access amongst the most vulnerable groups and disproportionately affecting preventative healthcare.[27] This debate affects primary care professionals daily. The importance of advocacy for vulnerable groups is just as important in Europe as it is in Africa. Advocacy can extend beyond a practitioner's direct patient population to a more global perspective. From casual conversations with colleagues and peers, posting on social media, writing articles for medical journals and the mainstream media to lobbying professional groups and MPs to take a more active role, there are multiple ways for individuals to improve other people's understanding of global health issues. And all this can be done without having to travel abroad.

For those who are in a position to travel and who are of a cosmopolitan bent, working overseas, particularly in low-income countries, allows the opportunity to not only model primary care through direct service provision but also to teach and develop longer-term partnerships. There are a variety of opportunities for overseas work at different career stages. Overseas electives in lower-income countries have been seen as the classic opportunity to actively participate in global health. In the past, there has been a certain lack of continuity, so important in primary care, and sometimes a missed opportunity to share learning and nurture it beyond the elective experience, but UK medical schools are now forming partnerships with healthcare institutions to foster continuity and reciprocity.[28]

During training, an out-of-programme experience provides an excellent opportunity to contribute to improving primary care capacity internationally. With modern technology, the contribution does not have to end once back on home soil. Ever increasing access to mobile phones and the internet globally means peer support can continue from afar. Several general practitioner (GP) schools and the Royal College of General Practitioners have organised placements with international partners for both trainees and qualified GPs.[29,30] The partnership model is gaining increasing attention as a way to share expertise in a way that develops capacity and long-term sustainability.[31,32] Later, in the career path, GP tutors, trainers and programme directors are well positioned to promote the global primary care agenda to students and trainees and to support them to partake in their own activism at whatever level they can.

CONCLUSION

A number of different normative theories can be relied upon to provide an ethical defence of the necessity of tackling the worst instances of global health inequalities. Indeed, there is now a broad and overlapping consensus in the bioethical community that something must be done about these inequalities. The evidence suggests that global health inequalities cannot be tackled without universal access to healthcare, incorporating primary care. There are a number of different ways that primary care professionals based in high-income countries can get involved in reducing global health inequalities. We hope that we have convinced readers that it is a moral necessity to remedy some global health inequalities, that affordable and effective primary care is an essential enabling tool to achieve this aim and that there are myriad ways in which primary care professionals in high-income countries can help make this aim a reality.

REFERENCES

1. World Bank. Statistics *WorldBank* [Internet]. 2015 [cited 2015 Feb 24]. Available from: http://data.worldbank.org/indicator/SP.DYN.LE00.IN
2. WHO. *World Health Organisation Health Statistics 2014* [Internet]. 2014 [cited 2015 Nov 28]. Available from: http://apps.who.int/iris/bitstream/10665/112738/1/9789240692671_eng.pdf?ua=1
3. World Bank. *Maternal Mortality Ratio (Modeled Estimate, per 100,000 Live Births) | Data | Table* [Internet]. 2015 [cited 2015 Nov 28]. Available from: http://data.worldbank.org/indicator/SH.STA.MMRT
4. Whitehead M. The concepts and principles of equity and health. *Int J Health Serv.* 1992;22(3):429–45.
5. UNICEF. *Levels and Trends in Child Mortality* [Internet]. 2014. 2014 [cited 2015 Nov 28]. Available from: http://www.unicef.org/media/files/Levels_and_Trends_in_Child_Mortality_2014.pdf
6. Singer P. Famine, affluence, and morality. *Philos Public Aff.* 1972;1(3):229–43.

7. Pogge TW. *World Poverty and Human Rights* [Internet]. 2nd ed. Polity; 2007 [cited 2016 Feb 24]. Available from: http://www.polity.co.uk/book.asp?ref=9780745641430

8. Risse M. Do we owe the global poor assistance or rectification? *Ethics Int Aff.* 2012;19(01):9–18. Cambridge University Press.

9. Rawls J. *The Law of Peoples.* Harvard University Press; 1999.

10. Rid A, Emanuel EJ. Why should high-income countries help combat Ebola? *JAMA.* 2014;312(13):1297–8.

11. Caplan A. Morality in a Time of Ebola [Internet]. *Lancet.* 2015 [cited 2016 Feb 24]. Available from: http://www.newsu.org/course_files/SRIpdfResources/Morality_in_a_Time_of_Ebola_The_Lancet.pdf

12. UN. *The Millenium Development Goals Report* [Internet]. 2015 [cited 2016 Feb 24]. Available from: http://www.un.org/millenniumgoals/2015_MDG_Report/pdf/MDG 2015 rev (July 1).pdf

13. Lee J-W, McKibbin WJ. *Estimating the Global Economic Costs of SARS* [Internet]. National Academies Press (US); 2004 [cited 2016 Feb 24]. Available from: http://www.ncbi.nlm.nih.gov/books/NBK92473/

14. Khan K, Arino J, Hu W, Raposo P, Sears J, Calderon F, et al. Spread of a novel influenza A (H1N1) virus via global airline transportation. *N Engl J Med* [Internet]. 2009 [cited 2016 Feb 24];361:212–14. Available from: http://www.nejm.org/doi/full/10.1056/NEJMc0904559

15. World Bank. *The Economic Impact of Ebola on Sub-Saharan Africa: Updated Estimates for 2015* [Internet]. 2015 [cited 2016 Feb 24]. Available from: http://www.preventionweb.net/files/42039_wbebola.pdf

16. World Bank. *The Short-Term Economic Costs of Zika in Latin America and the Caribbean* [Internet]. 2016 [cited 2016 Feb 24]. Available from: http://pubdocs.worldbank.org/pubdocs/publicdoc/2016/2/410321455758564708/The-short-term-economic-costs-of-Zika-in-LCR-final-doc-autores-feb-18.pdf

17. Beitz CR. *Political Theory and International Relations (Revised Edition) (eBook and Paperback)* [Internet]. Revised. Princeton University Press; 1999 [cited 2016 Feb 24]. Available from: http://press.princeton.edu/titles/6606.html

18. Marmot M, Bell R. Fair society, healthy lives. *Public Health.* 2012;126(Suppl):S4–10.

19. WHO. *Declaration of Alma-Ata in 1978.* Available from: http://www.who.int/publications/almaata_declaration_en.pdf

20. WHO. *Primary Health Care: Now More than Ever* [Internet]. 2008 [cited 2015 Nov 28]. Available from: http://www.who.int/whr/2008/whr08_en.pdf

21. CommonwealthFund. *Mirror, Mirror on the Wall* [Internet]. Commonwealth Fund; 2014 [cited 2015 May 25]. Available from: http://www.commonwealthfund.org/~/media/files/publications/fund-report/2014/jun/1755_davis_mirror_mirror_2014.pdf

22. WHO, World Bank. *Tracking Universal Health Coverage: First Global Monitoring Report* [Internet]. 2015 [cited 2016 Feb 28]. Available from: http://apps.who.int/iris/bitstream/10665/174536/1/9789241564977_eng.pdf

23. Macfarlane S, Racelis M, Muli-Muslime F. Public health in developing countries. *Lancet.* 2000;356(9232):841–6.

24. WHO. *One Year into the Ebola Epidemic: A Deadly, Tenacious and Unforgiving Virus* [Internet]. 2015 [cited 2016 Feb 28]. Available from: http://www.who.int/csr/disease/ebola/one-year-report/ebola-report-1-year.pdf

25. Starfield B, Shi L, Macinko J. Contribution of primary care to health systems and health. *Milbank Q.* 2005;83(3):457–502.

26. Keith L, van Ginneken E. Restricting access to the NHS for undocumented migrants is bad policy at high cost. *BMJ*. 2015;350:h3056.

27. Gertler P, van der Gaag J. *The Willingness to Pay for Medical Care: Evidence from Two Developing Countries*. 1990 [cited 2015 Jun 14]; pp. 1–154. Available from: http://documents.worldbank.org/curated/en/1990/11/440593/ willingness-pay-medical-care-evidence-two-developing-countries

28. King's College London. *King's College London—International Partners—Exchange & Elective Placements* [Internet]. 2016 [cited 2016 Feb 28]. Available from: http://www.kcl. ac.uk/lsm/education/meded/mbbs/electives/index.aspx

29. Reardon C, George G, Enigbokan O. The benefits of working abroad for British General Practice trainee doctors: The London deanery out of programme experience in South Africa. *BMC Med Educ*. 2015;15:174.

30. RCGP. *International Work* [Internet]. 2014 [cited 2016 Feb 28]. Available from: http:// www.rcgp.org.uk/support-our-work/international-work.aspx

31. Crisp N. *Global Health Partnerships: The UK Contribution to Health in Developing Countries* [Internet]. 2007 [cited 2016 Feb 28]. Available from: file:///C:/Users/Bridget/Downloads/ Global health partnerships - Crisp 2007 (1).pdf

32. Syed SB, Dadwal V, Rutter P, Storr J, Hightower JD, Gooden R, et al. Developed-developing country partnerships: Benefits to developed countries? *Global Health*. 2012;8(1):17.

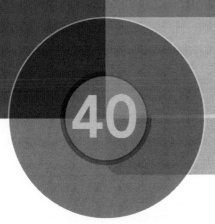

Primary care, the basic necessity: Part I: Explorations in economics

MALCOLM TORRY

INTRODUCTION

Healthcare systems come in all shapes and sizes: differently funded, and differently organised. This chapter employs the science of economics to explore different ways of paying for and distributing healthcare resources, and in particular evaluates the UK National Health Service (NHS) in terms of its economics. Throughout, we shall be particularly interested in the role of primary care practitioners, by which we mean general practitioners (GPs), practice nurses and all of the other members of primary care teams.

DIFFERENT METHODS OF FUNDING HEALTHCARE PROVISION

Healthcare absorbs resources, which must be provided as free gifts or in exchange for other resources – which, in a developed economy, means money. We'll come to the free gifts later. Here, we will explore a variety of different ways in which we might pay healthcare providers so that they can pay for the labour and other resources that healthcare requires. The funding mechanisms that we shall consider are donations, membership fees, payment per item, insurance premiums and taxation.

1. *Donations:* Poverty relief charities, churches and food banks rely almost entirely on donations. In past centuries, this is how many hospitals were funded. There are several drawbacks to this funding method: it is difficult to predict the amount of money that will come in, so planning is difficult; the amount coming in might be entirely inadequate to the demand that the organisation experiences; and people and organisations are more likely to donate to local provision rather than to national provision, so either national provision will be underfunded or local provision will be better in wealthier areas and worse in poorer areas. To pay for healthcare across the UK by inviting donations would be a risky option.

2. *Membership fees:* Trades unions, and roadside assistance organisations, obtain the money to pay for the resources that they need by charging membership fees. Leisure centres

and art galleries use a mixture of membership fees and payment per visit to fund their activities. These organisations are clubs,[1] which either exclude non-members from the services provided or include them on a pay-per-item basis (on which see below). In the UK, before the NHS was established, primary care gathered the majority of the resources that it needed by charging membership fees.

To fund today's healthcare via membership fees would mean that individuals who chose not to pay, or who were unable to pay, would be without healthcare; that it would be difficult to predict the amount of money coming in, so planning would be difficult; and that during an economic downturn, fewer people would be able to pay membership fees, so fewer resources would be available for healthcare and more people would be without it. Many organisations charge lower membership fees for groups of people likely to have less money, and the same mechanism could apply to healthcare; but the standard membership fee would still be higher than many employed adults could afford. In order to include every citizen, and to make the membership fee affordable, the fee would need to be made compulsory, and it would need to be calculated on an affordability basis. It would then be a tax (see below).

3. *Payment per item:* If I want to own a car, then I have to pay the price demanded by the vendor. Healthcare providers could obtain the resources that they need by charging per visit to a doctor or nurse, per day in hospital, per operation, and so on. There are two main problems connected with this method: the first is the additional costs generated by the administrative requirement to divide up healthcare into chargeable units; and the second is that the product being purchased is often difficult to define before the event. If I am ill, then it will often be far from clear how many visits to a doctor will be required, how many days I shall need to spend in hospital and precisely which operations will be needed. The situation will be more like that faced by someone instructing a lawyer in a civil case. Neither the litigant nor the lawyer will know how many hours of the lawyer's time will be required. The difference is that the litigant can decide to cut their losses and abandon the action if costs become unaffordable, whereas someone undergoing an operation might not be in a position to decline two weeks in a hospital bed. A more important problem is that the wealthy would be able to afford the healthcare that they need, whereas the poor would be unable to do so.

4. *Insurance premiums:* If I own a house, then I am wise to insure it. I pay premiums to an insurance company, and in return the company promises to pay any costs related to a variety of eventualities. If the house burns down, then the insurance company will pay to rebuild it – something that I would probably not be able to do myself. An insurance company is a mechanism for sharing risks. I cannot predict whether my own house will burn down or not. If the insurance company insures a sufficient number of houses, then it will be able to predict fairly confidently the number of houses that will burn down, and it will be able to set insurance premiums high enough to enable it to rebuild houses that burn down, as well as low enough to enable it to compete with other insurance companies.

Healthcare can be funded in the same way. An insurance company can charge premiums, and then pay the costs of healthcare for its customers. I cannot predict my own healthcare costs, but if an insurance company has a sufficient number of policyholders, then it will be able to predict the total healthcare costs fairly accurately and will be able to set the level of premiums accordingly. Risks will be shared.

However, the two situations are not the same. The task of rebuilding a house is well defined; what the insurer will pay for is generally well defined; and the householder, the insurance company and the builder rebuilding the house will all have access to similar information about what it takes to rebuild a house and about the cost of doing so. The task of solving someone's health problems is generally less well defined, the costs will be unpredictable, the scope for the interpretation of the terms of an insurance policy will be considerable, and the healthcare provider will possess more knowledge than either the individual or the insurance company,[2] and it is the healthcare provider that will be making the decisions as to what is to be done and paid for – and that provider might be influenced in their decisions by pharmaceutical company marketing techniques.[3] The healthcare provider will be tempted to undertake procedures and to provide drugs that might not be necessary, the insurance company will have little ability to question the decisions and their costs, and premiums will therefore be higher than they ought to be. If the company distributes profits to shareholders, then that will be an additional cost to be met by higher premiums, as will be the cost of the administrative controls required to restrain expenditure and to package the healthcare provided into chargeable units.[4] The result is premiums higher than they would be if everyone possessed the same information, if profits were not distributed to shareholders, and if no revenue-related administrative costs were being charged. Some people would be able to afford the premiums, but others would not be able to do so and would be deprived of healthcare.

A separate problem is that the insurance company will make its own decisions as to what it will pay for and what it will not. Such decisions will be taken on the grounds of the level and predictability of costs, rather than on the grounds of the individual's healthcare needs. The result will be that some insured individuals will find that they have healthcare needs that will not be met.

Insurance-based healthcare systems thus result in some people receiving more healthcare than they need, and often more than is good for them; some individuals having their simpler healthcare needs met, but not their more chronic and complex needs; and some individuals finding themselves entirely without healthcare.

Some of these problems are avoided by the kind of public insurance-based schemes found in such European countries as France and German, where the funds are managed by partnerships between government, trades unions and employers. Here, an added complication is the complexity of the relationship between the medical profession, the state and the other social partners.[5]

5. *Taxation:* To tax individuals according to the ability to pay, and to use some of the proceeds to provide healthcare free at the point of use for everyone, avoids all of the problems encountered with the four funding methods listed above. It provides a secure source of income for healthcare providers; the amount of healthcare available is relatively predictable; nobody is excluded from healthcare; everybody receives the healthcare that they need; provision can be consistent across the country; those who can afford to pay more are paying more, and those who can afford to pay little are paying little; and healthcare providers do not benefit financially by doing more than necessary for a patient, so they are not tempted to do so.

METHODS FOR RATIONING HEALTHCARE

There is one problem that tax-funded healthcare does not solve, but it is a problem that is common to every payment and distribution mechanism, so it should not be held against universal healthcare paid for through taxation. The problem is this: most individuals could absorb more healthcare than they currently do, so there will always be unmet demand. A growing and ageing population increases demand for healthcare provision, and new drugs and procedures are invented all the time, again increasing the demand. So the question is this: Given that resources are always limited, and that demand is already large and continues to grow, how is healthcare to be distributed?

Some funding methods function as rationing mechanisms. Membership fees might be unaffordable, so those who could not pay them would not consume healthcare resources. Similarly, insurance premiums and payment per item can be unaffordable for many, again restricting healthcare to those who can afford to pay. However, if healthcare is funded by donations or by taxation, and healthcare resources are free to every citizen, then how can distribution of limited resources be controlled so that the total amount provided remains affordable? There are several possible methods:

- Bulk purchasing can ensure that prices charged by such healthcare providers as pharmaceutical companies can be controlled, and can insulate practitioners from pharmaceutical company marketing techniques, thus reducing costs and enabling more healthcare to be provided for the same amount of money.[6]
- More expensive healthcare can be banned, so that more of the cheaper healthcare can be provided.
- Clinicians in both primary and secondary care can be trained and encouraged not to prescribe treatments that offer marginal or no benefit to the patient.[7,8]
- Time intervals between healthcare events can be lengthened, thus spreading demand into the future.
- A limited supply of a particular healthcare resource can be rationed (for instance, GP or practice nurse appointments).
- A gatekeeper can decide which healthcare resources will be available to each patient.

In the UK, the National Institute for Health and Care Excellence (NICE) is responsible for price control, and NICE and commissioners are responsible for deciding which treatments will be available on the NHS. Waiting times between appointments and for operations can be lengthened or shortened as supply falls or rises in relation to demand, and general practices will construct appointments systems to distribute a restricted supply of GP and practice nurse time. In relation to secondary care and other healthcare provision, GPs, nurses, receptionists and other primary care staff act as gatekeepers in most non-emergency circumstances, and in that capacity they make decisions about individual patient's consumption of healthcare resources. Many patients will experience all of these distribution methods in relation to a health problem: difficulty with getting a GP appointment, a GP deciding what treatment they need and what treatment they do not, a waiting list for consultants' appointments, a waiting list for operations, NICE deciding which drugs will be available, and the local commissioner deciding which healthcare resources will be commissioned and which will not be.

There are two new challenges to all of these rationing methods:

- 'Political consumerism': patient groups, including internet-based groups, demanding their own choice of treatment[9]
- An increasing understanding of healthcare as a commodity rather than as a public service.[10] Public services are understood to be subject to democratic control, whereas commodities are subject to consumer demand.

For the system to continue working, the mechanism by which rationing is applied must be trusted by patients. This requires the rationing agents – primary care practitioners – to be independent of the political process, so that their choices over which healthcare resources to employ are experienced as healthcare decisions and not as political ones. It is therefore essential for governments to permit the profession to self-regulate – a situation that the profession will generally achieve anyway, because it is in possession of a knowledge base (a 'technology') that government ministers and officials do not possess, and a situation that the government will in any case prefer because it leaves it free to make policy without too much interference from a self-interested profession.[11,12] Another requirement might be that government ministers and officials should avoid calling patients 'consumers'.

Already we are seeing how crucial primary care is to the economics of any healthcare system, and particularly to a universal tax-funded one, and how important it will be for primary care consciously to update its essential gatekeeping function in light of new challenges.

HYBRID SYSTEMS

The United States and various other countries have hybrid systems: insurance-based healthcare for those who can afford it, and a publicly funded system for those who cannot. As Richard Titmuss suggested, this results in a poor public service.[13] Only a service used by everyone will have the necessary democratic pressure behind it to ensure high quality and adequate funding.

But doesn't the UK have its own hybrid system? Yes, in two senses.

First of all, working-age adults have to pay towards the costs of prescriptions, dentistry and optician services, on a payment-per-item basis, unless they are deemed as not able to afford to do so. These are the parts of the healthcare system that it is possible to means test. We in the UK have been means-testing benefits since the Elizabethan era Poor Law, so we find it hard to resist giving a benefit and then withdrawing it as earnings rise, even though means-testing is highly inefficient. However, as we have seen, payment per item is a means of rationing healthcare provision, so for those who are earning sufficient to be paying for their prescriptions, spectacles, dentistry and visits to the optometrist, two rationing mechanisms are being operated: the primary care practitioner, dentist or optometrist deciding what healthcare is required, and the cost of the prescription, dentistry, eye test or spectacles.

Secondly, alongside the NHS we have a substantial private healthcare system, both insurance-based and paid per item, and often closely integrated with the NHS in terms of staffing and contracts (increasing numbers of NHS procedures are being contracted out to private healthcare providers). Is this a problem? In one sense no, and in another sense yes. As long as healthcare remains universal and free at the point of use, a parallel system is not a problem, but if too many people obtain healthcare through the private system, then there will be less political pressure – particularly from the middle classes – for the NHS to be adequately funded and of high quality. If too much NHS healthcare is provided by the private sector, and less by public sector organisations, and if the private sector does the easy bits and leaves the difficult bits to the public sector, then the public sector will cease to reap economies of scale, it will end up managing the more complex and more costly healthcare, and inefficiency will be the result, even if the price for each procedure looks similar in the public and private sectors. NHS healthcare has always involved private sector organisations – contracted out services in hospitals, and general practice partnerships, going back to the beginning of the NHS; but, as we shall see in chapter 41, there are good reasons for primary care being provided by partnerships, and there will clearly be efficiency savings if a private laundry is doing the laundry for lots of different hospitals rather than every hospital having its own laundry. It's the detail that matters, and it's the extent of private sector involvement that matters. So yes, the UK's dual system does matter.

A GIFT RELATIONSHIP

To return to the option of providing healthcare resources via voluntary donations, this method might be somewhat risky as the main source of resources, but that is no reason not to employ it as an important element. In the UK, blood is donated free of charge by millions of people in their own or their employers' time,[14,*] hospitals rely on armies of volunteers to undertake tasks for which paid staff are not available (in transport, shops, chaplaincy and much else) and hospices rely on massive voluntary effort for staffing and fundraising. It is of course difficult to calculate the value of this voluntary provision, simply because it is provided entirely free of charge; but it is clear that the withdrawal of all of this voluntary effort would impose substantial additional costs on healthcare providers. So, an important question is this: Would this voluntary effort be provided if the NHS was not a universal service free at the point of use? It is perhaps significant that in the United States blood is often paid for.

Let us suppose that in the UK healthcare resources were provided via insurance premiums, payment per item or membership fees. There would be no sense in which society as a whole was providing healthcare for society as a whole, and companies would be making profits and distributing them to shareholders. Volunteers would understand their donation of time and energy as a cost-saving to companies. Potential volunteers would be likely to donate their time and money elsewhere.

In the UK, healthcare is provided free to every legal resident. This invites a reciprocal response, particularly from those who have received high-quality, high-cost healthcare and haven't had to pay for it. The massive amount of voluntary activity that the NHS attracts is just one more reason for providing healthcare universally, and free at the point of use.

CONCLUSIONS

I have argued that a healthcare service that is universal and free at the point of use is economically efficient. This suggests that healthcare in the UK should remain universal and free at the point of use. I have also shown that primary care is an essential rationing mechanism. This means that any discussion of healthcare planning, NHS funding or the education of future healthcare professionals, should begin with primary care, and only then move on to the other parts of the service. The argument as a whole suggests that other countries should consider establishing healthcare systems that are universal and free at the point of use, and should ensure that primary care is at the heart of those systems.

REFERENCES

1. Hindriks J and Myles GD. *Intermediate Public Economics*. The MIT Press, Cambridge, MA, 2006, pp. 145–160.
2. Ibid., 251–291.
3. Brody H. *Hooked: Ethics, the Medical Profession, and the Pharmaceutical Industry*. Rowman and Littlefield, Lanham, MD, 2007.

---

* In the UK, there are 1.3 million registered blood donors: www.nhsbt.nhs.uk/what-we-do/blood-donation/

4. Hart JT. *The Political Economy of Health Care: A Clinical Perspective*. Policy Press, Bristol, 2006, pp. 28–29.
5. Salter B. *The New Politics of Medicine*. Palgrave Macmillan, Basingstoke, 2004, p. 29.
6. Hart, 2006, *op. cit.*, 28.
7. Brody H. From an Ethics of Rationing to an Ethics of Waste Avoidance. *The New England Journal of Medicine*, Vol. 366, no. 21, 2012, pp. 1949–1951.
8. Brody H. Talking with Patients about Cost Containment. *Journal of General Internal Medicine*, Vol. 29, no. 1, 2013, pp. 5–6.
9. Salter B, Zhou Y and Datta S. Hegemony in the Marketplace of Biomedical Innovation: Consumer Demand and Stem Cell Science. *Social Science and Medicine*, Vol. 131, 2015, pp. 156–163.
10. Hart, 2006, *op. cit.*, 7.
11. Salter, 2004, *op. cit.*, 26–7, 154–16.
12. Hasenfeld Y (ed.). *Human Services as Complex Organisations*. Sage, London, 1992, p. 10.
13. Titmuss R. *Commitment to Welfare*. George Allen and Unwin, London, 1968, p. 134.
14. Titmuss R. *The Gift Relationship: From Human Blood to Social Policy*. Allen and Unwin, London, 1970.

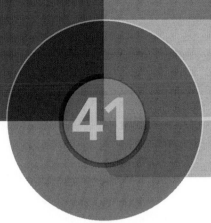

Primary care, the basic necessity: Part II: Explorations in ethics

41

MALCOLM TORRY

INTRODUCTION

The previous chapter employed the science of economics to evaluate healthcare systems. This chapter employs the ethical sciences to explore different ways of distributing and organising healthcare resources, and in particular evaluates the UK National Health Service (NHS) in terms of its ethics. Throughout, we will be particularly interested in the role of primary care practitioners, by which we mean general practitioners (GPs), practice nurses and all of the other members of primary care teams.

This chapter assumes a familiarity with the different funding and rationing methods discussed in the previous chapter.

We will begin by studying a variety of ethical theories that might be relevant to the distribution of healthcare.

HEALTHCARE AS A CATEGORICAL IMPERATIVE

For Immanuel Kant, a 'categorical imperative' is an imperative to 'act only in accordance with that maxim through which you can at the same time will that it become a universal law'.[1] Kant gives examples: I ought not to make a promise that I do not intend to keep, because if the practice were to become universal, then no promise would ever be believed, so the promise that I would make would not be believed and would be pointless[2];and I ought not to avoid helping those in need, because if that practice were to become universal then if I was in need, I would not receive the required assistance.[3] In similarly negative terms, a voter might formulate the maxim, 'healthcare should not be available free at the point of use'. They might one day need healthcare to be available free at the point of use, the people they know and love might need it to be available and the people on whom they rely might need it, so they ought not to act on that maxim. No voter should therefore vote for a political party that does not wish healthcare to be available free at the point of use. In all three cases – not making lying promises, not helping people in need and not voting for a party that would not wish healthcare to be available free at the point of use – the negative categorical imperative implies a positive obligation: to make promises that we intend to keep, to assist people in need and to establish or maintain a health-care system that is available to everyone free at the point of use. Payment per item, membership fees and insurance-based provision do not ensure such universal provision.

A donation basis for healthcare could potentially provide healthcare for all, but there is no guarantee that provision would be anything like adequate, and there will always be a free-rider problem. If I choose not to donate, then my failure to donate will have little effect on the total healthcare available, so the amount available to me will be little affected; but if most people choose not to donate, then the provision of healthcare will be inadequate. In order to provide an adequate amount of healthcare, we will need a social contract that requires everyone to contribute towards the cost. This suggests that taxation is the only secure method of funding healthcare that might in practice conform to a Kantian ethical principle.

ETHICAL HEALTHCARE FUNDING AND DISTRIBUTION

John Rawls, in his search for principles on which to build a just society, posits an 'original position' in which all parties are equal: 'all have the same rights in the procedure for choosing principles'. He envisages a 'veil of ignorance', that is, he asks us to envisage citizens choosing principles while not knowing which position they will hold in the society.[4] The two principles that emerge from this process are:

> [1] equality in the assignment of basic rights and duties … [2] social and economic
> inequalities, for example inequalities of wealth and authority, are just only if they result
> in compensating benefits for everyone, and in particular for the least advantaged members
> of society.[5]

One of the 'basic rights' that Rawls discusses is the right to 'primary goods'. We all have different aims in life, and need different resources to carry them out, and all of us require 'certain primary goods, natural and social' to enable us to do that. Rawls mentions some of them: 'rights and liberties, opportunities and powers, income and wealth'. He does not mention shelter, food and healthcare, which are clearly primary goods in terms of his definition. Presumably, he expects 'income and wealth' to enable everyone to provide such primary goods for themselves.[6] The requirement that everyone should have 'primary goods' available to them will only be met if this assumption is correct, which of course it might not be – particularly for 'the least advantaged members of society' – if income and wealth are not sufficient to provide necessary healthcare. Rawls does not discuss institutional arrangements in detail, but clearly, healthcare paid for via membership fees, insurance premiums or payment per item would be unlikely to provide the 'least advantaged members of society' with sufficient of the required primary good of healthcare. We have discounted healthcare funded by donations as a realistic option, which leaves healthcare free at the point of use and funded by taxation as the only method likely to meet Rawls' requirements.

We can arrive at the same conclusion via a Rawlsian thought experiment. If we were to extend Rawls' method from the formulation of principles to the construction of institutional arrangements, then behind the veil of ignorance, I would not know whether I would be able to afford healthcare membership fees, insurance fees or payment per item. I would therefore be most likely to choose a society in which healthcare was free at the point of use. This simple Rawlsian thought experiment therefore enables us to decide that a society that provides healthcare universally, and free at the point of use, is the most just and fair kind of society in terms of healthcare provision. Such a method might also be able to choose an appropriate structure for taxation. Two taxation methods are available: A flat tax system and a progressive tax system.[7] A flat tax system requires everyone to pay the same rate of tax on income, wealth or expenditure, whatever their income or wealth, whereas a progressive tax system charges higher rates on higher amounts of income or wealth. If I did not know how much income or wealth I would have, then I would need to suppose that I would not have very much income or wealth and would therefore wish to pay a low rate of tax. However, I would also wish to receive the maximum possible amount of public provision. This would require the maximum possible amount of tax revenue, and so higher tax rates on higher amounts of income and wealth. If I were to experience higher income and wealth, then I would be content to pay a higher rate of tax than individuals with lower income and wealth, but not much higher. So, this Rawlsian thought experiment suggests that a just and fair society would be one with a smoothly progressive tax system with a non-punitive top rate of tax.[*]

I have based this exposition and extension of John Rawls' method on the first expression of the two principles of justice that appears in his *A Theory of Justice*. Later on a somewhat different formulation is provided:

> First: each person is to have an equal right to the most extensive basic liberty compatible with a similar liberty for others. Second: social and economic inequalities are to be arranged so that they are both (a) reasonably expected to be to everyone's advantage, and (b) attached to positions and offices open to all.[8]

(This last proviso is later strengthened to require 'conditions of fair equality of opportunity' in relation to positions and offices.[9])

This more restricted formulation implies equality of opportunity, but only the universal provision of primary goods if we can argue that this is required for 'extensive liberty'. Here, we can take two different directions. A libertarian view regards the task of government as providing security for life and property, on the basis of an authority established by a covenant with the country's citizens,[10] but otherwise to leave citizens to make their own rational choices. Each of us has our own preferences and indifferences,[11] and should be free to employ our reason to 'maximise expected utility'.[†] This suggests that governments should collect taxes only to the extent that they are needed to fund the security and protective aspects of public services, but should otherwise leave everybody to make their own decisions as to how they spend their income and wealth. Funding healthcare through membership fees, insurance

---

[*] While the UK's income tax behaves in this way, other parts of the tax system do not. National insurance contributions are charged at 12% on lower earnings, and at 2% on higher earnings; and Value added tax is charged at the same rate whatever someone's income or wealth. For too many low-earning families, the payment of income tax and national insurance contributions at the same time as working and child tax credits, housing benefit, and council tax support are withdrawn, imposes a combined withdrawal rate of 96%, whereas the combined rate on higher earned incomes is only 47% (45% income tax and 2% national insurance contributions) (Ref. 12). The UK's tax system is far from just.

[†] That is, 'the weighted sum of the utilities of (particular decision's) possible outcomes weighted by their probabilities, which sum to 1': See Ref. 13. We can also use our reason 'to formulate new properties of reasons and to shape our utilisation of reasons to exhibit these properties. We can, that is, modify and alter the functions of reasons, and hence of rationality' (p. 132).

premiums and payment per item would therefore be indicated. The problems arise when we recognise that we are social beings, and that most of our decisions affect other people, and that theirs affect us and that your exercise of your liberty might reduce my ability to exercise mine. We therefore require a theory of 'social choice' that takes into account interpersonal comparisons of utility, which, given the differences between us, is difficult to discuss as well as to calculate.[14] We therefore find ourselves in the territory of the second direction that the pursuit of 'extensive liberty' might take: the view that we are only free to fulfil our preferences and indifferences if we already have sufficient primary goods to permit that – which requires that a certain level of healthcare should be provided for every citizen, including the least advantaged member of society. Only a tax-funded healthcare system free at the point of use can provide that.

Stuart White reaches a similar conclusion when he asks about the conditions for expecting citizens to contribute to the society's resources:

> Where institutions governing economic life are otherwise sufficiently just, e.g., in terms of the availability of opportunities for productive participation and the rewards attached to these opportunities, then those who claim the generous share of the social product available to them under these institutions have an obligation to make a decent productive contribution, suitably proportional and fitting for ability and circumstances, to the community in return. I term this the fair-dues conception of reciprocity.[15]

The condition for expecting a reciprocal contribution to the well-being of society is therefore a basic level of equality of resources administered in a way that does not treat some groups of people in condescending ways.[16] So, not only does a commitment to 'extensive liberty' imply a tax-funded healthcare system free at the point of use, but such a system also provides the basis for expecting the liberty thereby facilitated to be employed to the benefit of the society.

ETHICAL HEALTHCARE PROVISION MECHANISMS

We now turn from how healthcare should be funded to the institutions through which it should be provided.

A second useful element of Immanuel Kant's ethical theory is his insistence that human beings should always be an end and never a means to an end.[17] A human being should therefore never be treated as an object to serve some other end. Clearly, if we are to live together in society, the product of our labour will need to be treated as an object if we are to serve the good of society and of other individuals; but human beings themselves must never become such objects. Providing healthcare as a means to a profit gets quite close to treating the individuals to whom healthcare is provided as objects towards some other end. This suggests that private sector organisations that share profits with shareholders might not be the most ethical way to provide healthcare, and that public sector and not-for-profit voluntary organisations would cohere rather better with Kant's principle. (For the purpose of this discussion, organisations that do not share profits with shareholders, but that do share profits with managers in the form of high salaries, fall into the same category as private sector organisations that share profits with shareholders.)

But precisely what kinds of organisation will be the most ethical healthcare providers? Here, an ethical theory somewhat different from the Kant and Rawls tradition might help us.

Utilitarianism[18] asks the question: What should we do in order to provide the highest possible welfare for the greatest possible number? Here an entirely empirical approach needs to be taken. The Washington-based Commonwealth Fund has found that the UK NHS offers the highest quality of care out of the 11 Organisation for Economic Co-operation and Development healthcare systems that it studied, that it is the most efficient and the second cheapest per capita.[19] We have already come across some of the reasons for these findings in chapter 40. A healthcare system funded by taxation and free at the point of use is not tempted to do the unnecessary, primary care acts as a gatekeeper, the administrative systems required by insurance premium and payment per item systems are not required, profits are not shared with the shareholders of insurance companies, and nobody is excluded from healthcare.[20] As far as a utilitarian ethic is concerned, for everyone to have the benefit of high-quality healthcare is more ethical than for only a few to do so.[21] Quite simply, in terms of utilitarian ethics, a universal service that is free at the point of use is demonstrably the most ethical.

Somewhat more difficult to apply is a 'rights' ethical framework. If there is a right to healthcare, then clearly a universal health service free at the point of use will be required, because any other kind will restrict some people's access to healthcare. In the UK, a rights-based ethical approach is explicit in the rights of access defined in the *NHS Constitution for England*, 2013.[22] But is it healthcare that is a human right, or is it health? If the latter, then we will need to discuss the distribution of health outcomes, and because these depend on a wide variety of factors, including healthcare resources, diet, financial security, employment conditions, education and the quality of housing,[23] we shall find ourselves exploring the economics and ethics of social policy as a whole. In this short chapter such an exploration is clearly impossible, but one brief suggestion might be made. If, as I have shown, a universal healthcare system funded by taxation and free at the point of use is the most ethical and the most economically efficient, then the same might be true of other social provision.

PRIMARY CARE

In the previous chapter we have shown how crucial primary care is to the functioning of a universal healthcare system that is free at the point of use. We now employ the economic and ethical sciences to evaluate the ways in which it might be provided.

We have already employed Kant's principle that a human being is always an end, and never a means to an end, to suggest that public sector and not-for-profit voluntary sector provision are more ethical than provision by private sector organisations that distribute profits to shareholders. The same will be true of primary care. It would be more ethical to provide primary care through a public sector organisation or through a voluntary sector not-for-profit organisation than through a private sector organisation. But where does that leave the kind of general practice partnerships that we find in the UK? These are clearly in the private sector, and partners earn a share of profits rather than salaries. It is therefore both an ethical and an economic question as to whether the profit shares match the amounts that would be paid as salaries to individuals undertaking the same tasks and carrying out the same responsibilities. A practice manager might or might not be a partner, but the clinical partners will generally be both clinicians and managers, suggesting a high degree of organisational efficiency. Profit shares are often below the salary levels that would be payable for similar skills and responsibility levels in other organisations. This suggests that for primary care to be provided through general practice partnerships is both economically efficient and ethical. Given that private sector companies, public sector organisations and voluntary sector organisations would need to pay separately for clinical and management activity, it is difficult to see how any of them could be more economically efficient than partnerships; but might they be more ethical? A private sector company would not be, because it would share profits with shareholders and would therefore to some extent be treating patients as means to ends rather than as ends in themselves. Public sector organisations accountable to local or central government, and employing clinicians on the basis of employment contracts, might have a greater claim to ethical legitimacy, but they will always have their own ways of treating patients as means rather than ends. Hospital trusts will always serve a variety of political ends, which will inevitably turn patients into means rather than ends. Perhaps the most ethical kind of organisation would be a voluntary organisation managed by a board of trustees. Because this would be funded and regulated by government, it is doubtful that it would be any different from a public sector organisation in terms of ethical legitimacy. This gives us a further clue as to how we might understand general practice partnerships. They are closely regulated via their contracts with public sector organisations, and so in practice find themselves on the boundary between the public and private sectors, and with an ethical legitimacy close to that of any other public sector organisation. However, we are still unable to decide whether primary care is best provided via partnerships or via private, public or voluntary sector organisations employing only salaried GPs.

In order to break the tie between the different kinds of organisation, we might usefully study a further ethical theory.

VIRTUE WITHIN A COMMUNITY

Virtue ethics seeks the ethical individual rather than particular ethical actions, on the assumption that the ethical individual's actions will then be ethical.[24] So the question is this: Which kind of organisation is most likely to produce virtuous individuals? Public sector and voluntary sector organisations are bureaucracies in which a person's role in the organisation determines the task. The development of virtuous individuals is not impossible within such organisations, but there is nothing in their structures that actively encourages it. With partnerships, the situation is different. At the heart of a general practice partnership there is a community, not a hierarchy. While there might be a senior partner, they have no hierarchical status in terms of the management of the organisation. Communities can facilitate virtue in ways in which hierarchies cannot.[25] To take just one aspect of partnerships: in public sector organisations, governing bodies and managers manage clinicians, and clinicians' tasks are determined by contracts with governing bodies and are managed by managers. Virtue can be exercised within the role, and perhaps outside it, but the ways in which virtue can be exercised will be constrained by the organisation. General practice partners, because they function as individuals in community, are in an ideal position to develop and exercise virtue, towards their patients, towards their partners and towards their staff.[26] The staff of a practice will generally be hierarchically organised, but because there is a community at the heart of the practice, there will always be a certain amount of legitimate fuzziness in relation to lines of accountability. Bureaucratic aspects of the organisation will therefore function within a structure that is permanently characterised by aspects of community, allowing plenty of scope for the development of virtue. (The downside is that fuzzy lines of accountability can also allow organisational politics to subvert the organisation's purpose – but this is as true of the many public sector organisations that do not have structures appropriate to their tasks as it is of partnerships.)

The way in which a partnership can more easily facilitate virtue gives this kind of organisation the ethical edge over public and voluntary sector organisations, and because partnerships are more efficient in terms of their economics, they have to be the preferred option.

CONCLUSIONS

I have argued that a healthcare service that is universal and free at the point of use is ethical; that in most contexts, public sector providers are to be preferred to private sector providers, but that general practice partnerships are both ethically and economically efficient; and that primary care is necessarily at the heart of such a service.

The conclusions of this chapter therefore cohere nicely with the conclusions of the previous chapter, suggesting that healthcare in the UK must remain universal and free at the point of use; that public sector providers are in most circumstances to be preferred to private providers (and often to voluntary sector providers too), but that primary care should continue to be built around general practice partnerships; and that any discussion of health policy, healthcare planning, NHS funding or the education of future healthcare professionals should begin with primary care, and only then move on to the other parts of the service. It also suggests that other countries should consider establishing healthcare systems that are universal and free at the point of use.

REFERENCES

1. Kant, I., *Groundwork for the Metaphysics of Morals*, transl. A. W. Wood, Yale University Press, New Haven, CT, 2002, p. 37 (Ak 4.421: Ak numbers refer to the definitive German text, Immanuel Kants Schriften, Ausgabe der königlich preussischen Akademie der Wissenschaften, W. de Gruyter, Berlin, 1902).
2. Ibid., 39 (Ak 4.422).
3. Ibid., 40 (Ak 4.423).
4. Rawls, J., *A Theory of Justice*, The Belknap Press of Harvard University Press, Cambridge, MA, 1971, pp. 19, 136–42.
5. Ibid., 14–15.
6. Ibid., 93–5.
7. Tax by *Design: The Mirrlees Review*, Oxford University Press, Oxford, 2011, pp. 46–72; Hindriks, J. and Myles, G.D., *Intermediate Public Economics*, The MIT Press, Cambridge, MA, 2006, pp. 477–506.
8. Rawls, 1971, *op. cit.*, 60.
9. Rawls, 1971, *op. cit.*, 302.
10. John Locke, Leviathan, Wordsworth, Ware, 2014, first published in 1651.
11. Nozick, R., *The Normative Theory of Individual Choice*, Garland Publishing, New York, 1990, p. 312.
12. Murphy, R. and Reed, H., *Financing the Social State: Towards a Full Employment Economy*, Centre for Labour and Social Studies, 2013, pp. 25–7.
13. Nozick, R., *The Nature of Rationality*, Princeton University Press, Princeton, NJ, 1993, pp. 42–3.
14. Nozick, 1990, *op. cit.*, 322.
15. White, S., *The Civic Minimum: On the Rights and Obligations of Economic Citizenship*, Oxford University Press, Oxford, 2003, p. 59.
16. White, S., *Equality*, Polity Press, Cambridge, 2007, pp. 84, 93.
17. Kant, 2002, *op. cit.*, 36–8.
18. Mill, J.S. and Bentham, J., *Utilitarianism and Other Essays*, Penguin Books, London, 1987.

19. Karen Davis, Kristof Stremikis, David Squires, and Cathy Schoen, 'Mirror, Mirror, On the Wall: How the performance of the US healthcare system compares internationally', Washington, DC: Commonwealth Fund. www.commonwealthfund.org/publications/fund-reports/2014/jun/mirror-mirror.

20. Hart, J.T., *The Political Economy of Health Care: A Clinical Perspective*, Policy Press, Bristol, 2006, p. 172: The UK spends 6% of its GDP on healthcare, whereas other OECD countries spend an average of 9% and the USA spends 12%.

21. Smith, A., *The Theory of Moral Sentiments*, Penguin Books, London, 2009 (first published in 1759), pp. 325–6.

22. *The NHS Constitution for England: The NHS Belongs to Us All*, Department of Health, London, 2013, p. 6.

23. *Report of the Working Group in Inequalities in Health (the 'Black Report')*, Department of Health and Social Security, London, 1980; Townsend, P. and Davidson, N., *Inequalities in Health: The Black Report*, Penguin Books, Harmondsworth, 1982; Royal College of Nursing, *Health Inequalities and the Social Determinants of Health*, Royal College of Nursing, London, 2012; Dean, H., *Social Rights and Human Welfare*, Routledge, Abingdon, 2015, pp. 107–111.

24. Aristotle, *Nichomachean Ethics*, I, 8; II, 3; II, 6, in J.L. Ackrill, *A New Aristotle Reader*, Clarendon Press, Oxford, 1987, p. 372–3, 378–80, 382–4; Broadie, S., *Ethics with Aristotle*, Oxford University Press, Oxford, 1993, pp. 3, 7, 50; Hutchinson, D.S., Ethics, pp. 195–232 in Barnes, J., *The Cambridge Companion to Aristotle*, Cambridge University Press, Cambridge, 1995, pp. 199–219.

25. MacIntyre, A., *After Virtue*, 2nd edition, University of Notre Dame, Notre Dame, IN, 1984.

26. Toon, P., Setting boundaries: A virtue approach to the clinician-patient relationship in general practice, in D. Bowman and J. Spicer (Eds.), *Primary Care Ethics*, pp. 83–99. Radcliffe Publishing, Oxford, 2007.

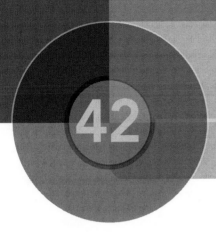

The special ethics of dentistry

42

DAVID OBREE AND ANDREW TRATHEN

Dentistry has always had a certain otherness about it in the UK. When the profession emerged from its barber surgeon origins, it kept its separation from mainstream healthcare and this independence was consolidated at the inception of the National Health Service (NHS) in 1948. Along with pharmacists and opticians, dentists became subcontractors of health care at the margins of the free-at-the-point-of-delivery enterprise.

Yet, whilst distinct, dentistry shares many of the ethical foundations of medicine and surgery such as the Hippocratic promise of best interest, confidentiality and respect for autonomy. The dentist–patient relationship is an intimate and personal one, demanding high levels of trust. Respect for autonomy, and its legal corollary consent, is as prominent in dentistry as other branches of healthcare, and the recent discourse on professionalism has been as enthusiastically debated within dentistry as it has in other spheres.[1] In common with all professions, it is the individual professional who fulfils the professional group's commitment to society and which generates public trust in the profession. Thus, the moral basis of the profession can be investigated on individual and societal levels.

Overall in the UK, dentistry is a primary care profession. Over 90% of dental treatment occurs in primary care and the bulk of this occurs in general dental practice. Around 58% of the annual £6 billion UK dentistry market is NHS spending and 42% is private spending.[2] The majority of dentists are paid for treatments carried out, whilst very few dentists are salaried. Most treatments involve a direct payment from the patient and this distinguishes dentistry from other areas of healthcare. In short, dentists have both a therapeutic and a financial relationship with their patients.

Thus, patients are increasingly seen as, and see themselves as, paying customers, with all the ramifications of demand, choice and expectation. Coupled with this, the availability of cosmetic treatment options such as bleaching, aesthetic crowns and orthodontics has created a market based on want rather than need. As patients progressively become consumers, we must ask if there is an ethical difference between treatment for pain relief and treatment to improve appearance.[3]

This chapter considers how these issues and the wider system of dentistry have shaped dentistry's distinct ethical environment.

ALTRUISM: DOES DENTISTRY PUT PATIENTS FIRST?

The conflicts that arise between best clinical outcomes, cost to the patient and remuneration for the dentist are daily ethical tensions. It is resource allocation, distributive justice, at the individual level. The more treatment dentists advise, the more they get paid, and this is dentistry's most conspicuous moral challenge.

Dentists' fee-for-service arrangement contrasts with much of the medicine in the UK, where under the NHS there are few patient payments, and puts dentistry closer to cosmetic surgery or the business professions such as law and accountancy. In all these professions, there can be an uncomfortable relationship between prescription of need and a presumption to supply, identified and criticised by sociologists in the 1970s:

> Merchants sell you the goods they stock. Guildsmen guarantee quality. Some craftspeople tailor their product to your measure or fancy. Professionals tell you what you need and claim the power to prescribe. They not only recommend what is good, but actually ordain what is right. Neither income, long training, delicate tasks nor social standing is the mark of a professional. Rather, it is his authority to define a person as a client, to determine that person's need and hand the person a prescription.[4]

Such criticism occurs in the context of the monopoly that dentists, and other professionals, have over their area of work.[5] The specialisation and expertise of dentistry ensure the quality and reliability of treatment and the benefit this brings to patient welfare. However, it also allows economic advantage to the professionals who are operating within a sheltered marketplace. This has implications for access to care for those who cannot afford treatment. The regulator does not concern itself with this group nor the dental profession's responsibility to them. Yet, the UK General Dental Council's (GDC) opening standard is 'Put patients' interests first', with the inference, from the apostrophe, that patients are a plurality and thus dentists should have a societal interest.[6]

The social contract that privileges the professional group in return for expertise is not always demonstrably balanced. In the United States, the Institute of Medicine estimated that in 2008, 4.6 million children had no access to dental care as their parents could not afford it.[7] They could not afford the services of one of the richest occupational groups[8] in the richest country in the world.

Children can have difficulties accessing services in the UK, albeit for different reasons. NHS dentistry is free to those under the age of 18, yet in 2013–2014, some 46,500 children were admitted to hospital for tooth extraction under general anaesthetic, a failure of the NHS to direct funding to preventive care.[9] Inequality can contribute to reduced uptake of services,[10] but allocation of funding is not uniform. Direct access to dental care professionals that do not demand the high income of dentists offers potential to address the problem,[11] but the profession has been opposed to their widespread use since the 1920s.[12–14]

DISTRIBUTIVE JUSTICE: DENTISTRY AS A BUSINESS

In contrast, it can be argued that there is an ethical imperative for a dental practice to be profitable. Without profit the business cannot survive and thus the beneficial healthcare facility is lost to the public.[15] Historically, the typical business model in the UK was an independent practice locally owned by a practising dentist with partners or associates, usually working on a percentage of their treatment income. Corporate groups were originally limited by the GDC regulation but this was deregulated, and by 2014 the number of practices operated by 'corporates' had risen to 22%.[16] To some, the rise of the corporates is an impersonal intrusion of hardline business into the personal matter of healthcare, to others it is the application of efficiency. Contrary to the perceived instinct to maximise profit by seeking the wealthiest patients, the corporates have been most active in the NHS sector of the market.[16]

The increase in corporate groups offering dental services would seem to fit with patients becoming 'consumers' of healthcare. Certainly, when the doctor–patient relationship is consumerist,[17] it emphasises the autonomy (or perhaps the choices) of a patient beyond all else. However, questions should be asked – is something lost if a consumerist relationship is pursued? Is healthcare a tradable commodity? The concerns expressed by the medical profession about the effect that commercialisation may have on public health,[18] or the corrupting effect that private practice can have on clinical decision making,[19] are being played out in a system of dentistry where the threat of commercialism to professionalism has long been recognised.[20]

Importantly, if the desires of the customer (patient) take precedence above all else, this leaves a dilemma for dentists' moral and professional duty of beneficence. When does respect for autonomy become respect for choice (choice perhaps motivated by external coercion or extreme selfishness)?

NHS DENTISTRY

At the inception of the NHS in 1948 dentistry was free to patients, but by 1952 a charge of £1 was introduced (at the same time as a one shilling (five-pence) charge for a general medical prescription). In 2016, that equated to £26.70 for dental treatment, and £1.34 for a prescription. Charges for dental treatment increased through the decades and in the 1970s became a percentage charge aligned with the amount of treatment required. In 2006, the system was overhauled and simplified so that only three bands of treatment existed, one for check-ups and cleaning, one for fillings and one for crowns and dentures.[21]

Whilst this has simplified matters for patients and the NHS commissioners, it creates perverse incentives that potentially harm the principle of patient-centric care. Some patients require complicated care, others little, but the system does not distinguish between the two. Thus, dentists are financially pressured to seek out patients requiring simpler treatments, or encourage them ignore more complex treatment options. It expands the moral question of how much should dentists be paid and what should they be paid for, prevention or cure? This is an important question in terms of the financial sustainability of future dental practice in the UK.

Dissatisfaction with NHS remuneration has driven more dentists into the expanding private sector.[2] Practices and individual practitioners can be wholly NHS, wholly private or a mix of the two. Whilst the majority of NHS adult patients contribute to the cost of their dental care by direct payments according to their band of treatment, there is also a significant low-income group exempt from charges along with all patients under 18. Some practices only see children and exempt patients on the NHS. In the private sector, best clinical interest versus cost negotiations occur directly between the dentist and patient who acts as both the recipient of the treatment and the (financial) resource allocator. In an NHS practice, the resource allocator (the NHS) is a restraining presence, limiting the availability of (clinical) resource to the patient and (financial) resource to the dentist. Thus, the NHS has an ethical role to play, a role ultimately controlled by government and healthcare finance ministers.

AUTONOMY AND SOCIAL JUSTICE: PERSONAL ACCOUNTABILITY FOR DENTAL HEALTH

A divisive ethical issue in healthcare economics that tends to split people along lines of political orientation is whether the society or the individual should pay for the population's dental care. The two principal dental diseases, caries (decay) and periodontal (gum) disease are common, but they are also largely preventable. Whilst the dental diseases can be framed as diseases of personal irresponsibility and failure to take responsibility for one's own health,[22] there is also the matter of social inequality and its damaging effect on individual agency.[23]

The fight against societal inequality may not be an obvious one for the clinical dentist, but as the tide of medical ethics turns from autonomy to social justice, the GDC's apostrophe may take on increasing significance. The principles of prevention over treatment and taking an 'up-stream' approach have wide agreement. Yet, successive governments have pursued a reparative policy rather than a preventive one, with dentists being paid for doing fillings on a fee-per-treatment basis rather than preventing them. Would a salaried or capitation service improve prevention? In theory, it could, but there is the worry that it would also disincentivise intervention and raise the incidence of supervised neglect. The concern is that if you pay dentists to treat, they over treat, if you pay them to prevent, they under treat.

Discussion about the least ethically corrosive method of financial incentive is not new in medicine. Papanikitas suggests that the discussion around payment for performance incentives (incentivised tasks) should not be separated from the general discussion of general practitioners' interests as employers, employees and citizens who themselves need to make a living from their vocation – this argument may also apply in the case of dentistry.[24] In the absence of professional ethics, any system of payment for clinical services can result in maximisation of income in preference to patient welfare. Roland.[25] illustrates this in Table 42.1.

The ethics of professional responsibility should limit excess and maintain patient best interest at its core. A separation of diagnosis and treatment could solve the worries articulated by the 1970s sociologists distrustful of professionals' power to prescribe and treat,[4] The model of the ophthalmic optician (diagnosing) and dispensing optician (treating) is an interesting model with merits, although largely unaccomplished since they commonly work together in the same business enterprise.

A potential source of funding for dental care that might simultaneously act as a 'nudge' for healthier behaviours is a tax on the causes. Recent debates about tax on sugar as a source of funds to tackle obesity-related disease can also be applied to dental decay,[25] The dental profession has sought to influence patients to improve oral hygiene and diet, whilst the political option to challenge soft drink and confectionary manufacturers has been largely avoided. Sugar taxes principally aim to raise revenue and influence consumer behaviour but manufacturers are also

Table 42.1 Payment methods for doctors and their potential consequences

Payment method		What doctors would do if they did not behave in line with their professional principles
Salary	Pay independent of workload or quality	As little as possible for as few people as possible
Capitation	Pay according to the number of people on a doctor's list	As little as possible for as many people as possible
Fee for service	Pay for individual items of care	As much as possible, whether or not it helped the patient
Pay for performance	Pay for meeting quality targets	A limited range of commendable tasks, but nothing else

Source: Roland, M., *BMJ*, 345, e582, 2012.

prompted to modify their products.[26] Debates between those suspicious of the 'nanny state' and those who want to rebalance the impact of corporate interests on people's health decisions continue to feature prominently in the media.[27]

GOVERNANCE

Crucial to any profession's interface with society is its organisation and governance. Recent trends have seen the ethical direction of the healthcare professions driven by government, either by controlling resource funding, as in the case of the NHS, or by dictating regulation, as in the case of the UK's newly constituted healthcare regulatory councils.

One role of professional councils is to produce guidelines, or standards, for members of the profession to maintain. These normative directives are broadly similar between the healthcare professions and share the same Hippocratic and philosophical origins. The current UK GDC guidelines are as follows: (1) Put patients' interests first; (2) communicate effectively with patients; (3) obtain valid consent; (4) maintain and protect patients' information; (5) have a clear and effective complaints procedure; (6) work with colleagues in a way that is in patients' best interests; (7) maintain, develop and work within your professional knowledge and skills; (8) raise concerns if patients are at risk; and (9) make sure your personal behaviour maintains patients' confidence in you and the dental profession.[28]

Whilst these standards are unremarkable, they are no longer formulated or enforced by dentists themselves. Historically, the majority of GDC council members were registered dentists, elected or nominated by their peer groups, in common with other healthcare professional councils. However, the political climate following Bristol children's heart, Alder Hey and Shipman scandals drove the government to reconstitute the healthcare councils into regulatory authorities with smaller government-appointed councils.[29] This change, in 2009, from democratically elected self-governance to government-orchestrated regulation has had a pronounced effect on professional morale.[30,31] Dentists no longer have any representation in how their profession is regulated and a significant increase in fitness to practise cases, with a concomitant rise in registration fees, has created anxiety about the new system.[32] Dentists are controlled not only by the GDC but also by the Care Quality Commission (CQC) and the Department of Health, a triumvirate whose roles significantly overlap with the result that dentists feel 'over-regulated'.[33] As in medicine, individual practitioners are increasingly subject to 'evidence-based' clinical guidelines from the Royal Colleges, NICE and specialist societies, not to mention the constant threat of litigation and inexpert media scrutiny. Along with other healthcare groups, there is a lament that governments have created a culture of compliance in place of a culture of conscience and that the virtue, or character, of the professional practitioner has been ignored in favour of box-ticking.

These concerns are not new. They were considered by Plato in the fourth century BC and rearticulated by Brian Hurwitz and others in the 1990s;[34] How do you balance the constraints of process-driven regulation with a personal, bespoke and ethical approach to patient care? Similarly, Eliot Freidson raised the sociological concern that without the involvement of individual professionals, whose disciplined knowledge has to be developed for the public good, the professions lose their moral legitimacy.[35]

Whilst enforcement of rule and regulation may not be the best way to foster the moral engagement of individual practitioners, there are also tangible economic concerns. Resources spent on regulatory compliance could be spent on patient care, and distributive justice is compromised when disproportionate attention is paid to regulatory obedience. A more nuanced and traditional approach, involving professionals in the organisation of their professional activities, would have a stronger claim for moral, sociological and economic legitimacy.

Professional regulation is about fairness to both sides of the partnership between patients and professionals. To command the confidence of both, it must also be seen to be fair, both to patients and health professionals.[29]

CONCLUSION

The difference between dentistry and medicine in the UK raises ethical questions perhaps less conspicuous in other areas of healthcare. Although economic concerns and issues of distributive justice are important in all fields, the direct financial transaction that occurs between the patient and the dentist creates a unique situation that other NHS clinicians in the UK will generally not have to face.

Despite changes made periodically since 1948, no government has successfully created a remunerative framework that incentivises a balance of prevention and cure, or that has met with approval from the profession itself. Perhaps this is an impossibility. Dentists exist simultaneously as altruistic professionals, placing the patient first, whilst also running a business that has to be kept viable. Reconciling duties to their business and their patient can be problematic and is a daily source of ethical tension.

Yet, this fundamental issue applies to other healthcare professions, albeit less obtrusively. Every pound spent on professional practitioners is a pound less to spend on healthcare equipment, on support staff, on buildings and on medicines. How much is enough? How should we balance our resources between funding a professional elite, and funding other elements of healthcare?

Dentistry also acts as a case study for the importance of good regulation. Regulatory costs have multiplied tenfold since the 1990s,[32] exacerbating the problems faced by dentists in balancing patient care and business. A concurrent increase in complaints and 'Fitness to practise' cases encourages dentists to think and practice defensively, rather than caringly. Tight regulation that protects the individual can thus have broader implications for the quality and accessibility of care that is given to the population.

As a microcosm for a number of important issues in medical ethics, dentistry can play a useful role. Part of the free-at-point-of-delivery philosophy for only a few years, money has dominated the ethical landscape of the profession. As governments push for greater influence of market forces on the commissioning and delivery of healthcare, a study of the ethics of dentistry can give us some insight into the pitfalls along that road.

REFERENCES

1. Zijlstra-Shaw, S., P.G. Robinson, and T. Roberts, Assessing professionalism within dental education: The need for a definition. *Eur J Dent Educ*, 2011; **15**: 1–9.
2. Office of Fair Trading, *Dentistry: An OFT Market study*. Office of Fair Trading; London, 2012.
3. Welie, J.V., Do you have a healthy smile? *Med Health Care Philos*, 1999; **2**(2): 169–80.
4. Illich, I., *Disabling Professions*. London: Marion Boyars; 1977.
5. Larson, M.S., *The Rise of Profesionalism: Monopolies of Competence and Sheltered Markets*. Transaction Publishers: Piscataway NJ; 2013.
6. Affleck, P., et al., What ethical difference does an apostrophe make? Balancing the interests of patients and dental professionals. *Brit Dent J*, 2013; **214**(2): 51–52.
7. Rivara, F., P. Erwin, and C. Evans, *Improving Access to Oral Health Care for Vulnerable and Underserved Populations*. Washington, DC: The National Academies Press; 2011.
8. Bureau of Labor Statistics, *May 2015 National Occupational Employment and Wage Estimates United States*. in Occupational Employment Statistics 2015 [cited 2016 August 17]; Available from: http://www.bls.gov/oes/current/oes_nat.htm#00-0000.
9. Faculty of Dental Surgery. *The State of Children's Oral Health in England*. Royal College of Surgeons England: London; 2015.
10. Gallagher, J.E., D.J. Cooper, and D. Wright, Deprivation and access to dental care in a socially diverse metropolitan area. *Community Dent Health*, 2009; **26**(2): 92–8.
11. Innes, N.P. and D.J. Evans, Evidence of improved access to dental care with direct access arrangements. *Evid Based Dent*, 2013; **14**(2): 36–7.
12. Larkin, G.V., Professionalism, dentistry and public health. *Soc Sci Med A*, 1980; **14**(3): 223–9.
13. British Dental Association, *Direct Access to Dental Care Professionals: BDA Submission to the General Dental Council*, London, 2012.
14. Welshman, J., Dental health as a neglected issue in medical history: The school dental service in England and Wales, 1900–40. *Med Hist*, 1998; **42**(3): 306–27.
15. Trathen, A. and J.E. Gallagher, Dental professionalism: Definitions and debate. *Br Dent J*, 2009; **206**(5): 249–53.
16. General Dental Council, *Patients Professionals Partners Performance*, London, 2016. p. 6.
17. Morgan, M.J., The doctor-patient relationship, in *Sociology as Applied to Medicine*, G. Scambler, Editor. London: Saunders; 2003, pp. 50–53.
18. McCoy, D., Commercialisation is bad for public health. *BMJ*, 2012; **344**: e149.
19. Dean, J., Private practice is unethical – And doctors should give it up. *BMJ*, 2015; **350**:h2299.
20. American Dental Association. *Ethics Summit on Commercialism*. in Ethics Summit on Commercialism. Chicago, IL: American College of Dentists; 2006.
21. NHS Choices. *NHS Dental Services Explained*. 2016 [cited 2016 August 17]; Available from: http://www.nhs.uk/NHSEngland/AboutNHSservices/dentists/Pages/nhs-dental-charges.aspx.

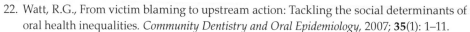

22. Watt, R.G., From victim blaming to upstream action: Tackling the social determinants of oral health inequalities. *Community Dentistry and Oral Epidemiology*, 2007; **35**(1): 1–11.

23. Watt, R. G., Listl, S., Peres, M., and Heilmann, A. *Social inequalities in oral health: from evidence to action*. International Centre for Oral Health Inequalities Research and Policy: London; 2015.

24. Papanikitas, A., Caught between the task and the vocation, in *From the Classroom to the Clinic: Ethics Education and General Practice* (PhD Thesis). Department of education and professional studies, Kings College London; 2013, pp. 315–18.

25. Roland, M., Incentives must be closely aligned to professional values. *BMJ*, 2012; **345**: e5982.

26. Welsh, J.A., E.A. Lundeen, and A.D. Stein, The sugar-sweetened beverage wars: Public health and the role of the beverage industry. *Curr Opin Endocrinol Diabetes Obes*, 2013; **20**(5): 401–6.

27. Moore, M., H. Yeatman, and R. Davey, Which nanny–the state or industry? Wowsers, teetotallers and the fun police in public health advocacy. *Public Health*, 2015; **129**(8): 1030–7.

28. General Dental Council, *Standards for the Dental Team*, London, 2013.

29. Donaldson, L., *Trust, Assurance and Safety: The Regulation of Health Professionals in the 21st Century.* London: Department of Health; 2007.

30. Hancocks, S., A profession no longer. *Brit Dent J*, 2007; **202**(5): p. 235.

31. Lewis, K., The curate's egg. *Brit Dent J*, 2010; **209**(4): p. 151.

32. Wilson, N. and S. Gelbier, *The Regulation of the Dental Profession by the General Dental Council: The John McLean Archive – A living history of Dentistry Witness Seminar 2*. John McLean history of dentistry witness seminars. British Dental Association, London, 2014.

33. Regulation of Dental Services Programme Board, *The Future of Dental Service Regulation.* Care Quality Commission [www.CQC.org.uk], London, 2015.

34. Hurwitz, B., Legal and political considerations of clinical practice guidelines. *BMJ*, 1999; **318**(7184): 661–4.

35. Freidson, E., The soul of professionalism, in *Professionalism – The Third Logic*. Polity Press: Cambridge; 2001, pp. 197–222.

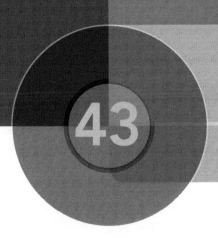

The ethics of administration

43

PETER TOON

INTRODUCTION

Consultations between individual patients and clinicians take up the largest part of the time of primary care clinicians, and are also usually the focus of ethical discussions. However, most clinicians also spend a significant part of their time on 'paperwork' – administrative tasks (increasingly carried out on computers rather than on paper) related to individual patients but carried out in their absence. These include dealing with prescription requests, correspondence to and from other clinicians and writing reports to non-clinicians.

Clinicians also spend a lot of time dealing with medical records – writing in them, summarising the records of new patients and updating existing summaries, and dealing with requests to see the records, with (or without) the patient being present.

It is easy to think of this as routine work posing no ethical challenges, but like all work involving patients, it means making decisions on both facts and values; decisions often made unconsciously. The decisions of different clinicians may vary widely according to what level of risk they find acceptable and how they trade-off risk against cost and inconvenience (to them and to patients), their view of the relative responsibilities of clinicians and patients in ensuring good medical care and their understanding of confidentiality. These examples of 'everyday' ethics are illustrated with reference to the National Health Service (NHS) in the United Kingdom.

REPEAT PRESCRIPTION REQUESTS

A peculiarity of the NHS in the UK is that while patients on long-term treatment often only need their medication reviewed every 6 or 12 months, prescribers in primary care are not allowed to prescribe medication to last for longer than 1, or (at the most) 2 months, except in the case of oral contraception (or are at least strongly discouraged from doing so).[1] Therefore, repeat prescriptions are often issued without seeing the patient.[2,3]

Whether this arrangement is actually necessary has been questioned.[4] On the positive side, it may reduce waste of medication dispensed but not used, and this is the reason usually given for this policy.[5] The cost of unused medication in the NHS is estimated at £300 million per year,[6] but whether this would increase if long-term treatments were dispensed for 6 months rather than 1 month is not clear.

Against possible saving in wasted medicines is the inconvenience to administrative staff who have to handle repeat requests and issue prescriptions, to clinicians who have to authorise them, and the cost of the time this takes them which might be more profitably employed, and to patients who have to request and collect their prescriptions and medication.

An advantage of the system less often publicly discussed is that although it creates work for community pharmacists and dispensing practices, they benefit financially from it, because they receive a fee for each prescription dispensed. Six-monthly or annual dispensing might destabilise the infrastructure of retail pharmacy, an important part of our healthcare system. Perhaps this is why no one has had the courage to try to reform this massive, costly paper chase.

Policy judgements on prescribing regulations depend on a value judgement of how much weight to be given to risk, convenience and cost, which will be affected by how well systems work and whether the labour involved can be reduced. Various stratagems have been introduced to improve the system.[7] These include websites which allow patients to request medication and collect it directly from the pharmacy,[8] and sometimes allow pharmacies to initiate the request as well, thus reducing the inconvenience to patients (although possibly leading to more unwanted medication being dispensed) and computer systems which make it easy (to varying degrees) to issue multiple, post-dated prescriptions when the patient is reviewed.[9]

Although the above 'electronic' prescriptions are beginning to change this, repeat prescription requests are typically accepted by administrative staff in primary healthcare teams, verbally, on paper or more recently by computer, and sometimes by telephone (although this is often discouraged for fear that a misunderstanding of what is required may arise – an ethical balance between risk management and patient convenience). Prescriptions are then prepared by administrative staff – at one time writing them by hand, but now usually by printing them from a computerised record system.

Other than whether this system is justified at all this doesn't seem ethically terribly complex, and although there is a significant literature on repeat prescribing suggesting how this might be done better[10–12] it is not usually seen as an ethical issue. In fact, however, signing of a repeat prescription involves a judgement with several implicit values, which are as follows:

- How long is it reasonable for a patient to have to wait for a repeat prescription?
- Should prescriptions always be authorised by the patient's usual clinician? If so, what happens on days-off and holidays?
- If authorisation is not by done by the usual doctor, can it be done only by a doctor who knows the patients or by any GP who happens to be around?

Practice on these matters varies considerably. Policy on 'turn round time' for prescription requests and who deals with them depends on how practitioners balance convenience to patients against convenience to themselves, and possible risks of mistakes if a prescription is authorised in a hurry or by someone unfamiliar with the patient; also on how important they consider the relationship between a particular clinician and patient even for acts done *in absentia*. It also depends on how happy they are to trust the management of risk to a system rather than to an individual clinician.

- Now that many nurses are authorised to prescribe, should they rather than the patient's doctor sign repeats, since if they review the patient's medication, as is common in many chronic diseases, they may be better placed to do this?

Decisions about allocation of jobs between doctors and nurses are based partly on judgements of fact. Who has the competence to carry out a task? How cost-effective is their respective use of time?

However, they also depend on evaluative issues about trust, status and merely what is traditional, which sometimes run counter to facts and reason.

- If the last medication review was satisfactory, the next review not due, and an appropriate quantity of medication has been requested, do clinicians need to check the prescription carefully or can they assume that the system will prevent any errors in prescribing?

Some practices separate 'routine' repeats from those which do not fit the rules of the system and require an explicit clinical decision. Meticulously checking every repeat takes a lot of time, with perhaps little benefit, but if clinicians sign such prescriptions without checking them against the patient record, they rely on the system being robust enough to prevent errors, which is not necessarily the case;[13] this is another evaluative balance between risk and workload.

Not all repeat prescription requests 'fit the rules'. Most of these fall into one of the four categories:

- The medication is authorised for repeat prescribing but review or the necessarily monitoring blood test is overdue.
- Too much or too little medication has been requested.
- The medication requested has been issued recently but has not been authorised for repeat prescription.
- The patient equates repeat prescribing with self-prescribing, and requests a medication not authorised for repeat prescribing but which for some other reason they think is appropriate for their condition.

In these cases, a judgement has to be made as to whether simply to refuse to sign the prescription, to authorise it but add a note asking the patient to discuss it soon, or to contact the patient before authorising the prescription. Again, the action taken depends on an assessment of risk and benefit (a factual judgement) and the balance of risk against extra work and inconvenience, to clinician and to patient (a judgement of values). The decision made about a drug with a high risk of harm if not adequately monitored (e.g. warfarin, lithium) or if abused (e.g. strong opiates) may be different from that with drugs where these risks are low.

It frequently also depends on our view of the respective responsibility of clinician and patient in the management of chronic illness. Clinicians have a legal as well as a moral responsibility to ensure that prescriptions do good, and even more that they do no harm, but they also need to consider how moral responsibility is divided between clinician and patient, and consider questions such as:

- How far does the prescriber's responsibility extend in ensuring that medical care is optimal? If, for example, a patient on treatment for epilepsy or asthma is happy to take it without the review that official guidance (from government organisations such as the National Institute for health and Care Excellence in the UK – NICE) recommends,[14,15] how much pressure should the clinician exert to persuade them to comply?
- How much too much or too little analgesia does a patient need to request before the clinician insists on discussing their treatment?
- If a medication has been prescribed previously as a therapeutic trial, or the patient has been taking it for a while but by accident or design it has not been authorised for repeat prescription, what should the clinician do before authorising it for long-term use?

CORRESPONDENCE

Primary healthcare care teams in the UK receive large numbers of letters, reports and discharge summaries from hospitals and other clinicians involved in patient care (physiotherapists, occupational therapists, social workers, etc.). Many of these just need filing in the patient's records in case they are needed in the future, but they all need to be looked at in case some immediate or future action is required. Usually this is clear, but sometimes it is not. For example:

I think the patient requires a CT scan to exclude the small possibility that the symptoms are due to a malignant lesion.

Has the specialist arranged this? Does he want the general practitioner (GP) to do so? What happens afterwards? What has the patient been told?

I have discharged the patient from my clinic but the problem will need to be kept under review.

How often? By whom? Who should arrange this?

As with repeat prescriptions, what clinicians decide to do depends on their evaluation of risk, benefit and cost: and where responsibility lies between the patient and the clinician, and in this case between other clinicians and themselves, as well as on the facts of the case.

Results of blood tests, microbiological cultures and radiographs and other imaging investigations may be dealt with separately from other correspondence, but similar issues arise. Are the results normal or abnormal? If they are normal, does the clinician need to inform the patient or can they just be filed? How intensively does a clinician need to ensure that an abnormal result is followed up if the patient does not come back to find it out?

With computerised laboratory systems, results requested by other clinicians are often copied automatically to the GP – if you see an abnormal result of a test you did not request do you have a responsibility to follow it up?

Again, this depends on a factual and evaluative assessment of the risks, and a judgement on how much responsibility for the patient's health lies with the clinician, and how much with the patient.

THIRD-PARTY REPORTS

GPs receive requests for medical reports in relation to insurance, employment and a variety of other issues. Some of these arise during consultations rather than in 'paperwork time' but the ethical issues are similar so that they are best considered together. The ethics of reports, particularly to insurance companies, have generated a significant literature and also legislation.[16,17] Toon[18] has classified medical reports and analysed the ethical issues they raise in detail. His conclusions, summarised in Table 43.1 are that the key moral issues are:

- Consent
- Whether the report benefits the patient
- Who pays for the report
- Whether the report poses a conflict of interest between responsibility to the person or body on whose behalf the clinician is acting, and responsibility to the patient.

Table 43.1 Categories of medical report and the key moral issues they raise

Purpose	Consent	Benefit to patient	Who pays?	Possible conflict of interest
Legal proceedings to advance patient care	Not obtainable	Yes	State	No
To advance the public good	Not required	No	State	No
Illness as an excusing factor or as grounds for entitlement	Required but sometimes constrained or inadequately informed	Yes	Patient or third party	Yes
		Yes	Patient or third party	Yes
Fitness to take part in dangerous sports	Yes but sometimes constrained	Yes	Patient	No
Fitness to engage in a particular occupation or profession	Yes but constrained	Little	Patient	Yes
Actuarial calculation		No	Third party	Yes

He suggested that clinicians faced with reports should ask the following questions:

- What class does the report fall into?
- Has the patient consented? Is the consent free and informed?
- To whose advantage is it that the report is given?
- Are there alternatives to giving the report, and what are their consequences?
- How valid is the information on which the report is based?
- Who will pay for the report, and is the fee appropriate?

WRITING IN THE PATIENT RECORD

Far more goes on in the shortest clinical contact than can be written down, and selecting what we write is a value judgement. Often, patients tell clinicians things they do not want to go any further – occasionally, they explicitly ask for something not to be written down, but do clinicians need to be sensitive when this is an implicit message? How much of the patient's social background and one's own opinions and suspicions should be written down? At one time, it was common practice to write derogatory remarks about patients in their records – this would not only be wrong but also very foolish now that in most legal systems patients have the right to see their records.

Similar issues arise in referral letters. Clinically, it may be helpful to share your concerns and suspicions about what is going on with specialist colleagues, but is it always right to share your concerns about a remote but serious possibility with an anxious or a suicidal patient, or your unsubstantiated suspicions about what is going on in their private life?

Some clinicians routinely write notes and dictate letters in the presence of the patient to emphasise that they are working in partnership and have no secrets; others do them later, not necessarily because they are withholding information but because it saves getting behind with appointments; another judgement on the balance of values, this time between patient involvement and timekeeping.

SUMMARISATION

Deciding what to include in the summary which is typically part of the medical record involves a factual decision on how likely issues are to impact on future care. Perhaps, more important is a factual psychological decision on how users process the information in a medical record. There is a trade-off between completeness and comprehensibility; the more the information, the smaller the chance that something important will be missing, but the greater the chance that something important that is there will be overlooked.

The main ethical problem with summaries involves clinically relevant but not strictly medical personal facts and sensitive medical information, particularly now records are on computers and once open, can be read by anyone in the consulting room. It might not be helpful for someone to see the record of their abortions or domestic or child abuse prominently on the screen every time they come to the doctor, even less so that their accompanying spouse or parent might see it. However, such matters are often of great importance and if not highlighted to clinicians; important issues may be missed. Here, the ethical balance is between risk and confidentiality. Some computer systems offer ways to hide sensitive data but post a flag which indicates they are there, and for ensuring that sensitive information is not transmitted when (as is increasingly common) records are shared or transferred electronically.

RELEASING MEDICAL RECORDS

In the UK both legislation[19] and professional guidance[20] provide a framework within which doctors asked to disclosure the medical records of patients to patients, to relatives and to other third parties must work. Many other countries have similar legislation,[21] although not all do so.

These regulations are based on the society's ethical judgements about the right of autonomous patients to see their records (a fairly recent view – 40 years ago, hospital records in the UK were often labelled 'Confidential – Not to be handled by the patient'[22]), the need to protect confidentiality and the need to avoid harm, although the ethical basis of the rules is rarely made explicit.

Practitioners however often have to make decisions within these frameworks which involve personal ethical judgements. There is sometimes provision in law to remove information which may seriously harm the patient or others; deciding what constitutes harm in such circumstances is one example of such a judgement. Disclosure of the records of children is a matter for parents (though the child should be involved as much as their age and maturity allows), and divorced or separated parents may both still be entitled to access to their children's records.[23] However, if one parent requests the record, the clinician may worry that the record is going to be used to demonstrate the inadequate parenting of the other party. Diplomatic as well as ethical skills may be needed to avoid getting sucked into a marital dispute.

There are also moral decisions on how to share information. Should autonomous patients just be handed their records to make what they will of, or do clinicians have a responsibility to guide them through them? Records are typically full of specialist terminologies not always clear to the lay person which they may need help to understand. They are not only a record of what happened but also an aide-memoire for clinicians and a way to share thoughts with other clinicians, and so they sometimes include notes about possible serious although unlikely diagnoses. However, if, for example, someone see 'cough and weight loss o/e NAD, need to consider TB, HIV, cancer' written 2 years previously, they may not realise that subsequent tests definitively exclude these possibilities. Is it paternalism or just good care to insist on seeing patients so that issues like these can be explained?

THE ETHICAL ANALYSIS OF ADMINISTRATIVE DECISIONS

Apart from the right to confidentiality, deontology is little help in administrative decisions – the issues are too complex and too subtle for this approach. It is important to be aware of the legal framework and the rights and responsibilities it implies, but many of the decisions needed are the sort where, if when clinicians seek advice from their medical indemnity provider (or medical-malpractice insurance provider outside the UK), they say 'You must follow your conscience and we will support you whichever way you decide'.

A sort of consequentialism, balancing up the costs and benefits of the different courses of action to the patient, the clinician and the practice population in general, is a possible approach. However, because so many of these judgements are common and have to be made rapidly detailed reflection on each occasion is not possible, and in practice they are often made without much conscious deliberation. A virtue approach, in which personal qualities of conscientiousness, respect for confidentiality and a courageous approach to risk, neither timid nor foolhardy, supplemented by a set of 'v-rules'[24] is probably the only practical way of dealing with the ethics of administration. Possible 'v-rules' for a UK GP might be things like:

- For patients on blood pressure medication add a reminder to come in to the first repeat request after review is due, a more strongly worded reminder to the second, and phone the patient after the third.
- Offer patients the chance to discuss what is in their records before sending them to a third party and give them two weeks to come and see you.
- Never sign a repeat prescription for warfarin without seeing a recent INR result.

These are merely examples, not necessarily the best v-rules to follow. Clinicians and groups of practitioners need to consider the problematic situations which commonly arise, devise their own policies to cover these and publicise them to patients and the public, something which is sometimes but not always done.

REFERENCES

1. Gilleghan, J. Prescribing in general practice. A review by the RCGP Prescribing Fellow in Scotland. *Occas Pap R Coll Gen Pract.* 1991. http://www.ncbi.nlm.nih.gov/pmc/articles/PMC2560319/pdf/occpaper00108-0002.pdf (accessed June 22, 2017).
2. Harris CM, Dajda R. The scale of repeat prescribing. *Br J Gen Pract.* 1996; 46(412): 649–53.
3. Drury M. *Repeat prescribing – A review. J R Coll Gen Pract.* 1982; 32(234): 42–5.
4. Scott T. Do we need to repeat prescribe? *J R Coll Gen Pract.* 1985; 35: 91–2.

5. Davies JE, Taylor DG. Individualisation or standardisation: Trends in National Health Service prescription durations in England 1998–2009. *Prim Health Care Res Dev.*2013 (accessed June 22, 2017). 14(2): 164–74.

6. Hazell B, Robson R. *Pharmaceutical waste reduction in the NHS*. 2015. https://www.england.nhs.uk/wp-content/uploads/2015/06/pharmaceutical-waste-reduction.pdf (accessed June 22, 2017).

7. Rothwell & Desborough Healthcare Group website. http://www.rdhg.co.uk/prescriptions1.aspx?p=K83021 (accessed June 23, 2017).

8. Bridge Practice website. http://www.bridgepracticechertsey.nhs.uk/health-services/prescriptions/ (accessed June 22, 2017).

9. NHS England *Electronic Repeat Dispensing Guidance*, 2015.Available at: https://www.england.nhs.uk/digitaltechnology/wp-content/uploads/sites/31/2015/06/electronic-repeat-dispensing-guidance.pdf (accessed June 23, 2017).

10. Bond C, Matheson C, Williams S, Williams P, Donnan P. Repeat prescribing: A role for community pharmacists in controlling and monitoring repeat prescriptions. *Br J Gen Pract.* 2000; 50(453): 271–5.

11. Zermansky AG. Who controls repeats? *Br J Gen Pract.* 1996; 46(412): 643–7.

12. Dreischulte T, Guthrie B. High-risk prescribing and monitoring in primary care: how common is it, and how can it be improved? *Ther Adv Drug Saf.* 2012 Aug; 3(4): 175–84.

13. McGavock H, Wilson-Davis K, Connolly JP. Repeat prescribing management – A cause for oncern? *Br J Gen Pract.* 1999; 49(442): 343–7.

14. Asthma Quality standard [QS25], 2013. National Institute for Health and Care Excellence (NICE)Asthma Quality standard [QS25] Published date: February 2013 National Institute for Health and Care Excellence (NICE). https://www.nice.org.uk/guidance/qs25/chapter/quality-statement-5-review (accessed June 22, 2017).

15. Epilepsies: diagnosis and management Clinical guideline [CG137], 2012. National Institute for Health and Care Excellence (NICE). https://www.nice.org.uk/guidance/cg137/chapter/1-guidance?un (accessed June 22, 2017). lid=75126157520164194129

16. Toon PD, Jones E. Serving two masters – A dilemma in general practice. *Lancet.* 1986; 328(8501), 1196–1198.

17. Access to Medical Reports Acts 1988. www.legislation.gov.uk/ukpga/1988/28/contents (accessed June 22, 2017).

18. Toon PD. Practice pointer. 'I need a note, doctor': Dealing with requests for medical reports about patients. *BMJ.* 2009; 338: b175.

19. Information Commissioner's Office – Health. https://ico.org.uk/for-the-public/health/ (accessed June 23, 2017).

20. GMC Confidentiality guidance. http://www.gmc-uk.org/guidance/ethical_guidance/confidentiality.asp (accessed June 23, 2017).

21. Mair J. Access and confidentiality of medical records: A legislative response inthe United States. *Health Inf Manag.* 1996; 26(1): 3340.

22. Toon PD. The resourceful patient. *J R Soc Med.* 2002; 95(9): 469–70.

23. GMC. *0–18 years guidance: Access to medical records by children, young people and their parents.* http://www.gmc-uk.org/guidance/ethical_guidance/children_guidance_53_55_access_to_medical_records.asp (accessed June 22, 2017).

24. Hursthouse R. *On virtue ethics.* Oxford: Oxford University Press, 1999.

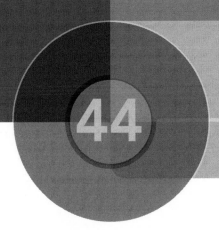

From professionalism to regulation and back again

SURENDRA DEO

INTRODUCTION

[General Practitioner] … struck off after running bootlegging racket while claiming to be a war hero.[1]

Nurse is struck off for faking patient records.[2]

Pharmacist struck off after serious and sustained misconduct.[3]

Social worker struck off after lie about child visit.[4]

Despite headlines such as these, and much publicised scandals involving healthcare professionals in the second half of the twentieth century and more recent years, the public still retains a high degree of trust in healthcare professionals. Polls in the USA show that the public rates honesty and ethical standards in healthcare professionals as very high, with nurses (85%) and pharmacists (68%) scoring above doctors (67%).[5] In the UK, among a group of professions, doctors retain the public's confidence with 90% of the public trusting them to tell the truth.[6]

In this chapter, I examine how this trust is maintained through the regulatory framework governing the healthcare professions involved in delivering primary care. I also look at the relevance of the codes as part of a wider ethical framework.

FROM PROFESSIONALISM TO REGULATION

Ethical conduct, professional integrity and moral probity have long been held to be central features of the 'professional', and traditionally, codes of ethics constituted one of the hallmarks and defining characteristics of the professions.[7] Less benignly, philosophers have taken the issue with a self-derived ethic that permits professionals to be guided by standards other than those of ordinary morality.[8] There is some ambiguity about who is a 'professional' but this is an increasingly irrelevant speculation because many occupations in healthcare are generally considered a profession or professional, especially if they are regulated.

In relation to professionalism and its assessment in medical training, Hilton and Slotnick suggested six domains in which evidence of professionalism can be expected: ethical practice, reflection/self-awareness, responsibility for actions, respect for patients, teamwork and social responsibility.[9]

In primary care, one would think of a professional as an individual possessing a superior knowledge base who can demonstrate competencies to apply this in a practical way to provide a special service, usually beneficial, to clients/patients. There is an expectation that professionals will observe norms and codes of conduct so that clients/patients will be assured of a good, competent level of service and will be held to account by a professional regulator to provide a reckless or unacceptable level of service.

HEALTHCARE REGULATORS

Traditionally, professions established early in their existence, a professional body (a professional regulator) which was intended to ensure high standards of education and conduct, regulate entry to the ranks of the profession, maintain a code of conduct (or ethical code), and, in some cases monitor and discipline their own members. This re-enforced the expectation of a high level of trust from patients and the state.[10]

Regulation formalises the idea of a contract between professionals and the public.[11] Professionals enjoy status and special privileges and in return are expected to uphold high standards not only of competence but also of behaviour and adhere to the traditional virtues of honesty, trustworthiness, reliability and fairness not only in relation to their work but also in their lives in general.

In the past (and perhaps even now), medical regulators appeared to be too protective of doctors and unwilling to tackle poor practice, putting doctors' interests before those of patients and being reactive rather than proactive. The mantra of patient empowerment now permeates the policy discourse, and the protection of traditional ethical codes administered by traditional professional bodies may not be sufficient to allay the anxieties of a public that has been persuaded by the media that professionals are not to be trusted.[12,13]

Recent trends stimulated by scandals widely publicised have included more lay representation and input into the regulatory function together with a proactive approach.[14] These have resulted in regulatory reforms, some of which directly challenge the concept of self-regulation. They include independent appointment processes to appoint members of regulatory bodies; greater lay participation in governance, policymaking and assessment procedures; and separation of disciplinary functions from registration and standard setting. There has also been sustained pressure on medical regulators and disciplinary bodies to become much more open about their processes and decisions. Public dissatisfaction with the veil of secrecy that shrouds much of the work of medical councils and tribunals is accompanied by calls from consumer groups and legislators for greater openness.[15] A contrasting argument is that external controls can be blunt instruments for finding the solutions in particular cases and require a functioning internal (professional) morality to interpret them.[16]

Medicine and healthcare also function in a political environment. Salter describes the three contracts between medicine, civil society and the state interlock to form a triangle of forces based on a mutual exchange of political benefits.[17] Commenting on medical regulation in the UK, Sir Donald Irvine, a past president of the General Medical Council (GMC), said that the GMC sits uneasily at the interface between the medical profession, the public, Parliament and the National Health Service. Herein lie the seeds of inertia and conflict.[18] Increasing openness, transparency and accessibility of information adds an additional fast-moving media interface.

In addition to professional regulation, primary healthcare practitioners work within a some-times confusing framework of responsibilities and advice. Many representative associations have a long history of providing ethical guidance, for example, The American Medical Association (AMA). In the UK ethical guidance may come from the GMC, the Royal Colleges, the Nursing and Midwifery Council (NMC), the British Medical Association and a variety of educational and medicolegal sources. Trainees also have a regulatory relationship with universities or other academic commissioners of training. Similarly, trainers will have to attain and maintain educational standards required for their role. Professionals also work within a contractual arrangement with employers or contractors. They may also work under constraints or restrictions imposed by commissioners of care (government, e.g., in the UK: National Institute for Health and Care Excellence, Care Quality Commission, National Health Service Codes of Practice and insurers).[19]

Finally, professionals are individuals with their own personal values and morals shaped by parental, religious, educational and societal influences. These influences can also cause some conflict.[20]

INTERNATIONAL COMPARISONS

A survey of medical regulators in 10 countries revealed that they all developed a number of different medical regulatory systems and, while all have departments of health, the development of standards and codes of ethics together with responsibility for the regulation of individual doctors has been devolved to other organisations. These range from a unitary state-authorised body such as the Egyptian Medical Syndicate (EMS), the Medical and Dental Council of Nigeria (MDCN), the Pakistan Medical and Dental Council (PMDC) or the Health Professionals Council of South Africa (HPCSA) to the decentralised polycentric Spanish, Indian, German and Italian systems. In two countries, Spain and Egypt, regulation and representation were delegated to the same body, prompting questions about conflict of interest. Nevertheless, there is a core set of regulatory functions to which all medical regulators subscribe with few exceptions.[21] In addition to upholding standards, regulators have the right to restrict practise or remove practitioners from the register. Relatively few regulators have the right to fine doctors, for example, Germany, Egypt and Nigeria.[22]

In the United States, 70 state and territorial medical boards are currently authorised to regulate physicians. In many states, other healthcare professionals are also licensed and regulated by medical boards in addition to physicians. Examples include physician assistants and acupuncturists. Some boards are independent and maintain all licensing and disciplinary powers, while others are part of a larger umbrella agency, such as a state department of health, exercising varied levels of responsibilities or functioning in an advisory capacity. Each state's Medical Practice Act defines unprofessional conduct within the state.[23]

In some countries such as the UK there is a single regulator for the traditional professions of medicine (GMC), nursing (NMC) and pharmacy (General Pharmaceutical Council). Another regulator, The Health and Care Professions Council (HCPC) currently regulates: arts therapists, biomedical scientists, chiropodists/podiatrists, clinical scientists, dietitians, hearing-aid dispensers, occupational therapists, operating department practitioners, orthoptists, paramedics, physiotherapists, practitioner psychologists, prosthetists/orthotists, radiographers, social workers in England and speech and language therapists.[24] All of these professions have at least one professional title that is protected by law, including those shown above. This means, for example, that anyone using the titles 'physiotherapist' or 'dietitian' must be registered with the HCPC. It is a criminal offence for someone to claim that they are registered with the HCPC when they are not, or to use a protected title that they are not entitled to use.[25] This is in contrast to the title 'doctor', which is not protected and is used by dentists, chiropractors and others.

Regulators have their own codes of conduct reflecting the values of each profession (as interpreted by the regulator) and standards required of registrants. Regulators implement their function to protect the public by deciding on the fitness to practise of practitioners judged against a standard usually published in a code. For instance, in the United Kingdom, the NMC's purpose is set out in a statutory order:

the principal functions of the Council shall be to establish from time to time standards of education, training, conduct and performance for nurses and midwives and to ensure the maintenance of those standards.[26]

PROFESSIONAL CODES

These have an ancient lineage, and perhaps the most well known is the oath attributed to the Hippocratic Corpus. They are cast in the language of trust and respect for the autonomous patient or, borrowing from principlism, autonomy, beneficence and non-maleficence.[27]

Primary care professionals have a variety of codes to refer to including the strictly regulatory ones they are governed by. International formulations include the World Medical Association Geneva Code of Medical Ethics (1949). This and the International Council for Nursing Code of Ethics for Nurses, most recently revised in 2012, provide a guide for action based on social values and needs.[28] This Code has served as the standard for nurses worldwide since it was first adopted in 1953. The American Nursing Association Code (2015) applies to nurses in the United States who are bound by the code as well as supported by it.[29]

Extant codes are articulated as a set of core values to which most regulators subscribe. They are deontological in nature, giving a guide to good (best) values and acceptable behaviour and help individuals to identify with 'their' organisation (professional group).[30] They are expressed however in a multitude of different ways. Most refer to respect for patients, for scientific knowledge and for colleagues. For instance, the German doctors' code, the *Berufsordnung*, requires doctors: to preserve and enhance the trust between doctors and patients; to ensure, in the interest of the whole population, the quality of doctors' work; to persevere the freedom and the reputation of the medical profession; to encourage worthy behaviour and to prevent unworthy behaviour of doctors. There are a few additional values arising out of culture or tradition. In Egypt, the first part of the code of ethics is an oath to God and there are references to Islam and pan-Arabic aspirations contained within the detail of the code, while in South Africa there is a strong emphasis on education as means of protecting the public.[31]

Clearly, the threat of sanction for breaching the code is a factor determining professional behaviour. However, this is not the only, or even the major, factor driving professional behaviour. Many professionals, especially in primary care, behave as they do because of role modelling and personal values (why they came into a caring profession in the first place).

The function of codes is threefold:

1. Providing normative occupation specific standards for the professional (competence).
2. Providing guidance for patients on what to expect of the professionals providing care.
3. Providing guidance on expected professional behaviour (aspirational).

It is important to recognise that codes should not be seen as primarily as tools to determine professionals 'who ought to be punished' (when standards are breached) but to provide standards that will protect the laity – patients in this case. As primary documents of regulators, they are explicit that their purpose is to protect patients.

Virtues are almost implied in the tone and content of the codes – the doctor or other primary healthcare professional is expected and considered to be honest, full of integrity, fair in all decisions and the protector of patients – even if it means blowing the whistle on colleagues. The codes broadly promote individual liberty as opposed to communitarian ideals of the common good. The coherence of broadly similar values and guidance lends strength to confidence that the codes are justified and should be accepted.[32]

Indeed, it can be seen that to adhere to the codes, the professional should be seen as a veritable beacon of virtue. However, in recent years, the overt emphasis on virtues has decreased, at least in the AMA code. Beauchamp and Childress point out the difference between the paternalistic virtues of benevolence, care and compassion versus the autonomy model where the virtue of respectfulness is more prominent.[33] They also point out the shift in traditional nursing virtues of obedience and submission (to doctors) to the more active virtue of advocacy.[34]

Ethical codes aim to promote 'ethical behaviour' and 'ethical standards of behaviour' specific to the context of practise.[35] Inevitably, these are formulated in general terms and are often supported by guidance. They are described as descriptive normative ethics.[36] They often include guidance on etiquette – relations between different subsets of the profession, rules on advertising, and so on, although this is less of a feature in recent editions. They have been referred to as 'ethics narrowly conceived'.[37] Similarly, they can be seen to aid substantive ethical reasoning in the form of 'quasi-legal ethics'.[38] They can therefore provide a framework to the moral environment in which healthcare is set, but they can never be so tightly drawn as to remove the need for the exercise of ethical choice by individual doctors, nurses or physiotherapists and others.[39] Beauchamp and Childress emphasise that no professional code has successfully presented a system of moral values free of conflicts and exceptions.[40]

O'Neill points out that the simplicities of older codes have been replaced with far more complex and detailed codes and by more formal certification of competence to perform specific interventions, and by many exacting forms of accountability. This replaces more traditional forms of trust with ideas of doctor's duties and patient's rights.[41] This movement is further captured in the need for measurement of standards in the form of audit and the recent introduction of revalidation for doctors and nurses in the UK.

ETHICS AND CODES

Many of the codes have a 'prime directive' (to borrow from the television series 'Star Trek') of *making the care of the patient the professional's first concern*. In the UK, this is contained in the codes governing the regulation of doctors and nurses. Sokol notes the Hippocratic flavour of this dictum that points to the sacred and timeless nature of the encounter between the healer and the sick person. He also critiques the simplicity of this phrase, bringing in practical considerations and other principles such as justice, saying that the rule could be revised too.

> In your professional capacity as a doctor, make the care of your patient your first concern, acting within morally and legally acceptable limits and bearing in mind your other patients, including at times future patients and their particular needs as well as any protective obligations to the broader community, your own obligations to develop your skills and knowledge as a clinician, and obligations you may have towards others for whom you are responsible.

He also points out the irony that too literal reading of the rule could lead to unethical conduct.[42]

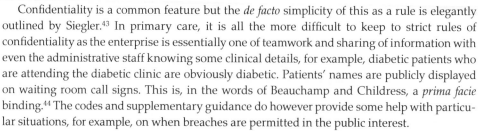

Confidentiality is a common feature but the *de facto* simplicity of this as a rule is elegantly outlined by Siegler.[43] In primary care, it is all the more difficult to keep to strict rules of confidentiality as the enterprise is essentially one of teamwork and sharing of information with even the administrative staff knowing some clinical details, for example, diabetic patients who are attending the diabetic clinic are obviously diabetic. Patients' names are publicly displayed on waiting room call signs. This is, in the words of Beauchamp and Childress, a *prima facie* binding.[44] The codes and supplementary guidance do however provide some help with particular situations, for example, on when breaches are permitted in the public interest.

The codes can come into conflict with obligations to an employer, the professionals' own values and the law. For instance, assisted suicide (but not euthanasia) is not illegal in either Germany or Switzerland, but a doctor's participation in Germany would violate the code of professional medical conduct and might contravene of a doctor's legal duty to save life.[45] At a more mundane level, primary care professionals are increasingly both commissioners and providers of care.[46] Regulators require practitioners to be open and honest with patients about financial arrangements and not to exploit their position in order to achieve monetary gain. Similar conflicts arise when physicians and other practitioners are given incentive payments for reduction in antibiotic prescribing and participation in research trials.[47]

Sometimes medical ethics (as embodied in codes) is more demanding than law; at other times, perhaps counter-intuitively, the law appears to ask more of doctors than does good medical ethics.[48] It would not be unlawful for a doctor to have a sexual relationship with a consenting, adult patient, but it would be unethical and breach code standards. This is contrasted with assessments on mental capacity which are condensed in ethical guidance but presented in much more detail in law. The concept of a patient's right to unwise decision-making faces institutional obstruction due to prevailing cultures of risk aversion and paternalism.[49]

However, the interplay and conflict between these influences can lead to ethical dilemmas for the primary healthcare practitioner. Obligations to regulatory standards reflect fitness for practise, whereas obligations to a job plan reflect fitness for purpose. These two aspects can occasionally intersect but on the whole, fitness for practise refers to higher-order qualities and capabilities.

In relation to personal values and beliefs, the codes have recently become more directive. In the UK the GMC has addressed these conflicts in its *Personal Beliefs and Medical Practice* (2013) guidance[50]:

> You may choose to opt out of providing a particular procedure because of your personal beliefs and values, as long as this does not result in direct or indirect discrimination against, or harassment of, individual patients or groups of patients. This means you must not refuse to treat a particular patient or group of patients because of your personal beliefs or views about them. And you must not refuse to treat the health consequences of lifestyle choices to which you object because of your beliefs.
>
> Employing and contracting bodies are entitled to require doctors to fulfil contractual requirements that may restrict doctors' freedom to work in accordance with their conscience. This is a matter between doctors and their employing or contracting bodies.
>
> If, having taken account of your legal and ethical obligations, you wish to exercise a conscientious objection to particular services or procedures, you must do your best to make sure that patients who may consult you about it are aware of your objection in advance. You can do this by making sure that any printed material about your practice and the services you provide explains if there are any services you will not normally provide because of a conscientious objection.

The codes cannot possibly provide the answer to every dilemma. This is recognised in the preamble to New Zealand's Good Medical Practice (2013):

> Good Medical Practice is not intended to be exhaustive. There may be obligations or situations that are not expressly provided for…Good Medical Practice is not a Code of Ethics – it does not seek to describe all the ethical values of the profession or to provide specific advice on ethical issues, ethical frameworks and ethical decision-making.[51]

Therefore, primary care professionals need to apply a more diverse range of ethical resources and tools to help decide on the right direction of travel. This is often simply a question of discussion with supervisors or colleagues and the patient/client to come to an agreed way forward. That is when the dilemma is recognised and hopefully addressed. The codes are useful in adding authoritative input to the discussion.

This is relatively easy with the more common issues of consent and confidentiality. Veracity has been a relatively recent addition to the codes.[52] Honesty is now a prime requirement of primary healthcare professionals and dishonesty, in any context, is viewed as serious as it may undermine trust.[53] The regulators seem to be finding their way in adapting to more recent issues such as use of social media, duty of candour, commissioning and end-of-life care. The codes have had some catching up to do to comply with these contemporary developments in technology, social mores and the law.

The published standards and expectations contained in the codes provide the common thread that runs through the policing function of regulators. Judging alleged breaches of the standards is not easy due to the constraints on definitive direction outlined above. Decision-makers are faced with a difficult task of balancing evidence and applying the standards to each case of alleged misconduct, health concern or poor performance. The role of the regulator is not to punish professionals but to protect the public. Therefore, if a professional has made a serious error but has remediated and there is little likelihood of repetition, it is unlikely that he or she will face regulatory action. It is understandable that this approach may not always sit well with a complainant who has suffered through incompetence or misconduct.

Scammell points out the limits of any code saying that professional (in this case nursing) codes are essentially about public protection and should embody the rights of users of health services to knowledgeable, competent and humane care and treatment, setting out core values and standards and embodying a set of expectations about the way nurses should behave and provide a touchstone for practitioners to model behaviour as well as to challenge others who fall short of standards laid out in the Code. However, any code, be it short and concise or long and detailed, is only a tool. What matters is whether the values embedded in a professional code reflect personal values, for only if this is the case will professionals' act according to those professional values.[54]

PROACTIVE VERSUS REACTIVE REGULATION

In the past, registration with a regulatory body would be all that was needed for a practitioner to prove his or her professional standing for the rest of their working life. The only stipulation was to pay the fees and stay away from any concerns about his or her fitness to practise. Recent scandals and the more open and transparent nature of information have led to calls for reform as this approach has been found wanting and is no longer fit for purpose.

Public inquiries into medical scandals such as the *Bristol* and *Shipman* inquiries in England, and the *Bundaberg* inquiry in Queensland, criticised the lack of oversight of healthcare professionals post registration. These and other concerns involving practitioners suggest that professionalism or the internal morality of medicine together with traditional models of regulation is not sufficient to ensure that practising doctors remain competent. A more proactive or agile regulation looking forward to anticipate change rather than looking back to prevent the last crisis from happening again is needed.[55]

Jurisdictions vary in their approach to addressing this aspect of regulation. In the UK, revalidation of practitioners (nurses and doctors) has recently been established.[56,57] Engagement and participation are required to retain a licence to practise. The process operates in a cyclical manner: doctors 5 yearly, and nurses every 3 years. It involves collecting evidence and essentially reflecting on practice through annual appraisals. The evidence includes continuing professional development, patient and colleague feedback, audit, case reviews and other learning.

New roles have emerged. General practitioners must connect to a 'designated body' and relate to a 'responsible officer', a clinician who is tasked with making a recommendation to the regulator at the end of every cycle.[58] It is hoped that this development will address some of the concerns outlined above.

CONCLUSION

Regulation and associated professional codes used in primary care are based on sound ethical foundations, mainly on traditional virtues and principles that have roots in the early establishment of the caring professions. They provide guidance and standards that are useful for practitioners, patients and the public. However, codes cannot operate in ethical isolation. Individual values prioritising humanised practices are needed to ensure that the care of the patient is truly the professional's first concern.[59]

The existence of multiple regulators has been criticised. Primary healthcare is increasingly an integrated team exercise with the patient at its heart. The agreement of a professional ethos in a unified code would encourage inclusivity and sharing of values and focus.[60] A transdisciplinary code of ethics applicable to all health professionals and created with public input would be the first step towards generating a social contract that can meet the contemporary needs of health professionals and the patients and communities they serve.[61,62]

REFERENCES

1. Kent Online. 2016. Available at http://www.kentonline.co.uk/malling/news/gp-struck-off-after-running-48897/ (accessed July 10, 2017).
2. Sunday Herald (Scotland). 31 October 2014. Available at http://www.heraldscotland.com/news/13187159.Nurse_is_struck_off_for_faking_patient_records/ (accessed July 10, 2017).
3. *The Pharmaceutical Journal*. 2012. Available at http://www.pharmaceutical-journal.com/news-and-analysis/pharmacist-struck-off-after-serious-and-sustained-misconduct/11105141.article (accessed July 10, 2017).
4. Southern Daily Echo. Available at http://www.dailyecho.co.uk/news/14114459.Social_worker_struck_off_after_lie_about_child_visit/ (accessed July 13, 2017).
5. Gallup Poll (USA). 2015. Available at http://www.gallup.com/poll/1654/honesty-ethics-professions.aspx (accessed July 10, 2017).

6. ipsos-mori Poll. 2015. Available at https://www.ipsos-mori.com/researchpublications/ researcharchive/3504/Politicians-trusted-less-than-estate-agents-banker s-and- journalists.aspx (accessed July 13, 2017).

7. Lunt I. Ethical issues in professional life. In: Cunningham B, editor. *Exploring Professionalism.* London: Bedford Way Papers, IoE; 2008. p. 73.

8. Chapman R. The future of professional ethics. *Ethical Perspect.* 1997; 4(2): 291.

9. Hilton S, Slotnick H. Proto-professionalism: How professionalisation occurs across the continuum of medical education. *Med Educ.* 2005; 39(1): 58–65.

10. Irvine D. A short history of the General Medical Council. *Med Educ.* 2006; 40: 202–211.

11. Lunt, 2008, *op. cit.,* 77.

12. Salter B. *The New Politics of Medicine.* Basingstoke: Palgrave Macmillan; 2004. p. 66.

13. Ibid., 87.

14. Irvine, 2006, *op. cit.*

15. International Revalidation Symposium: Contributing to the evidence base. 2010. Available at http://www.gmc-uk.org/International_Revalidation_Symposium_ Publication_of_proceedings.pdf_44014486.pdf (accessed July 10, 2017).

16. Paul C. Internal and external morality of medicine: lessons from New Zealand. *BMJ* 2000; 320: 499.

17. Salter, 2004, *op. cit.,* pp. 6–7.

18. Irvine, 2006, *op. cit.*

19. Beauchamp T, Childress J. *Principles of Biomedical Ethics.* 5th ed. Oxford: OUP; 2001. p. 317.

20. Chapman, 1997, *op. cit.*

21. General Medical Council. *International Comparison of Ten Medical Regulatory Systems.* London: General Medical Council; 2009.

22. General Medical Council. *State of Medical Education and Practice.* London: General Medical Council; 2015. p. 144.

23. Federation of State Medical Boards. *U.S. Medical Regulatory Trends and Actions Report.* 2014. Available at https://www.fsmb.org/Media/Default/PDF/FSMB/Publications/us_ medical_regulatory_trends_actions.pdf (accessed July 10, 2017).

24. Health and Care Professions Council. Available at http://www.hcpc-uk.co.uk/aboutus/ (accessed July 10, 2017).

25. Ibid.

26. Select Committee on Constitution Written Evidence: Memorandum by the Nursing and Midwifery Council. http://www.publications.parliament.uk/pa/ld200304/ldselect/ ldconst/68/68we53.htm

27. Randall F, Downie RS. *Palliative Care Ethics A companion for All Specialties.* Oxford: OUP; 1999. p. 3.

28. International Council of Nurses. *The ICN Code of Ethics for Nurses.* 2012. Available at http://www.icn.ch/who-we-are/code-of-ethics-for-nurses/ (accessed July 10, 2017).

29. American Nurses Association. *Code of Ethics for Nurses with Interpretive Statements.* 2015. Available at http://www.nursingworld.org/MainMenuCategories/EthicsStandards/ CodeofEthicsforNurses/Code-of-Ethics-For-Nurses.html

30. Miller S. What use are ethical codes? An analysis of three possible rationales for the use of ethical codes in medical schools and a review of the evidence relating to them. *Med Educ.* 2000; 34: 428–9.

31. General Medical Council. *International Comparison of Ten Medical Regulatory Systems.* London: General Medical Council; 2009.

32. Beauchamp and Childress, 2001, *op. cit.,* 401.

33. Ibid., 31.
34. Ibid., 33.
35. Lunt, 2008, *op. cit.*, 79.
36. Beauchamp and Childress, 2001, *op. cit.*, 2.
37. Randall and Downie, 1999, *op. cit.*, 2.
38. Fulford K, Dickenson D, Murray T, editors. *Healthcare Ethics and Human Values, an Introductory Text with Readings and Case Studies.* Oxford: Blackwell; 2002. p. 162.
39. Butler J. *The Ethics of Healthcare Rationing, Principles and Practices.* London: Cassell; 1999. p. 122.
40. Beauchamp and Childress, 2001, *op. cit.*, 15.
41. O'Neill O. *Autonomy and Trust in Bioethics.* Cambridge: Cambridge University Press; 2002. pp. 20–21.
42. Sokol D. Make the care of your patient your first concern. *BMJ.* 2011; 342: 312.
43. Siegler M. 'Confidentiality in Medicine' – A decrepit concept. *NEJM.* 1982; 307: 1518–21.
44. Beauchamp and Childress, 2001, *op. cit.*, 284.
45. Bosshard G, Broeckaert B, Clark D, Materstvedt LJ, Gordijin B, Müller-Busch HC. A role for doctors in assisted dying? An analysis of legal regulations and medical professional positions in six European countries. *J Med Ethics.* 2008; 34: 28–32.
46. Beauchamp and Childress, 2001, *op. cit.*, 319.
47. Ibid.
48. Jackson E. *J Med Ethics.* 2015; 41: 95–8.
49. Ibid.
50. General Medical Council - Conscientious Objection. Available at http://www.gmc-uk.org/guidance/ethical_guidance/21177.asp
51. Medical Council of New Zealand. Available at https://www.mcnz.org.nz/assets/News-and-Publications/good-medical-practice.pdf
52. Beauchamp and Childress, 2001, *op. cit.*, 283.
53. General Medical Council. *Making Decisions on Cases at the End of the Investigation Stage: Guidance for the Investigation Committee and Case Examiners.* GMC; 2014. Available at http://www.gmc-uk.org/DC4599_CE_Decision_Guidance___Making_decisions_on_cases_at_the_end_of_the_investigation_stage.pdf_58070536.pdf (accessed July 10, 2017).
54. Scammell, *op. cit.* See case of Scammell at https://www.nmc.org.uk/globalassets/siteDocuments/FTPOutcomes/2015/Mar/Reasons-Scammell-CCCSH-039698-20150309.pdf (accessed July 10, 2017).
55. General Medical Council. *International Revalidation Symposium: Contributing to the Evidence Base.* 2010. Available at http://www.gmc-uk.org/International_Revalidation_Symposium_Publication_of_proceedings.pdf_44014486.pdf (accessed July 10, 2017).
56. NMC. *Welcome to Revalidation.* Available at http://revalidation.nmc.org.uk/welcome-to-revalidation/ (accessed July 10, 2017).
57. General Medical Council. *The GMC Protocol for Making Revalidation Recommendations: Guidance for Responsible Officers and Suitable Persons* (Fourth edition). GMC; London, 2015.
58. Ibid.
59. Scammell, *op. cit.*
60. Butler, 1999, *op. cit.*, 121.
61. Wynia MK, Kishore SP, Belar CD. A unified code of ethics for health professionals. Insights from an IOM workshop. *JAMA.* 2014; 311(8): 799–800.
62. Institute of Medicine. *Establishing Transdisciplinary Professionalism for Improving Health Outcomes.* Washington, DC: The National Academies Press; 2013.

Index